MEDICAL Music Therapy:
Building a Comprehensive Program

Edited by Lori F. Gooding, PhD, MT-BC
University of Kentucky

MEDICAL Music Therapy:
Building a Comprehensive Program

Edited by Lori F. Gooding, PhD, MT-BC
University of Kentucky

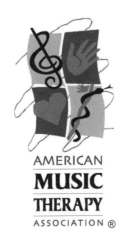

American Music Therapy Association
www.musictherapy.org

ISBN: 978-1-884914-31-7

Copyright Information: ©American Music Therapy Association, Inc., 2014
                              8455 Colesville Road, Suite 1000
                              Silver Spring, MD 20910 USA
                              www.musictherapy.org
                              info@musictherapy.org

Technical Assistance: Wordsetters
                              Kalamazoo, Michigan

Cover Design and Layout: Tawna Grasty, Grass T Design

Printed in the United States of America

List of Contributors

Virginia Barragan, FACHE, PT, DPT, MOMT
Service Line Director of Rehab/Developmental Services
Palomar Health
San Diego, CA

Andrea Cevasco-Trotter, PhD, MT-BC
Associate Professor of Music Therapy
University of Alabama
Tuscaloosa, AL

Darcy DeLoach, PhD, MT-BC
Director of Music Therapy
University of Louisville
Louisville, KY

Alexandra Fields, MS, MT-BC
Family Centered Care Support Services
Children's Hospital Los Angeles
Los Angeles, CA

Lori F. Gooding, PhD, MT-BC
Director of Music Therapy
University of Kentucky
Lexington, KY

Dianne Gregory, MM, MT-BC
Associate Professor of Music Therapy
The Florida State University
Tallahassee, FL

Miriam Hillmer, MM, MT-BC
Music Therapist
Tallahassee Memorial Hospital
Tallahassee, FL

Brianna Negrete, MM, MT-BC
Music Therapist
Tallahassee Memorial Hospital
Tallahassee, FL

Michelle Pellito, MM, MT-BC
Music Therapist
Capital Music Therapy
Tallahassee, FL

Jennifer Jarred Peyton, MM, MT-BC
Music Therapist
University of Kentucky Healthcare
Lexington, KY

Jessica Rushing, MM, MT-BC
Music Therapist
University of Kentucky HealthCare
Lexington, KY

Jayne M. Standley PhD, MT-BC
Robert O. Lawton Distinguished Professor
Colleges of Music and Medicine
The Florida State University
Tallahassee, FL

Natalie Wlodarczyk, PhD, MT-BC
Assistant Professor of Music Therapy
Drury University
Springfield, MO

Olivia Swedberg Yinger, PhD, MT-BC
Assistant Professor of Music Therapy
University of Kentucky
Lexington, KY

A Note from the Editor

As the efficacy of music therapy treatment for patients with a wide range of diagnoses grows, so do the opportunities for medical music therapy. As someone who has had the privilege of developing a medical music therapy program, I can speak first hand of the value that we, as music therapists, add for patients, families, and staff in the healthcare setting. My own program at the University of Kentucky went from a staff of one, to a staff of 5 music therapists in four years, and we were honored to add music therapy as a covered service under the University of Kentucky Insurance Plan in July of 2014.

While I am proud of what we have been able to accomplish, I also want to recognize the many pioneers who have come before us that worked tirelessly to promote medical music therapy. In particular I would like to thank Dr. Jayne Standley, whose book *Medical Music Therapy: A Model Program for Clinical Practice, Education, Training, and Research*, was the inspiration for this text.

I would also like to thank the many authors of this book for their invaluable contributions to the practice of medical music therapy. I am honored to know each one of you and thrilled to have had the opportunity to work with you on this project. I would also like to thank the students whose questions inspired this book; I hope that it serves as a valuable resource for you. Finally, I would like to thank my husband and son for their support and patience. I would not have been able to do this without you.

Contents

Section 1: Foundations of Medical Music Therapy

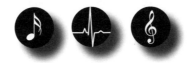

Chapter 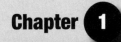 1

An Introduction to Medical Music Therapy
Jayne M. Standley, PhD, MT-BC

Medical music therapy is a rapidly developing career area with programs in hospitals, rehabilitation facilities, clinics, hospices, and child care settings for medically fragile infants and toddlers. Evidence-based music therapy is the approach that best fits the medical, neurologic, and child development models incorporated in such facilities and has become a highly specialized, referral-based, reimbursable treatment option within these venues.

Research demonstrates that individuals respond differently to music therapy depending upon their gender, age, type of treatment, or music preferences. The study of medical music therapy requires synthesis of awareness of the effect of music on individuals, along with knowledge in psychology, biology, and neurology. It also requires competence in the rules of the U.S. health care services at the federal, state, and local levels.

The participating authors for this volume are experienced in the incorporation of academic training and research with the management of an ongoing model for evidence-based clinical music therapy (MT) treatment in an affiliated hospital. This approach synthesizes innovative clinical demonstration with piloted reimbursement development, practica and internship training, and research innovation. In 2005, a description of the original program was published as a resource for future medical MT clinicians—*Medical Music Therapy: A Model Program for Clinical Practice, Education, Training, and Research* (Standley et al., 2005). This new work updates and supplants that text and provides information that we hope will prove helpful to others striving to develop the field of medical MT.

Ten years ago the Institute for Infant and Child Medical Music Therapy was created at The Florida State University with the mission of improving medical services to children through evidence-based music therapy. It successfully combined research, innovative clinical demonstration, and specialized training functions. In 2003, specialized training in NICU-MT for premature infants was developed with requirements for both textbook and in vitro clinical instruction in affiliated hospitals. The first evidence-based music therapy clinical text for premature infants was published (Standley, 2003) and is now in the second edition (Standley & Walworth, 2010). Additionally, research into music for reinforcement of feeding problems led to the development of an FDA-approved commercial medical device to teach feeding skills to premature infants, the PAL©. Today, the Institute has grown into a research/training network of multiple university music therapy programs and affiliated hospitals, including:

- The Florida State University

- The University of Alabama

- The University of Kentucky

- The University of Louisville

- Tallahassee Memorial HealthCare, Tallahassee, FL

- Florida Hospital for Children, Orlando, FL

- DCH Regional Medical Center, Tuscaloosa, AL

- Kosair Children's Hospital, Louisville, KY

- University of Louisville HealthCare, Louisville, KY

- University of Kentucky HealthCare, Lexington, KY

In the last 10 years, many research projects and publications have been completed and hundreds of music therapists have been trained in NICU-MT. Recently, the first European NICU-MT training program was conducted in London, and further international dissemination of this evidence-based specialized music therapy is planned. The Institute is also affiliated with *imagine*, the online magazine for early childhood music therapy.

The use of medical music therapy with children has grown across the nation. At the current time, there are over 200 MT-BCs employed in medical settings serving children. They are primarily located in the Southeastern, Great Lakes and mid-Atlantic regions and many provide NICU-MT (Tabinowski, 2013). Likewise medical music therapy in general has grown, with 12% of respondents to the 2013 American Music Therapy Member Survey and Workforce Analysis working in medical/ surgical settings (AMTA, 2013).

Our intent is to further the field of medical music therapy in general with special emphasis on the needs of children. With that in mind, we sought to provide the most up-to-date, complete information on innovative MT medical programs; how to organize, implement, and document them; and even how to do a cost/benefit analysis to propose a new position or document outcomes of an existing program. Therefore, our mission and purpose for this book are:

1. To synthesize research results into evidence-based clinical music therapy practice;

2. To provide a model for the development of cutting-edge, evidence-based medical music therapy programs that meet health care standards for third party reimbursement;

3. To develop specialized medical MT protocols for children;

4. To provide a pedagogy for training students in medical music therapy techniques; and

5. To demonstrate how volunteer artists and musicians can be effectively incorporated into an evidence-based music therapy clinical program.

We have a vision for the future where medical MT is used in every major medical setting; where hospital standards for ratio of music therapists per number of hospital beds have been established; where multiple MT-BCs in each facility meet patient needs 24 hours a day, 365 days a year; where MT is a separate department no longer supervised by child life, the chaplain, or other non-therapeutic specialty areas; where MT is differentiated from efforts of all other musicians in the medical setting; where hospital-wide reimbursement exists for all MT services; and where specialized training for medical counseling, emergency department MT, and medical gerontology services is a standard within the profession. We hope this book helps further that vision. With implementation of the Affordable Care Act in October 2013, and its emphasis on reducing medical costs while maximizing patient satisfaction, our profession stands on the brink of major growth in medical MT. Evidence-based medical music therapy is the epitome of the therapeutic service that enhances highly effective medical treatment, reduces cost of care, increases patient satisfaction across all areas of the hospital, and increases quality of life of patients, especially children.

References

American Music Therapy Association (AMTA). (2013). *2013 AMTA member survey and workforce analysis.* Retrieved from http://www.musictherapy.org/documents/

Standley, J. (2003). *Music therapy with premature infants: Research and developmental interventions.* Silver Spring, MD: American Music Therapy Association.

Standley, J., Gregory, D., Whipple, J., Walworth, D., Nguyen, J., Jarred, J., Adams, K., Procelli, D., & Cevasco, A. (2005). *Medical music therapy: A model program for clinical practice, education, training, and research.* Silver Spring, MD: American Music Therapy Association.

Standley, J. M., & Walworth, D. (2010). *Music therapy with premature infants: Research and developmental interventions* (2nd ed.). Silver Spring, MD: American Music Therapy Association.

Tabinowski. K. (2013). *A survey of current music therapy practices in pediatric hospitals and units* (Unpublished master's thesis). Florida State University, Tallahassee.

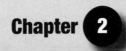

Chapter 2

Understanding Neuroscience within the field of Medical Music Therapy
Olivia Swedberg Yinger, PhD, MT-BC

Music therapists are frequently asked the question, "What is music therapy?" The brief answer to this question often depends on who is asking the question and in what context, as well as the music therapist's own experiences and theoretical orientation. Often, examples of music therapy applications with specific populations are given to provide a glimpse into what music therapists do. Although many people who ask the question "What is music therapy?" are satisfied with a description of *what* a music therapist does and *for whom,* it has been my experience that health care professionals are often also interested in *why* music therapy is effective and *how* the process works. This chapter attempts to describe the mechanisms by which certain music therapy interventions affect the organ through which sensory input is processed: the brain.

Recent research on the effects of music on the brain has shed light on how music therapy can enhance treatment in medical settings. There is no single center for musical processing in the brain; rather, music listening engages multiple areas of the brain. By understanding more about how music affects the brain and staying current on research in cognitive neuroscience in music, music therapy clinicians and researchers can better understand how to provide individualized, evidence-based treatment. In order to understand how music therapy affects neural processes, one must first have a basic understanding of human neuroanatomy and neurophysiology, knowledge of methods by which neural processes may be studied, including neuroimaging and electroencephalography, and familiarity with key studies on the cognitive neuroscience of music. Coursework in human anatomy and physiology, psychology of music, medical music therapy, and music perception and cognition typically covers these areas in greater detail; therefore, information in this chapter is meant as an overview only. A glossary at the end of the chapter contains definitions of neuroanatomical terms frequently used when discussing cognitive neuroscience of music, as well as descriptions of neuroimaging and electroencephalography techniques.

Music therapy intersects with other disciplines, including music perception and cognition, which seek to understand the impact of music on human functioning. Music perception and cognition is a subdiscipline of cognitive psychology, which focuses on understanding the mental mechanisms involved in humans' appreciation of music (Justus & Bharucha, 2002).

Topics of interest within the field of music perception and cognition include perceptual organization of musical elements such as pitch and time, musical performance and ability, musical universals and origins, and cognitive neuroscience of music. Whereas a basic understanding of all of these areas is helpful for music therapists, the area of cognitive neuroscience of music is of particular interest to music therapists working in medical settings. Cognitive neuroscience of music commonly focuses on neuropsychology, neuroimaging, and measurement of electroencephalography. Figure 2.1 shows the organization of subspecialties related to the study of music and the brain.

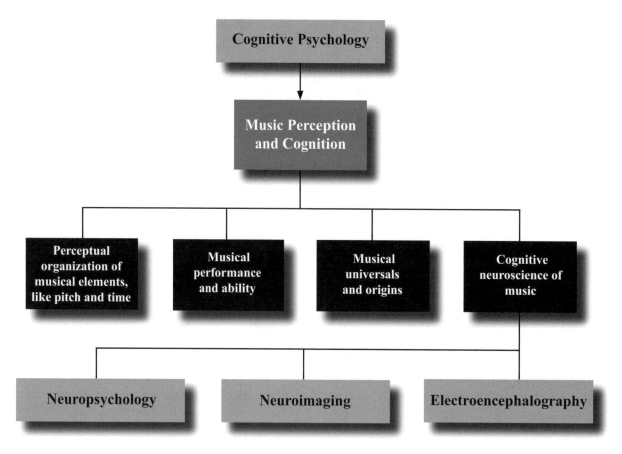

Figure 2.1. Organization of subspecialties related to music and the brain (based on taxonomy described by Justus & Bharucha, 2002).

An unknown author once said, "The half of knowledge is knowing where to find it." This statement seems to be particularly true in the field of cognitive neuroscience of music, where research related to the effects of music on the brain may be published in various journals across numerous fields of study, often outside of the music therapy journals with which readers may be the most familiar. Knowing where to look for up-to-date research is crucial in a field that is growing rapidly. The latter part of this chapter will provide a list of journals in which key studies were found, as well as a description of ways in which evidence-based practitioners can use technology to conduct effective literature searches and receive electronic notifications when new studies of interest are published.

The purposes of this chapter are to provide an overview of neuroimaging techniques and neuroanatomical structures pertinent to music perception, to highlight key recent studies using neuroimaging techniques to study these processes, and to provide information on ways in which music therapists can stay current on research related to music and the brain.

Understanding Neuroimaging Procedures

Various neuroimaging procedures are currently used to measure both brain structure and function. Given the number of brain imaging techniques now available, it is important for readers of neuroscience research to have a basic understanding of the differences among various imaging techniques and how they are frequently used. Descriptions of several commonly used neuroimaging procedures are given below. In addition, pros and cons of each procedure are listed. A more in-depth description of brain imaging techniques and neuroanatomical can be found in chapter 20 of Bhatnagar's (2008) helpful text, *Neuroscience for the Study of Communicative Disorders*.

Structural Imaging Procedures

• *Computed Axial Tomography (CT or CAT) scan*: The CT scan uses a series of x-rays that show the head from different angles. *Pros:* Can create cross-sectional images quickly. *Cons:* Does not provide information about brain functioning.

• *Magnetic Resonance Imaging (MRI)*: A magnetic field and radio waves create high resolution, two- or three-dimensional cross-sectional images of internal organs. *Diffusion Tensor Imaging (DTI)* is one type of MRI that maps the diffusion process of molecules of water in tissues. DTI is especially useful in mapping brain abnormalities of individuals who have experienced strokes. *Pros:* No radioactive tracer is necessary. High in precision and able to detect structural changes over time. *Cons:* Does not provide information about brain functioning.

Functional Imaging Procedures

• *Electroencephalography (EEG)*: Electrodes are placed on the scalp to detect and record the brain's patterns of electrical activity. Scale electrodes can compare the strengths and positions of electrical activity from various parts of the brain. *Pros:* Records timing of activity precisely. *Cons:* Poor resolution. Only measures exterior brain activity directly.

• *Electromyography (EMG) and Transcranial Magnetic Stimulation (TMS)*: TMS applies an electrical pulse to the motor cortex, while EMG uses electrodes on the skin or inserted intramuscularly to detect the *motor evoked potential (MEP)* produced by muscle cells when they are stimulated. Using the two procedures together allows for examination of the corticospinal pathways and the motor cortex. *Pros:* Produces useful information about the motor cortex. *Cons:* EMG may cause pain or discomfort.

• *Functional Magnetic Resonance Imaging (fMRI)*: fMRI maps blood flow using magnetic properties of blood. Changes in signal strength produced by the magnetic field of blood are called *blood oxygen-level dependent (BOLD)* contrasts. Subjects perform repetitive motions during the test, such as tapping a finger or a foot. Images of the brain are produced every second. *Pros:* High resolution and able to provide information about brain functioning. *Cons:* Time-consuming and requires the subject to remain completely still for long periods of time. Noise and other internal and external factors may affect interpretation of results.

• *Magnetoencephalography (MEG)*: MEG uses magnetic fields produced by the brain's electrical currents to map brain activities and is able to measure functioning of various parts of the brain. *Pros:* Better resolution and more accurate than EEG. *Cons:* Not as sensitive as EEG to activity occurring in gyri.

• *Positron Emission Tomography (PET)*: A chemical tracer is injected into the bloodstream and travels to the brain. The PET scan sensors detect radioactivity from the tracer in different regions of the brain. Two- or three-dimensional images show blood flow, oxygen, and glucose metabolism. Findings in neuroimaging research are often reported in terms of *regional cerebral blood flow (rCBF)*. *Pros:* Can show blood flow, oxygen, and glucose metabolism in functioning brain tissues. High resolution and provides quick results. *Cons:* Useful only for short tasks, since the radioactivity decays quickly.

• *Single Photon Emission Computed Tomography (SPECT)*: A chemical is injected into the bloodstream and travels to the brain. A gamma camera moves around the head to capture multiple images of the brain. The distribution of the chemical shows which areas of the brain are activated by measuring increased blood flow. *Pros:* Tracers last longer so it is able to measure longer tasks than PET. Requires less equipment and fewer staff than PET. *Cons:* Has poorer resolution than PET and records fewer types of brain activity.

Modern brain imaging techniques allow researchers to better understand how brain structures function in real time and how its structure changes over time. Long before imaging techniques were available, understanding of brain structure was accomplished by dissecting cadavers. Many of the brain's individual regions and structures were given Greek or Latin names based on their appearances. At times it can be helpful for those studying neuroanatomy to know the derivation of terms, which may at first seem very foreign. For this reason, the derivation of neuroanatomical terms is included in Tables 2.4–2.10). A complete glossary of anatomical terms, originally created by Dr. Toby Arnold, is available at http://www.anatomy.usyd.edu.au/glossary/ (Arnold & Bryce, n.d.). In addition, the results of selected recent studies on neuroimaging and music are summarized in Tables 2.2–2.10 to show how music listening or music performance affects the brain regions described here.

An Overview of Neuroanatomy

The human brain is often grouped structurally into three large sections: the *forebrain* (prosencephalon), the *midbrain* (mesencephalon), and the *hindbrain* (rhombencephalon). These three large sections are further broken down into the structures listed in Table 2.1. An image of the major sections of the brain is shown in Figure 2.2.

Table 2.1 Organization of the Human Brain				
FOREBRAIN (Prosencephalon)		MIDBRAIN (Mesencephalon)	HINDBRAIN (Rhombencephalon)	
Telencephalon	Diencephalon		Metencephalon	Myelencephalon
Cerebral cortex	Thalamus	Tectum	Cerebellum	Medulla oblongata
Hippocampus	Hypothalamus	Tegmentum	Pons	
Amygdala	Subthalamus	Basis pedunculi		
Basal ganglia	Epithalamus			
Fiber tracts				

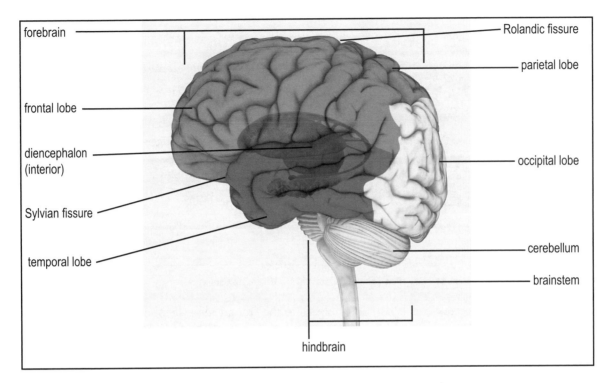

Figure 2.2. Major parts of the human brain and lobes of the cerebral cortex. Taken from
http://www.thinkstockphotos.com/image/stock-illustration-digital-illustration-of-areas/98359362

Forebrain

The forebrain, or prosencephalon, consists of the telencephalon and the diencephalon. The *telencephalon*, also known as the cerebrum, is the largest part of the brain. It consists of (a) the cerebral cortex, (b) the hippocampus, (c) the amygdala, (d) the basal ganglia, and (e) fiber tracts. The *cerebral cortex* is the outer surface of the brain, consisting of two cerebral hemispheres (the right and left hemispheres), which are connected by a fiber tract called the *corpus callosum.* The exterior surface of the cerebral cortex consists of *gyri* (or elevations; singular = gyrus) and *sulci* (or grooves; singular = sulcus). The presence of gyri and sulci help fit the large surface area of the cortex within a relatively small space.

Telencephalon. *Cerebral cortex. Brodmann's areas* (BA) are a set of numbers based on the work of German anatomist Korbinian Brodmann that are used to define specific areas within the cerebral cortex. Using Brodmann's areas can be helpful, since different sources sometimes have different names for certain areas of the cerebral cortex, but the numbers remain constant. Lateral (from the side) and medial views (toward midline) of the cerebral cortex with Brodmann's areas labeled are shown in Figure 2.3.

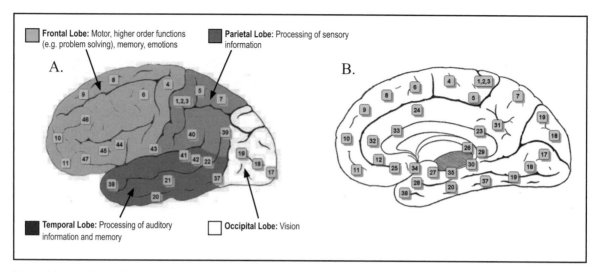

Figure 2.3. Lateral (A) and medial (B) views of the cerebral cortex, showing Brodmann's areas.

The cerebral cortex consists of four lobes: (a) the frontal lobe, (b) the parietal lobe, (c) the temporal lobe, and (d) the occipital lobe. The *frontal lobe* is bounded inferiorly by the lateral sulcus (Sylvian fissure) and posteriorly (tail/ hind end) by the central sulcus (Rolandic fissure). Several components of the motor cortex are located in the frontal lobe, including the primary motor cortex, the premotor cortex, and the supplementary motor area. The posterior portion of the frontal lobe, or precentral gyrus, is also known as the *primary motor cortex* (BA 4), since it works with other parts of the brain to plan and carry out movements.

The *primary motor* cortex is activated during musical activities that involve movement, such as foot-tapping, dancing, or playing a musical instrument (Levitin & Tirovolas, 2009). The portion of the cortex anterior (head/ front of) to the precentral gyrus is called the *premotor cortex* (BA 6), which also plays a role in planning movements. It is called the *pre*motor cortex because it is activated before the movement occurs and is involved in selecting movements based on occurrence of internal and external cues or events (Purves et al., 2001). The *supplementary motor area* (BA 6) is located anterior to the primary motor cortex and medial to the premotor cortex. The supplementary motor area helps with planning movements that are more complex and organizing movements that involve both hands (Dubuc, 2013). See Table 2.2 for more information on these areas and their connection to music.

Table 2.2. Motor Areas of the Brain		
Region of the brain	**Response to music**	**Source(s)**
Medial supplemental motor area	Increases in cerebral blood flow when participants listened to music that gave them "chills" (PET).	Blood & Zatorre, 2001
Premotor cortex	Activated only with trained melodies and learned patterns (fMRI)	Lahav et al., 2007
	Increased activation when listening to pleasant music (fMRI).	Koelsch et al., 2006
Primary motor cortex	Size of motor evoked potential was greater when listening to fear-related music compared to neutral music or a control stimulus (TMS/EMG).	Giovanelli et al., 2012

The anterior portion of the frontal lobe is known as the *prefrontal cortex*. It is often subdivided into the dorsolateral (BA 9, 46), orbitofrontal (BA 11, 12, 47), and frontopolar (BA 10) regions. The prefrontal lobe is involved in thinking, behavior, and personality. Areas of the prefrontal cortex are involved with creation, violation, and satisfaction of expectations in music (Levitin & Tirovolas, 2009). The anterior frontomedian cortex (BA 9, 10) is part of the "Theory of Mind" network (Steinbeis & Koelsch, 2009), which is activated when one is trying to interpret the thoughts or feelings of another person. Table 2.3 provides an overview of the frontal areas and their response to music.

Table 2.3. Frontal Areas		
Region of the brain	**Response to music**	**Source(s)**
Anterior frontomedian cortex (Medial prefrontal cortex)	Activated during nontonal music that listeners thought was composed by people rather than computer-generated (fMRI) Decreases in cerebral blood flow when participants listened to music that gave them "chills" (PET). Ventromedial prefrontal cortex involved in valuation during music listening (fMRI).	Steinbeis & Koelsch, 2009 Blood & Zatorre, 2001 Salimpoor et al., 2013
Left medial/superior frontal gyrus (10)	Positive correlation between BOLD signal difference and Snaith-Hamilton Pleasure Scale for participants with depression (fMRI).	Osuch et al., 2009
Medial orbital frontal cortex (BA 11); also BA 24	Activated in non-depressed (but not depressed) individuals when listening to their favorite music (fMRI).	Osuch et al., 2009
Right frontal lobe	Increased activity in the right prefrontal lobe has been noted in people who are depressed. Shifts in frontal lobe activity toward the left were found in depressed adolescents who listened to preferred music (EEG).	Field et al., 1998

Broca's area (BA 44, 45) is the third frontal convolution of the frontal lobe, also called the inferior frontal gyrus. Broca's area is involved with phonological processing (BA 44) and semantic components of language (BA 45). Damage to Broca's area, often due to a stroke, commonly results in expressive (non-fluent) aphasia, in which one is unable to produce spoken or written language. The speech of those with expressive aphasia is frequently halting and hard to initiate, although they can comprehend what is said to them and know what they intend to say.

The *parietal lobe* is bounded anteriorly by the central sulcus, inferiorly by the posterior end of the lateral sulcus, and posteriorly by the parietooccipital sulcus. The postcentral gyrus is commonly known as the *primary somatosensory cortex* (BA 1, 2, 3), since it is the primary cerebral area that receives information from the thalamus related to the sense of touch. The primary sensory cortex includes a cortical representation of various parts of the body, referred to as a *homunculus*.

The *secondary somatosensory cortex* (BA 40) works with the primary sensory cortex to respond to sensory stimuli. Located posterior to the primary sensory cortex, the *somatosensory association cortex* (BA 5, 7) integrates information from the primary somatosensory cortex. The primary sensory cortex and the somatosensory association cortex are involved with interpretation of tactile feedback from playing a musical instrument or dancing (Levitin & Tirovolas, 2009). The inferior portion of the somatosensory association cortex, known as the *inferior parietal lobule* (BA 7), works with the posterior superior temporal gyrus, or *Wernicke's area* (BA 22), to derive meaning from speech. The *arcuate fasciculus* is a fiber tract connecting Wernicke's and Broca's areas within the left hemisphere and is responsible for conveying expressive and receptive information related to speech. Damage to the arcuate fasciculus results in conduction aphasia, in which one lacks communication but is able to repeat the speech of others. More information on these structures and their connection to music can be found in Table 2.4.

Table 2.4. The Secondary Somatosensory Cortex		
Region of the brain	**Response to music**	**Source(s)**
Arcuate fasciculus (Latin: arcuate = curved; fasciculus = small bundle; thus, a curved bundle of fibers)	Increased volume of arcuate fasciculus fibers was found in patients with left hemisphere strokes who received 75–80 daily Melodic Intonation Therapy sessions (DTI).	Schlaug, Marchina, & Norton, 2009
Broca's area (named after French anatomist, Paul Broca)	Activated while listeners heard a sequence of chords (fMRI). Activated bilaterally during singing and speaking (fMRI).	Koelsch et al., 2002 Özdemir et al., 2006
Inferior parietal lobule (Latin: parietal = wall)	Activity was correlated with increases in rhythmic complexity of a tapping task when listening to previously heard rhythms of varying complexity (fMRI).	Chen et al., 2009
Wernicke's area (named after German anatomist, Carl Wernicke)	Activated while listeners heard a sequence of chords (fMRI).	Koelsch et al., 2002

The *temporal lobe* is bounded superiorly (above midline) by the lateral fissure and is involved with auditory comprehension, memory, and certain speech/language functions. As mentioned above, *Wernicke's area* (BA 22) in the dominant hemisphere (usually the left hemisphere) is involved with understanding language. Damage to Wernicke's area frequently results in receptive (fluent) aphasia, in which the rhythm and syntax of speech are preserved but the utterances are mostly meaningless. The superior temporal plane consists of the *auditory cortex* (BA 41, 42). The auditory cortex is involved with listening to sounds and perception and analysis of tones (Levitin & Tirovolas, 2009). The *temporopolar area* (or temporal pole; BA 38) is the most rostral part of the superior and middle temporal gyri. The *superior temporal sulcus* is located between the middle and superior temporal gyri (BA 21, 22). The temporal poles and the superior temporal sulcus are both part of the Theory of Mind network. Visible only in medial sections of the cortex, the *parahippocampal gyrus* (BA 34) is involved with memory encoding and retrieval. More information on the temporal lobe areas and their response to music can be found in Table 2.5.

Table 2.5. The Temporal Lobe		
Region of the brain	**Response to music**	**Source(s)**
Right middle temporal gyrus	Negative correlation between BOLD signal difference and Snaith-Hamilton Pleasure Scale for participants with depression (fMRI).	Osuch et al., 2009
Parahippocampal gyrus	Increased BOLD when listening to unpleasant music (fMRI).	Koelsch, et al., 2006
	BOLD activation of the left parahippocampal gyrus correlated with higher BDI scores for participants with depression (fMRI).	Osuch et al., 2009
Superior temporal sulcus	Activated during nontonal music who listeners thought were composed by people rather than computer-generated (fMRI).	Steinbeis & Koelsch, 2009
Temporal poles (Latin: temporal = time; hence the temporal area of the scalp, where grey hair first appears, marking the process of aging)	Increased BOLD when listening to unpleasant music (fMRI).	Koelsch, et al., 2006
	Activated during nontonal music that listeners thought was composed by people rather than computer-generated (fMRI).	Steinbeis & Koelsch, 2009

The *occipital lobe* is bounded anteriorly by the parietooccipital sulcus. Located in the occipital lobe, the *primary visual cortex* (BA 17), *secondary visual cortex* (BA 18), and *associative visual cortex* (BA 19) are responsible for processing visual information. The visual cortex is activated when reading music or looking at a performer's movements (including one's own) (Levitin & Tirovolas, 2009).

Folded within the lateral sulcus, between the temporal, parietal, and frontal lobes, is an area called the *insula* (BA 13), which is sometimes referred to as the insular cortex or the insular lobe. The insula is involved with awareness of body states, including heartbeat, blood pressure, pain, and warmth. It is also involved with motor control and emotional awareness.

Located on the medial surface of the cerebral cortex, the *cingulate gyrus,* also called the cingulate cortex (BA 23, 24, 26, 29, 30, 31, 32), can be seen in medial cross-sections of the brain, superior to the corpus callosum. The cingulate gyrus is an important part of the limbic system and is involved with emotional responses and motivation. See Table 2.6 for response to music.

Table 2.6. The Insular Cortex and the Cingulate Cortex		
Region of the brain	**Response to music**	**Source(s)**
Insula (Latin: island)	Correlations between delta activity and pain intensity ratings during a painful experience were found when listening to preferred music (MEG).	Hauck et al., 2013
	Increased BOLD when listening to pleasant music (fMRI).	Koelsch, et al., 2006
Cingulate gyrus (Latin: belt like gyrus)	Increases in cerebral blood flow to the medial anterior cingulate cortex when participants listened to music that gave them "chills" (PET).	Blood & Zatorre, 2001
	Correlations between delta band power and unpleasantness ratings during a painful experience were found in the mid cingulate gyrus when listening to preferred music (MEG).	Hauck et al., 2013

Hippocampus. The hippocampus is located in the medial temporal lobe. It plays an important part in consolidating information from short-term to long-term memory. Memory loss in Alzheimer's disease is partly related to damage to the hippocampus. The hippocampus is involved in memory for music, musical experiences, and contexts (Levitin & Tirovolas, 2009).

Amygdala. The amygdala is a group of nuclei that is also located in the medial temporal lobe, superior to the hippocampus. The amygdala plays an important part in processing memory and emotional reactions and is involved with emotional responses to music (Levitin & Tirovolas, 2009). See Table 2.7 for each region's response to music.

Table 2.7. The Amygdala and Hippocampus		
Region of the brain	**Response to music**	**Source(s)**
Amygdala (Greek: almond)	Increased BOLD when listening to unpleasant music (fMRI). Decreases in cerebral blood flow to the left amygdala and increases in cerebral blood flow to the right amygdala when participants listened to music that gave them "chills" (PET). Involved in valuation during music listening (fMRI).	Koelsch, et al., 2006 Blood & Zatorre, 2001 Salimpoor et al., 2013
Hippocampus (Greek: sea horse)	Increased BOLD when listening to unpleasant music (fMRI). Decreases in cerebral blood flow to the left hippocampus when participants listened to music that gave them "chills" (PET).	Koelsch, et al., 2006 Blood & Zatorre, 2001

Basal ganglia. The term *basal ganglia* is somewhat of a misnomer. Ganglia are groups of nuclei in the peripheral nervous system. Since the basal ganglia are part of the central nervous system, a more accurate term for this collection of structures would be *basal nuclei*, but the name basal ganglia is used frequently. The basal ganglia are positioned at the base of the forebrain and actually include structures of the telencephalon (amygdala, striatum, and globus pallidus), as well as structures of the diencephalon (subthalamic nuclei) and the mesencephalon (substantia nigra). The dorsal *striatum* consists of the *caudate nucleus* and the *putamen,* whereas the ventral striatum is made up of the *olfactory tubule* and the *nucleus accumbens.* The nucleus accumbens plays an important part in reward, pleasure, and learning and is involved with emotional responses to music (Levitin & Tirovolas, 2009). The basal ganglia are involved in a variety of functions, including motor control and emotional functioning. The basal ganglia are shown in Figure 2.4, and more information on responses to music is provided in Table 2.8.

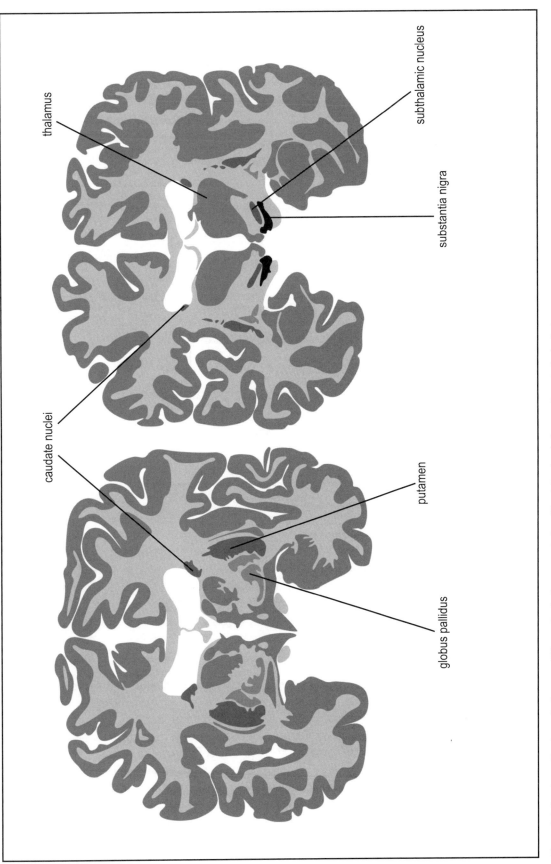

Figure 2.4. Basal ganglia, shown both at two different depths in a coronal view. The right view is deeper, closer to the brainstem.
Taken from http://commons.wikimedia.org/wiki/File:Basal_ganglia.svg

Table 2.8. The Basal Ganglia		
Region of the brain	**Response to music**	**Source(s)**
Caudate nucleus (Latin: cauda = tail; thus, tail-like nucleus)	Involved in anticipation of peak emotional experiences during music listening, (PET/fMRI).	Salimpoor et al., 2011
Right globus pallidus (Latin: globus = globe; pallidus = pale; thus, pale globe)	Negative correlation between BOLD signal difference and Snaith-Hamilton Pleasure Scale for participants with depression (fMRI).	Osuch et al., 2009
Nucleus accumbens (Latin: accumbens = reclining or leaning; thus, the nucleus leaning on the septum)	Activated in non-depressed (but not depressed) individuals when listening to their favorite music (fMRI).	Osuch et al., 2009
	Activated during listening to researcher-selected classical music (fMRI).	Menon & Levitin, 2005
	Involved in peak emotional experiences during music listening (PET/fMRI).	Salimpoor et al., 2011
	Activity in the nucleus accumbens was the best predictor of how much participants were willing to pay to hear music again (fMRI).	Salimpoor et al., 2013
Ventral striatum (Latin: furrowed; hence, the furrowed or striped appearance of the striatum)	Increases in cerebral blood flow to the left ventral striatum when participants listened to music that gave them "chills" (PET).	Blood & Zatorre, 2001 Koelsch, et al., 2006
	Increased BOLD when listening to pleasant music (fMRI).	
Ventral tegmental area	Activated during listening to researcher-selected classical music (fMRI).	Menon & Levitin, 2005

Fiber tracts. The *arcuate fasciculus* is a fiber tract that connects Wernicke's and Broca's areas within the left hemisphere. Another important fiber tract is the *corpus callosum*, which connects the right and left hemispheres. *Projection fibers* within the cerebrum are afferent and efferent tracts that connect cortical and subcortical structures. The *fornix* is a C-shaped fiber tract that carries signals from the hypothalamus to the hippocampus. It is also a key structure within the limbic system.

Diencephalon. The diencephalon consists of the thalamus, hypothalamus, subthalamus, and epithalamus. The pineal gland and the posterior portion of the pituitary gland are also part of the diencephalon. The *thalamus* is the largest structure in the diencephalon and serves as a relay center, conveying motor and sensory signals from the midbrain to the cerebral cortex. In addition, the thalamus helps regulate body states such as consciousness, sleep, and alertness. The *hypothalamus* links the nervous system to the endocrine system through the pituitary gland. It is responsible for controlling basic functions such as body temperature, sex drive, hunger, thirst, sleep, and circadian cycles, in addition to secreting hormones that stimulate or inhibit secretion of pituitary hormones. It contains the *medial* and *lateral geniculate bodies*, which serve as relay centers for auditory and visual information, respectively. The *subthalamus* (also called the prethalamus) contains *subthalamic nuclei*, which are part of the basal ganglia. The *epithalamus* secretes melatonin via the pineal gland, which helps regulate circadian rhythms. It also serves as a connection between the limbic system and the basal ganglia. Responses to music by the hypothalamus and thalamus are outlined in Table 2.9.

Table 2.9. Diencephalon		
Region of the brain	**Response to music**	**Source(s)**
Hypothalamus (Greek: under the thalamus)	Activated during listening to researcher-selected classical music (fMRI).	Menon & Levitin, 2005
Thalamus (Greek: bedroom or chamber; hence, the central chamber within the brain)	Increases in cerebral blood flow to the right thalamus when participants listened to music that gave them "chills" (PET).	Blood & Zatorre, 2001

The *Limbic system* consists of portions of the cerebrum (cingulate gyrus, hippocampus, amygdala, and corpus callosum) and the diencephalon (thalamus and hypothalamus). The fibers of the *fornix* carry signals from the hippocampus to the hypothalamus. The limbic system is the network that plays an important role in emotional processing. The limbic system is shown in Figure 2.5.

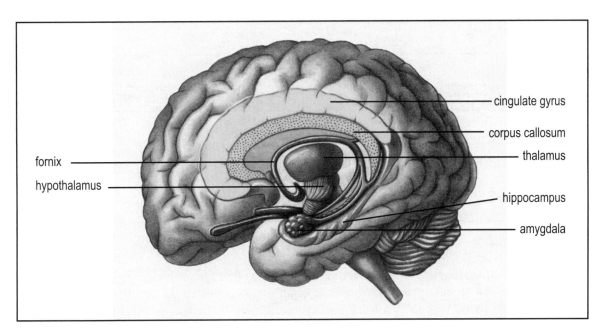

Figure 2.5. Structures of the limbic system. Taken from http://www.thinkstockphotos.com/image/stock-illustration-cross-section-illustration-of-human/98955099

Midbrain

The *midbrain*, or *mesencephalon*, is continuous with the diencephalon. The dorsal part of the midbrain is called the *tectum*; the central part of the midbrain is called the *tegmentum*; and the ventral part of the midbrain is called the *basis pedunculi*. The tectum contains the *superior colliculus* (which is involved with vision), the *inferior colliculus* (which is involved with hearing), and the *periaqueductal gray matter* (PGA), which is related to perception of pain. The tegmentum also contains motor tracts called the *red nucleus*, and the basis pedunculi contains motor tracts called the *substantia nigra* (which are also considered part of the basal ganglia).

Hindbrain

The *hindbrain*, or *rhombencephalon*, consists of the medulla oblongata, the pons, and the cerebellum. The hindbrain is frequently subdivided into the *myelencephalon* (medulla oblongata) and the *metencephalon* (pons and cerebellum). Together, the midbrain, pons, and medulla oblongata are sometimes referred to as the *brainstem*.

Myelencephalon. *Medulla oblongata.* The medulla oblongata is continuous with the spinal cord. It is the control center for cardiac, respiratory, vomiting, and vasomotor functions. The medulla contains a pair of bulges called the olivary bodies, which are part of the auditory pathway. The pyramids are the anterior ridges of the medulla, containing the cortico-spinal tract (pyramidal tract). The decussation of the cortico-spinal tract occurs in the medulla.

Metencephalon. *Pons.* The pons contains tracts of axons called peduncles that serve as bridges from the medulla oblongata to the cerebellum. Certain nuclei in the pons send signals from the forebrain to the cerebellum, whereas others are involved with basic functions such as sleep, respiration, swallowing, bladder control, hearing, taste, and eye movement.

Cerebellum. The cerebellum is attached to the posterior side of the pons via the superior and inferior peduncle. The cerebellar cortex consists of gray matter. The cerebellum plays an important part in motor control. It is involved with movements such as foot tapping, dancing, and playing an instrument, as well as emotional reactions to music (Levitin & Tirovolas, 2009). More information, including responses to music, is provided in Table 2.10.

Table 2.10. The Cerebellum and Midbrain		
Region of the brain	**Response to music**	**Source(s)**
Cerebellum (Latin: little brain)	Increases in cerebral blood flow to the left cerebellum when participants listened to music that gave them "chills" (PET).	Blood & Zatorre, 2001
Midbrain	Increases in cerebral blood flow to the left dorsomedial midbrain when participants listened to music that gave them "chills" (PET).	Blood & Zatorre, 2001

Auditory Pathways

Although areas of the limbic system or the motor cortex may be engaged by listening to certain types of music, there is a specific pathway within the brain that is activated during the process of music perception itself. What follows is a brief description of how the central nervous system processes sound (Figure 2.6).

1. Sound is first processed via the *cochlear nuclei*, which decodes the frequency, intensity, and duration of the auditory stimulus. The cochlear or auditory nerve is one branch of the *eighth cranial nerve* (also called the vestibulocochlear nerve). The cochlear nerve begins in the spiral ganglia of the cochlea, where afferent receptors are activated through the process of auditory conduction. A complete description of auditory transduction can be found at http://www.youtube.com/watch?v=PeTriGTENoc

2. Auditory impulses then move both ipsilaterally (on the same side) and contralaterally (on the opposite side) to the *superior olivary complex* in the hindbrain. Differences in the strength of signals between the two hemispheres assist with localization of sound.

3. The impulse then travels via the *lateral lemniscus* to the *inferior colliculus* in the *tectum*, where auditory and visual input is coordinated.

4. Next, the impulse goes to the *medial geniculate nucleus* in the thalamus, which coordinates preparation of motor responses.

5. Finally, the impulse is transferred to the *primary auditory cortex* (BA 41, 42) and integrated with voluntary responses. From the auditory cortex, commands are sent to other cortical areas via efferent nerve signals. The auditory cortex is inferior to the Sylvian fissure in the temporal lobe, where sound is organized tonotopically.

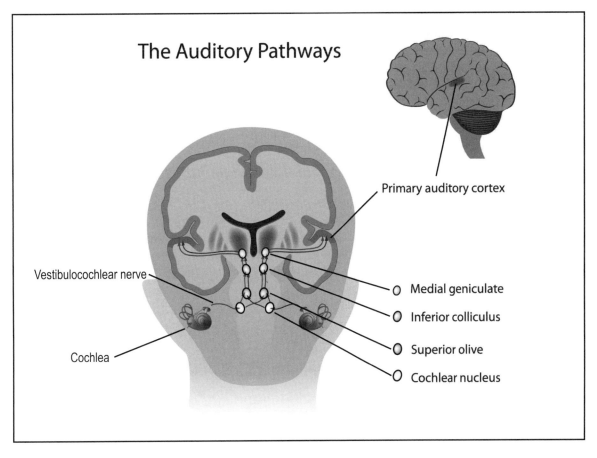

Figure 2.6. Auditory pathways. See http://www.123rf.com/photo_15313015_the-auditory-pathways.html

Following Current Research in Cognitive Neuroscience of Music

The preceding summaries of key studies on music and the brain are not meant to be exhaustive. New studies in the field of cognitive neuroscience are being published regularly in a wide variety of journals, some of which music therapists may not regularly read. How then can music therapists stay informed about current research on the effects of music on the brain? Figure 2.7 lists journals in which studies in this review have been published, as well as others that this author has encountered.

Journal Resources

Annals of the New York Academy of Science
Brain Research
Brain: A Journal of Neurology
Cerebral Cortex
Cognition and Emotion
Cognitive Brain Research
Cortex
European Journal of Neuroscience
Journal of Cognitive Neuroscience
Journal of Neurology, Neurosurgery, & Psychiatry
Journal of Neurophysiology
Journal of Neuroscience
Journal of the Acoustical Society of America
Nature Neuroscience
Neurobiology
Neuroimage
Neuron
Neuropsychologia
NeuroReport
Neuroscience Letters
Pain
Proceedings of the National Academy of Sciences (PANAS)
Psychology of Music
Psychomusicology
Psychophysiology
Science

Figure 2.7. Journal resources.

A simple way to stay up-to-date on music in the field of cognitive neuroscience of music is to sign up for electronic alerts through a database for scholarly publications. ERIC, Google Scholar, PsycINFO, and PubMed all offer services through which users can receive e-mail alerts when new articles containing specific search terms are published. The Pierfranco and Luisa Mariani Foundation also compile a biweekly e-mail newsletter called Neuromusic News, which highlights recent studies on music neuroscience. It is free of charge and those interested may register on their website (http://www.fondazione-mariani.org/en/register.html) in order to receive Neuromusic News.

Conclusion

The field of cognitive neuroscience of music is a fascinating one and has much to offer the field of music therapy. Through an understanding of the neuroscientific bases of music perception and music performance, music therapists can provide better care for their clients. Having a basic knowledge of neuroanatomy and physiology and following current research in cognitive neuroscience of music are of special importance for medical music therapists, who are frequently called upon to explain how music therapy works from a neurological standpoint.

References

Arnold, M. A., & Bryce, D. (n.d.). *Arnold's glossary of anatomy*. Retrieved from http://www.anatomy. usyd.edu.au/glossary/

Bhatnagar, S. C. (2008). *Neuroscience for the study of communicative disorders* (3rd ed.). Baltimore, MD: Lippincott Williams & Wilkins.

Blood, A. J., & Zatorre, R. J. (2001). Intensely pleasurable responses to music correlate with activity in brain regions implicated in reward and emotion. *Proceedings of the National Academy of Sciences, 98,* 11818–11823.

Chen, J. L., Penhume, V. B., & Zatorre, R. J. (2009). The role of auditory and premotor cortex in sensorimotor transformations. *Annals of the New York Academy of Science, 1169,* 15–34.

Dubuc, B. (2013). *The brain from top to bottom*. Retrieved from http://thebrain.mcgill.ca/intermediaire. php

Field, T., Martinez, A., Nawrocki, T., Pickens, J., Fox, N. A., & Schanberg, S. (1998). Music shifts frontal EEG in depressed adolescents. *Adolescence, 33,* 109–116.

Giovannelli, F., Banfi, C., Borgheresi, A., Fiori, E., Innocenti, I., Rossi, S., … Cincotta, M. (2012). The effect of music on corticospinal excitability is related to the perceived emotion: A transcranial magnetic stimulation study. *Cortex, 49*(3), 702–710. doi:10.1016/j.cortex.2012.01.013

Hauck, M., Metzner, S., Rohlffs, F., Lorenz, J., & Engel, A. K. (2013). The influence of music and music therapy on pain-induced neuronal oscillations measured by magnetencephalography. *Pain, 154,* 539–547.

Justus, T. C., & Bharucha, J. J. (2002). Music perception and cognition. In S. Yantis & H. Pashler (Eds.), *Stevens' handbook of experimental psychology, volume 1: Sensation and perception* (3rd ed., pp. 453–492). New York: Wiley.

Koelsch, S., Fritz, T., Cramon, D. Y., Müller, K., & Friederici, A. D. (2006). Investigating emotion with music: An fMRI study. *Human Brain Mapping, 27,* 239–250.

Koelsch, S., Gunter, T. C., Cramon, D. Y., Zysset, S., Lohmann, G, & Friederici, A. D. (2002). Bach speaks: A cortical "language-network" serves the processing of music. *NeuroImage, 17,* 956–966.

Lahav, A., Saltzman, E., & Schlaug, G. (2007). Action representation of sound: Audiomotor recognition network while listening to newly acquired actions. *The Journal of Neuroscience, 27,* 308-314.

Levitin, D. J., & Tirovolas, A. K. (2009). Current advances in the cognitive neuroscience in music. *Annals of the New York Academy of Science, 1156,* 211–231.

Menon, V., & Levitin, D. J. (2005). The rewards of music listening: Response and physiological connectivity of the mesolimbic system. *NeuroImage, 28,* 175–184.

Osuch, E. A., Bluhm, R. L., Williamson, P. C., Théberge, J., Densmore, M., & Neufeld, R. W. J. (2009). Brain activation to favorite music in health controls and depressed patients. *NeuroReport, 20,* 1204–1208.

Özdemir, E., Norton, A., & Schlaug, G. (2006). Shared and distinct neural correlates of singing and speaking. *NeuroImage, 33*, 628–635.

Purves, D., Augustine G. J., Fitzpatrick, D., Katz, L. C., LaMantina, A. S., McNamara, J. O., & Williams, M. S. (2001). *Neuroscience* (2nd ed.). Sunderland, MA: Sinauer Associates. Retrieved from http://www.ncbi.nlm.nih.gov/books/NBK10796/

Salimpoor, V. N., Benovoy, M., Larcher, K., Dagher, A., & Zatorre, R. J. (2011). Anatomically distinct dopamine release during anticipation and experience of peak emotion to music. *Nature Neuroscience, 14,* 257–264.

Salimpoor, V. N., van den Bosch, I., Kovacevic, N., McIntosh, A. R., Dagher, A., & Zatorre, R. J. (2013). Interactions between the nucleus accumbens and auditory cortices predict music reward value. *Science, 340*(6129), 216–219.

Schlaug, G., Marchina, S., & Norton, A. (2009). Evidence for plasticity in white matter tracts of chronic aphasic patients undergoing intense intonation-based speech therapy. *Annals of the New York Academy of Science, 1169*, 385–394.

Steinbeis, N., & Koelsch, S. (2009). Understanding the intentions behind man-made products elicits neural activity in areas dedicated to mental state attribution. *Cerebral Cortex, 19*, 619–623.

Glossary of Neuroanatomical Terms		
Term	**Language of Origin**	**Derivation**
Basis pedunculi	Latin	Small foot
Cerebral Cortex	Latin	Cortex means bark; thus, the outer covering of the brain.
Cerebrum	Latin	Brain
Cochlea	Latin	Snail
Colliculus	Latin	Small tail
Corpus callosum	Latin	Hard body
Diencephalon	Latin	Between brain
-encephalon	Greek	Brain
Fornix	Latin	Arch
Frontal	Latin	Related to the forehead
Ganglion	Greek	Swelling
Geniculate	Latin	To flex the knee
Gyrus	Greek	Circle, coil; describes the coiling appearance of the gyri.
Homunculus	Latin	Miniature human
Lemniscus	Greek	Band or ribbon
Limbic	Latin	A margin, usually curved
Medulla oblongata	Latin	Marrow; Oblong
Mesencephalon	Greek	Midbrain
Metencephalon	Greek	Behind brain
Myelencephalon	Green	Marrow brain
Nucleus	Latin	Kernel or nut
Occipital	Latin	Prominent head
Olivary	Latin	Related to the olive
Periaqueductal	Latin	Situated around the aqueduct of the brain
Pineal	Latin	Pine cone
Pons	Latin	Bridge
Prosencephalon	Latin/Greek	Pro = in front of; thus, the forebrain
Putamen	Latin	Peel, husk, or shell of a fruit or seed
Rhombencephalon	Greek	Rhomboid brain; encloses the rhomboid fossa
Substantia nigra	Latin	Black substance
Sulcus	Latin	Groove
Tegmentum	Latin	Covering
Telencephalon	Greek	Tele = end; thus, the hindbrain

Section 2: Program Development

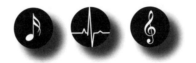

Chapter 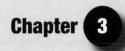 3

Medical Music Therapy Program Development
Jessica Rushing, MM, MT-BC, and Virginia Barragan, FACHE, PT, DPT, MOMT

> *For music therapists who embrace change, unlimited opportunities exist to actively participate in the redefinition of health care and the transformation of practice settings.*
> (Reuer, 1996)

Music therapy as a field has its roots in the medical community. Following World War I, musicians began performing for veterans experiencing physical and emotional trauma. Patients' positive responses to music prompted hospitals to hire musicians, which in turn created the need for specialized training. This then led to the creation of the first music therapy degree program in 1944 (Dileo & Bradt, 2009). Today, some 70 years later, music therapy is again becoming a valued part of the medical community.

Music therapy is a versatile and flexible discipline used for both habilitative and rehabilitative purposes. Music therapists systematically target nonmusical outcomes in a variety of domains (Dileo & Bradt, 2009). Music therapists regularly enhance communication and innately practice patient- and family-centered care. Skills used regularly by music therapists include:

- planning and organizing,
- developing preventative measures,
- adapting in the moment to change,
- encouraging problem solving,
- anticipating challenges,
- breaking down tasks to meet individual needs, and
- evaluating outcomes.

While these skills are fundamental to competent music therapy services, they are also foundational skills necessary for program development. Through this chapter, music therapists will learn how to apply these skills to program development. Specifically, this chapter covers (a) approaching program development, (b) reviewing strategic planning elements, (c) identifying resources, (d) developing/submitting proposals, and (e) highlighting considerations for program implementation. (The Program Development Checklist found in Appendix A can be used as supplemental guide to this chapter.)

Approaching Program Development

Levels of Care

Levels of care dictate both the quantity of patients served and the specialization of services available. The first level of care is *primary care*. This includes primary care physicians (PCP) or other subspecialties necessary for routine care and initial symptom analysis. *Secondary care* encompasses referrals outside of the PCP needed for diagnosis and treatment. Much of secondary care includes specialized equipment, lab work, and medical professionals with specific areas of expertise. Secondary care may take place in a hospital or ambulatory care center. Ambulatory care centers (outpatient-based centers) often provide both secondary and tertiary care, provided the procedures can be completed in one calendar day. *Tertiary care* primarily involves hospitalization and incorporates highly specialized expertise and equipment.

What levels of care are you interested in working with? What level of care is provided at the facility that has expressed interest in you, or you in them? It is likely that the facility provides a variety of care levels. As you research facilities, it is important to identify their levels of care, populations they serve, and areas of need. It is also important to identify each facility's mission and values. In fact, a facility's *MISSION* can provide tremendous insight as you develop a music therapy program.

Focus on Mission

Simply put, a mission statement is a "formalized document defining an organization's unique and enduring purpose" (Bart & Tabone, 1999, p. 19). Mission statements are closely aligned with an organization's (a) philosophy and values, (b) services delivered, (c) geographical area served, (d) self-image, and (e) public image (Bart & Tabone, 1999). Executives and administrators do not lightheartedly develop mission statements or values. They reflect on them. They gather feedback from the community, focus groups, and employees. Health care facilities care deeply about their mission statements. *Mission statements drive programming and decision-making processes.*

What type of mission do YOU want to be a part of? Consider your approach as a medical music therapist. Why is working for a particular hospital important to you? What will music therapy services bring to patients and the health care community? Does music therapy enhance a facility initiative? Does it address a gap in patient care? How does the introduction of music therapy add value to the service provided at this hospital? How does it align with the hospital's values and philosophy of care? Remember: *you are asking them to integrate a new service, so you must also be willing to invest and integrate with them.*

What Role Does Music Therapy Play?

When developing a medical music therapy program, it is necessary to reflect on the role of music therapy within the medical model. In the health care setting, music therapists work to assess, treat, and evaluate patients based on medical, psychosocial, and emotional needs within the context of a discharge timeline (American Music Therapy Association [AMTA], 2012; Magee & Andrews, 2007). Music therapists work in children's hospitals, cancer centers, and general medical facilities, among others. Clinical music therapy services are provided in response to medical referrals in a variety of inpatient medical units, including (a) newborn intensive care units; (b) pediatrics/pediatric intensive care units; (c) pediatric rehabilitation; (d) oncology; (e) heart and vascular units; (f) geriatric units, extended/long-term care; and (g) labor and delivery. Outpatient units served by music therapists include (a) neuroscience programs (Parkinson's), (b) neurorehabilitation, (c) pediatric rehabilitation, (d) cardiac outpatient, and (e) adult day care (Walworth, 2005). Given the wide range of possibilities, it is important to understand the continuum of care and to be able to communicate where music therapy can add the most value.

Music Therapy Treatment in the Medical Setting

Music therapy treatment in a health care setting can differ substantially from services provided in other areas. For example, consider educational settings; music therapy services in an educational setting are often IEP-based (Individualized Education Program). For a child to receive IEP music therapy services, he or she must be identified, evaluated, and found eligible. A meeting must be held and IEP goals written. Services are then provided, and progress is documented and reevaluated according to a set timeline. The whole process can last months or even years. In a health care setting, a patient's stay typically consists of days or weeks, at most. Therefore, assessment, treatment, and evaluation occur rapidly, possibly even multiple times a day. Medical music therapists must be able to quickly identify potential referrals and/or have a standardized referral system. They must be able to quickly identify patient goals and expected outcomes. Unlike an IEP meeting where information is gathered and presented, it is often up to the medical music therapist to gather relevant information as well as consult with interdisciplinary team members as necessary. These team members may include nursing, other therapies, case managers, social workers, chaplains, unit managers, physicians, and more.

Another difference lies in reports, both formal and informal. Again, consider the educational setting. IEP reporting follows a standardized format, and music therapy is simply incorporated into the existing structure. If music therapy is new to a health care organization, there are likely no set standards for program reporting. *The communication of information is essential for (a) creating, (b) developing, (c) sustaining, and (d) expanding services.* Written data collection ensures an ability to conduct program assessment, and it is up to the servicing music therapist to develop protocols consistent with the facility medical records system.

While educational and medical settings differ, medical music therapy has marked parallels with the private practice setting, particularly in relation to logistics. Private practitioners may contract hours with a hospital to provide services on specific units. Hours at a hospital may be developed unit by unit, much like a private practice approaches various facilities individually. Assessment of needs and implementation of services may be very different for each unit. A number of music therapists have had success contracting by the hour with hospitals, and their practice has grown substantially by doing so. However, it is important to remember that a contract can be terminated or cut swiftly from a budget. Although an employee can be cut as well, there is a certain level of investment put forth for hospital employees that may or may not occur for a contractor. On paper, an employee is an entity of the hospital. They (a) participate in ongoing training, (b) undergo performance evaluations, (c) maintain a certain level of competency, and (d) have the opportunity to participate on committees (e.g., advisory boards, practice councils, performance improvement projects, and more).

Educating the Interdisciplinary Team

A music therapist must assist potential colleagues and administrators in creating an understanding of what music therapy services will "look" like. During the initial communication process, an administrator will likely consider two things: the monetary impact of new services, and the benefit to patients and the enterprise. The more administrators truly understand what happens in a music therapy session, the more support they will bring to budget meetings, unit meetings, executive meetings, and perhaps most importantly, to hallway conversations.

As your program development moves forward, you must take advantage of all opportunities to interact with staff at all levels, creating both a horizontal and vertical flow of information throughout the organization (see Figure 3.1). *Interdisciplinary involvement is vital for the introduction of music therapy into a health care system.* From frontline health care workers such as nurses to C-suite executives, a music therapist must be willing to educate all about potential new services and opportunities for patients and families. Presentations, inservices, and other opportunities may or may not arise during the initial phases of program proposal and development. However, they play a vital role as services are being implemented.

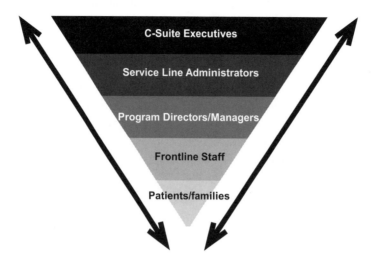

Figure 3.1. Communication flow.

Consider Your Audience

When communicating with various staff, it is important to consider each staff member's education, training, and career background. Consider the best delivery strategy for each individual; be prepared to describe a session, share news footage, or bring an article that highlights a specific music therapy technique related to (a) individuals' personal background, (b) their unit's goals, and/or (c) one of the hospital's initiatives. Speak to them in their language whenever possible. (In Appendix B you will find terms commonly used in health care.)

Strategic Planning Elements

According to the *2013 American Music Therapy Survey and Work Force Analysis* (AMTA, 2013), "medical/surgical" is the third largest population served by music therapists, preceded by "mental health" and "developmentally disabled." The medical setting is also the third largest setting in which music therapists work. Though these statistics suggest that music therapy in health care settings has grown tremendously, services are not yet integrated uniformly. Programs often vary in:

- structural organization (administration),

- funding sources, and

- student impact.

The following information outlines various approaches to these three areas of program development. One approach is not necessarily better than another, as all have proven successful. It is important to recognize all options and be willing to work with administrators to promote program start-up, program growth, and program sustainability.

Structural Organization

Health care facilities typically employ individuals at three different levels: benefited employee, per diem employee, or contractor. Each has its pros and cons, and the benefits of each should be considered in advance of any discussions with an administrator.

Benefited employee. A benefited employee is usually an employee of the facility. Typically benefited employees are guaranteed a certain number of hours per pay period, dependent on part- or full-time status. Benefits such as health care, a 401k, and paid time off (PTO) are usually provided. In exchange, the employee is dedicated to the facility and must be available for the agreed-upon hours. Approval must be granted for time off. The hourly wage is fixed and might be slightly lower to factor in the cost of benefits provided. According to Walworth (2005), the most beneficial use of a music therapist in a health care setting is a full-time employee who serves a variety of medical units and is able to be on call for procedural support needs.

Per diem. A per diem employee is also an employee of the hospital, but typically there is no guarantee of hours or benefits. In exchange, the employee receives a slightly higher hourly wage and, in many cases, permission for time off is not needed (although an absent employee with no replacement could impact program growth).

Contractor (non-benefited employee). An independent contractor negotiates a rate for provision of services but must ensure there is someone to serve as a replacement if he or she takes time off. The employee is also responsible for his or her own liability insurance and benefits. Independent contractors often have some flexibility when setting hours.

Funding Sources

Administrators work tirelessly to ensure their hospital's welfare and financial security. When reviewing potential avenues for funding, the music therapist must be mindful of financial concerns within the structure of the health care setting. Hospitals work on a fiscal year (FY) system, which generally runs either from July 1–June 30 or January 1–December 31. Major budget planning tends to occur approximately 3 to 4 months prior to the start of the fiscal year. This does not mean that the introduction of new services is limited to any particular time frame. However, administrators must consider the current fiscal year as well as future progress when contemplating implications of a new cost item (e.g., a music therapist). Being sensitive to this may open doors to future discussions, if barriers arise.

Try asking, "Do you think music therapy is something that could be considered during budgeting this coming year?" or "In relation to budgeting for a music therapist, is there a particular time when you would be reviewing current services and considering opportunities for piloting music therapy?"

Music therapy positions are funded in many ways. Direct funding from one or more contributing departments or areas is common. Possibilities include:

- individual units (oncology, rehabilitation, etc.),

- endowments or private donors,

- grants,

- reimbursement (generating revenue),

- revenue retention (cost savings/patient satisfaction), or

- university affiliations.

At times you may find that even a supportive administrator is hesitant to bring on a new full-time employee (FTE) music therapist. There are still options. Administrators may need quantitative data to increase their confidence and demonstrate to their supervisors a return on investment (ROI)—YOU. Consider this up front and determine the amount of time and pay for which you are willing to pilot a program. Music therapists are trained, credentialed clinicians. It is highly recommended that they be compensated as such for all services provided.

Individual units. After researching and assessing a facility's needs for your services, you should be ready to discuss how music therapy can be a value-added service. If necessary, a pilot project can provide data for a targeted population or unit. Although one department alone may not be able to fund a 1.0 FTE music therapy position, it is likely that multiple departments could split percentages of the cost based on hours worked on the individual unit and demand for services.

Pinpointing the best option for initial funding can be complex, so it is important to ask yourself, "Who should I approach first?" The best option is likely to vary drastically with each proposal, contacts made, expertise of the therapist, and nature of circumstances. *If you are at a starting point, we suggest approaching the rehabilitation administration as a first point of contact.* Table 3.1 highlights a few reasons behind this line of thought.

Table 3.1. Reasons for Approaching Rehabilitation as a Starting Contact Point	
Reason	**Rationale**
Therapists	Music therapists think like therapists. They communicate like therapists. They function as therapists. They relate to therapists.
Documentation	Functional, objective outcomes are adjunctive and in line with other therapy goals. Goals often address barriers to progress in therapy such as mood or pain, therefore directly aiding in the continuum of care.
Co-Treating	Therapists value co-treating. It is supportive and fosters creative problem solving. It also allows colleagues to see firsthand the effects of music therapy, therefore enhancing interdisciplinary support and communication.
Reimbursement	Rehabilitation administrators are keenly versed in both reimbursement practices and the coding that music therapists commonly use. As reimbursement continues to evolve toward a standard in music therapy practice, this type of administrator may be key in the expansion of music therapy in inpatient settings.
Research	A growing body of music therapy research is targeting *specific* rehabilitation-related areas such as aphasia, traumatic brain injuries, gait training, and more. Specific, measurable outcomes can easily be targeted.
System-wide Service	The rehabilitation team is already set up to provide services across a health care system, making logistics of expansion to other units potentially more fluid and natural.

Endowments and donations. Donors and investors often play key roles in developing or sustaining new programming. Many music therapy programs are funded through endowments, either solely or as a supplement to other funding resources. Working with hospital-specific foundations to promote community contributions can be a successful funding strategy. These foundations often provide web support and marketing materials. They may be also able to assist with fundraising and promote program needs through "instrument wish lists." Likewise, hospitals with existing arts in health care or arts-in-medicine programs may already have a strong arts-funding base. Are the directors of those programs positioned as possible advocates for music therapy services? Clinical music therapy services can work well with existing arts-based programs; conversely, there may be role ambiguity and barriers to access for both. Always enter into discussions with existing programs with respectful caution, looking for ways to foster cooperation whenever possible.

Grants. Grants are another possible funding option for program development. Grants may be tied to the facility itself, community-based, or connected with research. Be willing to approach facility development or grants officers about possible funding resources. Likewise consider approaching community organizations (corporations, city/county governmental entities, etc.). Finally, look for music therapy-specific funding opportunities like those available from the American Music Therapy Association. (Note: Be aware that some grants will not fund start-up expenses; work carefully with grants coordinators to determine eligibility.)

Prior to my first meeting with a service line administrator, she was provided with various requested research materials and a full program proposal. Of all the materials provided, the first word she picked out to discuss with me was "reimbursement."

Reimbursement. Along with cost benefit/cost savings and patient satisfaction, Robertson (2009) suggests reimbursement as a major area of focus to ensure program permanence and sustainability within the current system. Reimbursement focuses on generating actual revenue, while cost benefit/savings and patient satisfaction focus on retaining funds received. All three options have merit, but the appropriateness of the option will often vary based on the type of facility (inpatient vs. outpatient) and funding source (insurance, Medicaid, etc.). It is important to be able to address ways in which music therapy can impact revenue generation and retention.

In order for a medical treatment to be reimbursable, it must be physician ordered. In some cases, Advanced Practice Registered Nurses (APRN) can also "drop" orders, as can additional medical staff on behalf of a physician. While some medical music therapy programs require physician referrals, others do not. The music therapist, along with the facility, must determine whether the program requires physician orders for music therapy treatment as part of standard operating protocol. *It is highly recommended that clinical music therapy services should be set up as physician-referred whenever possible.* This contributes to the continuum of care, placing music therapy on equal footing with other forms of treatment. It also establishes the referral process for future reimbursement possibilities. Medical music therapy is a clinical service; positioning it as such is vital.

A working knowledge of reimbursement practices is necessary for music therapists when seeking employment in health care. Regardless of whether a hospital decides to pursue reimbursement for music therapy services, reimbursement is the language of health care. As a health care clinician, it is important to understand how reimbursement functions as well as the impact it has on the health care system. The Centers for Medicare & Medicaid Services (CMS) is considered the gold standard in reimbursement practices across the United States. CMS is a valuable resource for information on current reimbursement practices.

CPT codes. Music therapists should also be familiar with Current Procedural Terminology (CPT) codes. CPT codes are governed by the American Medical Association. Each code defines a specific service or unit of time spent providing a service. Any services rendered reimbursable must be submitted using a CPT code. CPT codes are not discipline-specific but instead are service-specific. Multiple therapies may be working toward similar goals, and thus the services provided are reported using the same CPT code. Multiples of the same code may not be billable in the same day, as that may indicate duplication of services. Insurance plans also often have limits on therapeutic services, with caps on therapeutic services. Music therapists should research the codes they plan to use and consult with facility billing experts, who will set up the behind-the-scenes actions needed to attach codes to services. The financial staff will also put in place the modifier, revenue codes, and charge masters to make it all happen smoothly. In general, as a music therapist, you should be able to

- clearly define your services,

- have a general understanding of common CPT codes used by music therapists, and

- have a basic understanding of reimbursement as a driving force in health care.

An increasing number of resources, specific to music therapy practices on reimbursement as well as the use of CPT codes, are available. See the *CPT Code Fact Sheet 2012* found at http://www.musictherapy.org/documents/ for more information. (Additional information on reimbursement can be found in Appendix C.) Information specific to reimbursement in the NICU can be found in Standley and Walworth's (2010) *Music Therapy with Premature Infants: Research and Developmental Interventions.*

Insurance options. In the United States, there is no universal health insurance system (see Table 3.2). A music therapist will most likely encounter the following insurance formats: (a) Health Maintenance Organization (HMO), (b) Participating Provider Option (PPO), (c) Consumer Directed Health Plan (CDHP), and/or (d) Health Savings Account (HSA). CMS reimbursement operates using a Prospective Payment System (PPS). A Prospective Payment System is a "method of reimbursement in which Medicare payment is made based on a predetermined, fixed amount" (www.cms.gov). Frequently, reimbursement is based on diagnosis-related groups (DRGs). DRG-based reimbursement is calculated based on diagnosis and associated care; payment rates are set according to individual diagnoses. Various situations may come into play but, in general, if a patient has X diagnosis, the hospital receives X dollars despite length of stay and course of treatment.

Table 3.2. Basics of Insurance Plans		
Type of Program		**Highlights**
HMO	Health Maintenance Organization	Primary Care Physician (PCP) is your first point of contact prior to referrals to specialists. Low out of pocket expenses. Limited to no coverage for out of network providers.
PPO	Participating Provider Option	PCP referral not required to see a specialist. Increased access to out of network providers. Higher out of pocket expenses up front.
CDHP	Consumer Directed Health Plan	May involve a combination of a PPO and HSA. High deductibles, lower premiums.
HSA	Health Savings Account	Tax-advantage account to which you contribute money that covers deductibles or other gaps in coverage.
PPS	Prospective Payment System	CMS's primary system of payment to providers based on fixed amounts per diagnosis.

In a recent conversation with a service line administrator, the question was posed, "What are the one or two most valuable change outcomes you look for as an administrator?" Length of stay (LOS) and pain were quickly her first responses. She went on to discuss the impact of these two outcomes and their relationship to reimbursement.

Cost benefits/cost savings. Current health care revenue is largely based on PPSs and DRGs. In these models, the facility receives a set payment amount regardless of services rendered. As a result, administrators and hospital financial experts may be hesitant to pursue music therapy reimbursement. Given that payment amounts are set, it may be difficult to advocate for the addition of new services when payment amounts are fixed, i.e., when the facility will not receive additional revenue when adding a new service. In these situations it may be best to argue that music therapy can provide cost benefits or savings, thereby allowing the facility to retain a higher percentage of any revenue generated.

For example, consider one factor that often impacts funding—length of stay (LOS). Perceived pain can lead to increased length of stay (LOS). Increased LOS can result in decreased reimbursement. Standley (2000) reported that music can have an even greater effect when some pain is present. Perhaps by reducing perception of pain, music therapists can also reduce length of stay, improving reimbursement. By documenting the effect of music therapy services on patients' pain levels, music therapists can demonstrate outcomes that impact the bottom line. W*ell versed health care clinicians should be able to speak to reimbursement practices in their field and provide resources to their administrator to determine the best course of action.* For more information on cost benefits of music therapy, see Robertson (2009).

In addition to length of stay, there are a number of other factors that impact revenue retention. Pain management, reductions in medication, and repeat admissions are just a few examples. For a concise review of music therapy cost-benefit literature, see *Music Therapy in Texas: A Fact Sheet* (http://www.swamta.com/texas%20task%20force/TexasFactSheet.pdf), or the *Music Therapy in Illinois Fact Sheet* (http://musictherapyillinois.org/wp-content/uploads/2010/12/Illinois-Music-Therapy-Fact-Sheet.pdf).

Patient satisfaction. Another contributing factor is patient satisfaction, which is increasingly tied to reimbursement. Patient satisfaction is frequently measured through surveys like the Press Ganey or the Consumer Assessment of Healthcare Providers and Systems program (CAHPS). A study by Yinger and Standley (2011) found that patients who received music therapy rated their overall satisfaction an average of 3.4 points higher than those who did not receive music therapy. Improving patient satisfaction can be another cost-benefit of music therapy services. Additional possibilities for assessing patient satisfaction may include (a) post-service simple surveys, including a question about music therapy during post-discharge follow-up calls; (b) logging comments made by patients, family, and staff; or (c) other forms of tracking feedback implemented at the facility.

Student Impact

Many health care facilities value research and student training. Partnering with a university program may provide benefits to both the music therapy program and the health care facility. Academic institutions have ready access to the latest research and can be an ongoing resource for manpower. Working with an academic institution can also be an excellent way to promote community engagement, an element often incorporated into the mission of many health care facilities. Finally, partnering with an academic program can promote music therapy research, which will in turn enhance the field of music therapy. A complete review of a university-affiliated program can be found in *Medical Music Therapy: A Model Program for Clinical Practice, Education, Training, and Research* (Standley et al., 2005).

Identifying Resources

Making Contacts

Program development often requires making contacts and networking. Have no fear of the "cold call." It is simply a conversation that needs warming up. As a therapist, you build rapport with each of your clients by presenting your expertise and responding to their needs. You can approach various contacts at a hospital in much the same way. Focus on your knowledge and expertise as a music therapist when making initial contacts. Assess responses, anticipate needs, and develop strategies for implementation of services. When strategizing whom you should contact, consider the following:

- Possible funding sources

- Your interest and clinical expertise

- Decision makers

- Hospital initiatives

- History, if any, of previous attempts to establish music therapy

Service line administrators are the budget gatekeepers for the various units of a health care facility. They are also highly influential as they work directly with key personnel (e.g., CEO, administrators, unit managers, etc.). Head physicians are also important decision makers and can champion your referral process. Finally, other staff (administrators, other therapists, etc.) may be included in the discussions. Be prepared to present to a variety of people when proposing a program including administrators, physicians, program directors, managers, board members, and others.

During the initial communication phase, it is helpful to identify the contact's preferred mode of communication. Phone calls are personable, allowing real-time exchange of ideas as well as insight regarding responses. Reaching someone by telephone can prove to be difficult, so be prepared to leave a voice mail. In your message you should include a brief introduction, clearly stated contact information at the beginning and end of the message, and a specific response you would like to receive, such as

- a return phone call;

- a meeting;

- a response to an email you will be sending with more information;

- an opportunity to present the idea of music therapy to people within their facility; or

- a simple response as to their level of interest in learning more about music therapy.

Be sure to let your contact know why you are communicating with them, why their facility stood out to you, and why music therapy as a clinical service could fit into their mission as a leading health care provider in the area. Quickly highlight your expertise in music therapy and the services you can offer their facility.

Tip: When leaving a phone message, provide multiple ways to be contacted and repeat your preferred way twice at the end so there is no need to replay the message, which may or may not happen immediately. For example, "My name is Sarah Smith, my phone number is xxx-xxxx; again the number is xxx-xxxx. I look forward to talking with you in regard to music therapy at your facility."

Review of music therapy program development at a multi-campus regional not-for-profit hospital in southern California revealed an average of 100 days once pursuit of expansion to a new unit was initiated to acquiring hours on that unit. This is approximately 3 months. Initial pursuit was defined as a meeting, conversation, or presentation involving focused consideration of implementing music therapy on the unit. Some units took well over 100 days and multiple meetings. Some units took small hallway conversations and one logistics conversation, following which services were implemented.

Developing the Proposal

Timing

Timing plays a large but often uncontrollable factor in program development. Market research and speaking with your contacts can be invaluable tools in terms of timing. Factors that contribute to timing include, but are not limited to:

- *Strategic initiatives* – Align your programming with hospital initiatives, if possible.

- *Budgeting* – Consider fiscal year concerns, as well as budgeting for the next FY.

- *Physical development* – Are there major renovations occurring? Is budget tight with no wiggle room, or is it the perfect opportunity to consider innovative programming and requests for storage/office space.

- *Productivity* – All forms of business are run on productivity. Units are constantly striving for high productivity, as defined by each, often related to efficient staffing-to-patient services ratios. Can music therapy services influence productivity at your facility?

- *Outcome measures* – Hospitals are paid based on outcome measures. Are they meeting them or exceeding them? Are they innovative in their approaches? If your services can influence outcomes measures, you will be extremely valuable. HCAHPS (Hospital Consumer Assessment of Healthcare Providers and Systems), Press Ganey (patient satisfaction) surveys, mortality rates, and clinical outcomes are large determinants of value-based purchasing.

Selling Music Therapy: The Proposal

Head, heart, and wallet. These are the three elements that will sell music therapy to a hospital. You must present all three in concise, confident language that is familiar to your audience.

Head. Proposing music therapy to a health care facility requires evidence-based research to support consideration of services. Randomized control trial (RCT) studies are the gold standard, as are systematic reviews and meta-analyses. It may be advantageous to create a table that summarizes the latest research related to your proposal. Options for accessing research include: (a) university libraries, (b) public library databases, (c) medical libraries, (d) journals like the *Journal of Music Therapy* and *Music Therapy Perspectives*, and (e) Cochran reviews.

Heart. Health care professionals care deeply about the patients they serve. Many administrators started out as clinicians. In addition to research and budget information, share the impact that music therapy can have on the human experience. Be prepared to play a video, share a vignette, or show a card you once received from a patient. Share personal stories on a regular basis as they help remind administrators of the impact that music therapy has on patients.

I once shared a six-month program report with the head physician on my unit. It included great quantitative information about how many patients had been seen, average number of sessions, reasons for referrals, program development highlights, and other information supporting music therapy as a value-added service. At the end of the report, I included a small number of standout quotes from patients and staff. After spending a few minutes reviewing the document, the physician smiled at me and said, "I really like that quote from Mr. Smith."

Wallet. A music therapy position is an investment, and an administrator will likely ask about the return on investment (ROI) when hiring a music therapist. Ideally, the return is in cost savings. Be familiar with research related to medical cost benefits and music therapy. (See http://www.swamta. com/texas%20task%20force/ TexasFactSheet.pdf for a concise summary.) Return can be discussed in terms of outcome measures, such as reduction in measurable pain, anxiety, length of stay, or medications used. It can also be discussed in terms of music therapy's impact on patient-centered care and patient satisfaction. In other words, music therapy can be considered a "value added" service. Determine what the most important outcomes are for the types of patients you are proposing to work with.

The written proposal. A proposal may include but is not limited to:

- cover letter

- executive summary

- population-specific research and benefits

- cost benefits

- program costs/budget (annual expenses)

- testimonials

- letters of support

- contact references

- ideal short-term and long-term goals

When preparing a proposal, offer more than one option for implementation of services, as well as your vision for the future. Prepare to speak their language by reviewing terms in Appendix B at the conclusion of this text. Be certain you have done targeted research on the facility. Be prepared to offer a pilot program with a target population(s); pilot programs help minimize the risk for administrators. Let the administrator know you would like to work together to develop a strategic plan to implement music therapy services in stages. Define measurable outcomes for program evaluation. Data collection possibilities include:

- patient surveys

- post-discharge questionnaire with music therapy questions

- research projects

- specific objective outcome measures

Ultimately it may be necessary to have both a full proposal and a "two-page" version as many administrators prefer a summary for easy dissemination. Be equipped with both options, making sure the essential information is conveyed regardless of format.

Considerations for Program Implementation

Program Assessment and Documentation

As you develop your music therapy program, you will find it necessary to provide regular updates to administrators and/or decision makers. Updates should contain current information on services, program goals, accomplishments, and issues that arise. *Remember, program updates provide administrators information that can be used during daily conversations/meetings.*

Just as music therapy services will need support from the administration, the administration needs support from the music therapist in the form of information, vignettes, program data, and any information that may be helpful for them to know. Documentation and communication related to program events are the music therapist's responsibility; the administration and colleagues may or may not ask for that type of information. If there has never been a music therapist in the health care system, the logistics of the role and expectations of a music therapist will likely not be defined. The music therapist is the expert and should help by establishing standards of music therapy clinical services on par with clinical services throughout the hospital.

Regardless of the amount of hours or services provided, program progress must be tracked and evaluated. In collaboration with your supervisor, determine the most appropriate data to be tracked. By establishing the data tracking process from the very beginning, you will be able to regularly evaluate the clinical services being provided. Never underestimate the power of a well thought-out spreadsheet, as it will provide easy access to supporting evidence when opportunities such as grant funding, unplanned presentations, or possibilities of service expansion arise. This will also allow administrators to speak confidently about music therapy services. At a very minimum, quarterly and annual program evaluation is recommended. In particular, productivity data can be crucial information, and all services lines are regularly required to report productivity measures. Productivity measures include:

- *Number and type of patients seen*—This information could be representative of diagnoses, unit, age, type of situation, etc. Determine what would be the most valuable based on your services.

- *Referral reasons*—For example, 45% of patients are referred for psychosocial needs, 40% for pain management, 10% for increased anxiety, and 5% for difficulty coping with hospitalization.

- *Who is referring patients*—Monitor where referrals are coming from—physicians, nursing, self/family, or other. Which units are generating the most referrals? Expand on this information.

- *Outcomes*—Changes can be determined through pre/post measures of pain, anxiety, or other.

- *Length of session and interventions used*—This information can help provide a complete picture of what is happening. It could also be used for potential research or reporting on medical music therapy services in general. Length of session (client contact and related tasks represent employee productivity).

- *Impact on families*—Track the number of family members/visitors present or affected by services.

- *Hot comments*—Keep a running log of comments made that particularly stand out. These can come from patients, family, visitors, and staff. All are important.

- *Service*—These can include presentations, community events, or other. Note the number of participants. Be able to report on how many of each event you participated in.

- *All program development or happenings*—Keep a log of successes and barriers.

As you consider your program's forward movement, it may help to keep in mind the *Plan–Do–Check–Act* cycle widely used for process improvement (Figure 3.2). Development of a program is very much an ongoing process. *Plan*—Identify the needs or opportunities and develop a plan. *Do*—Through a pilot or sample data collection, test the plan. *Check*—Evaluate the outcomes and check the progress or lack thereof. *Act*—Implement services and process based on pilot results and make adjustments based on outcomes, as needed.

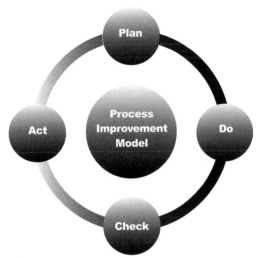

Figure 3.2. The Plan–Do–Check–Act cycle.

Integrating into the Medical Setting

As part of a medical team, a music therapist will develop (a) policies and procedures, (b) infection control protocols, (c) a documentation system, (d) referral guidelines, (e) ongoing staff education, (f) a data collection system, and (g) progress data demonstrating music therapy as a value-added service. Depending on your facility, you may be expected or encouraged to participate in research, Performance Improvement projects (PI), or facility initiatives like a memorial celebration. In many cases, taking on or creating such opportunities can be highly valuable for the development and sustainability of a medical program.

When you are part of a hospital, you are part of a system. Hospitals are large, breathing, changing, and challenging bodies. Things move rapidly, timing is critical, opportunities are abounding. Go in with your eyes and ears open. Be sensitive to the culture of your hospital; relationships are important; hierarchies are important. Remember the foundational skill set a music therapist possesses and look for opportunities to share it with the hospital as a whole, not just in direct clinical services.

Patient-Centered Care

The final section of this chapter focuses on patient-centered care, a concept of growing importance in the American health care system. Health care facilities are increasingly exploring ways to expand patient-centered care, and music therapy is uniquely positioned to meet this need. Focusing on patient-centered care can be an excellent way to promote music therapy program development and expansion.

The experience of care, as perceived by the patient and family, is a key factor in health care quality and safety.

(Institute for Patient- and Family-Centered Care, 2011, p. 3)

With the passage of the Affordable Care Act in 2010, patient-centered care became increasingly important when patient satisfaction was directly tied to reimbursement. Patient-centered care was further stressed by The Joint Commission in 2012 with the inclusion of patient-centered communication standards (The Joint Commission, 2010) in the accreditation process for hospitals.

(The Joint Commission accredits over 20,000 health care organizations, representing quality and commitment to standards in health care.) Today, patient-centered care is an important concept in health care, one that music therapy is uniquely equipped to address. Figure 3.3 highlights the core concepts of patient- and family-centered care.

Concepts

Dignity and Respect of patients and families, taking into account culture, knowledge, values, and beliefs.

Information Sharing that is complete, accurate, unbiased, and timely.

Participation in care as desired.

Collaboration across all levels of care and implantation of care.

(Institute for Patient- and Family-Centered Care, 2011)

Figure 3.3. Core concepts.

Patient- and family-centered care concepts are the standards of practice that music therapists adhere to. According to Magee and Andrews (2007), music therapy can be a platform for addressing multiple needs simultaneously. While patients are the primary focus of music therapy services, many, if not all, music therapists in medical settings document regularly on family involvement in sessions. A medical music therapist may even provide services to family members separate from the patient, if applicable. Specific family needs can be targeted either through explicit referral reasons, demonstration of needs, or expression of needs. It is not uncommon for music therapists to be asked to work with patients and families who have barriers to standard care such as (a) special needs comorbidities, (b) inability to verbalize or express needs, (c) agitation, (d) pain and depression, or (e) general dissatisfaction with hospitalization experience.

Integration with Music Therapy

Music therapy is inherently a patient-centered service, regularly integrating aspects of the eight dimensions of patient care. Figure 3.4 provides the eight dimensions of patient-centered care.

---

8 Dimensions of Patient-Centered Care

Patients' Preferences   Emotional Support   Physical Comfort   Information & Education

Community & Transition   Coordination of Care   Access to Care   Family & Friends

Note. Developed by Harvard Medical School and Picker Institute researchers, based on thousands of interviews, commonly known as the Picker Surveys. This is a tool currently used in America by the National Research Corporation.

Figure 3.4. Eight dimensions of patient-centered care.

The American Music Therapy Association's *Standards of Clinical Practice: Medical Settings* (2012) outline standards for music therapy services within medical settings. The following standards specifically address aspects of patient-centered care:

2.1 The music therapy assessment will include the general categories of psychological, cognitive, communicative, social, and physiological functioning focused on the client's needs and strengths. The assessment will also determine the client's responses to music, music skills, and musical preferences.

2.2 The music therapy assessment will explore the client's culture. This can include but is not limited to race, ethnicity, language, religion/ spirituality, social class, family experiences, sexual orientation, gender identity, and social organizations.

3.0 The music therapist will prepare a written individualized program plan based upon the music therapy assessment, the client's prognosis, and applicable information from other disciplines and sources. The client will participate in program plan development when appropriate.

As music therapists align with the advances in health care delivery, they should consider the presented elements of patient- and family-centered care. The following are suggested ideas to reflect on:

- Are you involving patients and families in decisions about their music therapy treatment?

- Are they informed about the treatment they are receiving?

- Do they have access to resources related to music therapy?

- Are they given information that meets their needs in a timely manner?

- Is there an effective line of communication between health care providers and persons receiving music therapy services?

- Are there any gaps in the delivery of care or initiatives at your facility that music therapy could target?

Additional considerations include:

- Do patients and families have opportunities to participate in all levels of decision making from strategic planning to evaluation?

- Do you believe that patients' and families' participation in these processes is essential to the safety and quality of health care?

- Do patients and families you serve have access to information in appropriate and easy-to-access formats, such as Web-based opportunities, written materials, and community-based forums? Are literacy levels, primary language needs, and other cultural considerations taken into account?

Figure 3.5 provides a checklist that can be used by music therapists as they consider their own approach to care.

A Checklist for Attitudes About Partnering with Patients and Families

Do I believe that patients and family members bring unique perspectives and expertise to the clinical relationship?

Do I encourage patients and families to speak freely?

Do I listen respectfully to the opinions of patients and family members?

Do I encourage patients and family members to participate in decision making about their care?

Do I encourage patients and family members to be active partners in assuring the safety and quality of their own care?

(Institute for Patient- and Family-Centered Care, 2011, p. 29)

Figure 3.5. A checklist for attitudes about partnering with patients and families.

Patient- and family-centered care is an approach to the planning, delivery, and evaluation of health care that is governed by collaborative partnerships among health care providers, patients, and families.

(Sodomka, 2006)

Additional information on patient-centered care can also be found in Table 3.3.

Table 3.3. Resources That Highlight Patient Centered Care	
Source	**Description**
Institute for Patient- and Family-Centered Care	Seeks to advance the understanding and practice of patient- and family-centered care. It seeks to serve as a central resource for all aspects of integrating patient- and family-centered care principles into health care. http://www.ipfcc.org
The Joint Commission	Health care accrediting not-for-profit organization. The Joint Commission defines the Core Measures Sets aligned with the Centers for Medicare & Medicaid Services (CMS). http://www.jointcommission.org
Picker Institute	Non-profit sponsoring research and education in promoting patient-centered care. Producer of the Picker Survey. http://www.pickerinstitute.org
Planetree	Consults with organizations to promote patient-centered care by transforming the health care experience from national quality strategies to environment and the arts. A system can receive the Planetree Designation representing the "highest level of achievement in patient-/person-centered care. http://www.planetree.org
Patient Centered Outcome Research Institute	Developed by a federal mandate; funds research related to patient centered outcomes. http://www.pcori.org

Conclusion

The information in this chapter can be highly useful when developing a medical music therapy program. However, you must decide what you want your program to look like. What do you want it to feel like? What are your short-term and long-term goals for the program? Are you looking for a few hours on a unit or two, an entire music therapy department with multiple interns and services across the system, or something in between? Be prepared, have a focused plan and vision as you meet with administration, but remain flexible to adapt to the needs of the hospital.

References

American Music Therapy Association (AMTA). (2012). *AMTA standards of clinical practice: Medical settings.* Retrieved from http://www.musictherapy.org/about/standards/

American Music Therapy Association (AMTA). (2013). *2013 AMTA member survey and workforce analysis.* Retrieved from http://www.musictherapy.org/documents/

Bart, C. K., & Tabone, J. C. (1999). Mission statement content and hospital performance in the Canadian not-for-profit health sector. *Health Care Manage Review, 24,* 18–29.

Dileo, C., & Bradt, J. (2009). Medical music therapy: Evidence-based principles and practices. In I. Söderback (Ed.), *International handbook of occupational therapy interventions* (pp. 445–451). New York, NY: Springer.

Institute for Patient- and Family-Centered Care. (2011). *Advancing the practice of patient- and family-centered care in primary care and other ambulatory care settings: How to get started.* Bethesda, MD: Author. Retrieved from http://ipfcc.org/tools/downloads.html

The Joint Commission. (2010). *Advancing effective communication, cultural competence, and patient- and family-centered care: A roadmap for hospitals.* Oakbrook Terrace, IL: Author.

Magee, W. L., & Andrews, K. (2007). Multi-disciplinary perceptions of music therapy in complex neuro-rehabilitation. *International Journal of Therapy and Rehabilitation, 14*(2), 70–75.

Reuer, B. (1996). Posturing for the changing world: Consulting as a career option. *Music Therapy Perspectives, 14,* 16–20.

Robertson, A. (2009). *Music, medicine and miracles: How to provide medical music therapy for pediatric patients and get paid for it.* Orlando, FL: Florida Hospital.

Sodomka, P. (2006). Engaging patients and families: A high leverage tool for health care leaders. In *Institute for Patient- and Family-Centered Care* (Ed.), *Advancing the practice of patient- and family-centered care in hospitals* (pp. 9–10). Retrieved from http://www.ipfcc.org/pdf/getting_started.pdf

Standley, J. M. (2000). Music research in medical treatment. In AMTA (Ed.), *Effectiveness of music therapy procedures: Documentation of research and clinical practice* (pp. 1–64). Silver Spring, MD: American Music Therapy Association.

Standley, J. M., Gregory, D., Whipple, J., Walworth, D., Nguyen, J., Adams, K., … Cevasco, A. (2005). *Medical music therapy: A model program for clinical practice, education, training, and research.* Silver Spring, MD: American Music Therapy Association.

Standley, J. M., & Walworth, D. (2010). *Music therapy with premature infants: Research and developmental interventions* (2nd ed.). Silver Spring, MD: American Music Therapy Association.

Walworth, D. D. (2005). Procedural-support music therapy in the healthcare setting: A cost-effectiveness analysis. *Journal of Pediatric Nursing, 20,* 276–284.

Yinger, O. S., & Standley, J. M. (2011). The effects of medical music therapy on patient satisfaction as measured by the Press Ganey inpatient survey. *Music Therapy Perspectives, 29,* 149–156.

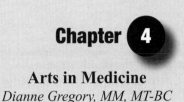

Chapter 4

Arts in Medicine
Dianne Gregory, MM, MT-BC

Defining "Arts in Medicine"

Information about "Arts in Medicine" (AIM), a program offered by many hospitals, is included in this book to help readers differentiate between an arts-therapy program like music therapy and an AIM program. The chapter begins with a definition of AIM and categorizes options for implementing AIM programs in hospitals. Several alternative names for AIM programs that are currently used in hospital programs are listed, and issues related to the absence of a uniform name are discussed. The chapter's primary focus is to articulate the differences between AIM programs and arts-therapy programs and to provide resources for examples of AIM and practical suggestions for implementing an AIM program. The chapter concludes with a description of a unique service learning course (Arts in Medicine Service) offered by a university to students in all majors and managed by collaboration between an on-site hospital music therapist and a music therapy faculty member.

When considered separately, the key words *arts* and *medicine* are easily defined, but when combined to describe a specific program, they require clarification. In a very practical sense, *medicine* refers to, and is limited in this case, to a general hospital setting. "Arts in the Hospital" is perhaps a more accurate program title. Patients' rooms, hospital units, general waiting areas, and possibly designated arts activity rooms are typical hospital venues for Arts in Medicine (AIM) program implementation. The all-encompassing word *medicine,* which includes services like diagnostic imaging and treatment procedures, is misleading in this context. AIM programs, unlike arts-therapy programs, are not directly connected to specific individualized medically related interventions and outcomes. (Other chapters in this book provide examples of medically related interventions and outcomes provided by music therapists in a hospital.) AIM services are primarily connected to hospital administrations' concerns for the well-being of patients and their families during hospital stays. Direct services, for the most part, are provided by community volunteers, not employed, credentialed arts therapists. Both AIM and arts-therapy programs are necessary and valuable services in today's hospitals, but each has a different role in a hospital.

Examples of options for Arts in Medicine (AIM) programs help limit the word *medicine* to *hospital* in this context. Some AIM contributions in the hospital are stationary. Community artists' donations of paintings, sculptures, and other visual art products are placed in strategic places to enhance and beautify the hospital environment for everyone. Another stationary contribution includes live performances by community musicians and actors in different hospital venues. A performance occurring in an atrium, cafeteria, or large waiting room provides an entertaining diversion for visitors, staff members, and patients. Viewing art work and watching and listening to live performances are stationary representations that, without question, change and enhance a hospital's *physical* environment. Other AIM program options are interactive and are designed to actively engage at least one person in an arts project during that person's time in the hospital. Interactive examples include a volunteer and a patient working on a painting together, a volunteer working a puzzle with family members in a waiting room, or a group of volunteers and staff members writing motivating songs together during a break. Positive human interactions in non-medical arts-related activities are effective humanizing enhancements of a hospital's *social* environment.

Hospitals' physical and social environments are changed by people who volunteer in an AIM program. Most programs have someone who knows and works well with community organizations and artists and manages the on-site AIM volunteers. Implementing stationary contributions in a hospital requires a knowledgeable and arts-minded staff member who maintains contacts with a local community's visual and performing artists' coalitions to solicit art product donations and to recruit performers. Implementing interactive contributions in a hospital requires a staff member who selects, schedules, and supervises volunteers who offer entertaining distractions for patients, visitors, and staff members.

While limiting the word *medicine* to *hospital* in the phrase "arts in medicine" provides clarity, the definition of *arts* requires expansion beyond the traditional use of the word. The word *arts* is usually associated with a concept that includes fine and performance arts such as (a) music, (b) dance, (c) drama, (d) visual arts, and (e) literary arts. In fact, AIM programs began as efforts to humanize the relatively sterile, if not inhibiting, hospital environments through the addition of fine and performing arts contributions. These efforts continue and are important parts of today's AIM programs, but the "arts" concept is expanding beyond traditional meanings to include offerings like acrobatic performances, digital media, and juggling. Can the "art" of conversation be added to the list of possibilities? The Oxford Dictionary defines *arts* as "the expression or application of human creative skill and imagination producing works to be appreciated primarily for their beauty or emotional power." If we use the tried-yet-true cliché "Beauty is in the eye of the beholder" while acknowledging at the same time the vastly wide range of feelings people of all ages have related to "emotional power," then defining an art "work" or "product" becomes less problematic for AIM programs. A volunteer in the pediatric playroom helps a child make a puppet, while observant parents genuinely "ooh" and "aah" during every step of the process. A volunteer helps patients in the oncology unit design and construct personal thank you cards that bring tears to the receiving nurses' eyes. A volunteer "chats" with a very anxious patient in the neurology unit and thoughtfully improvises with topics that gradually divert the patient's attention and calms him to the point of shared smiles and brief chuckles. These examples are "products" that can be appreciated for their "beauty or emotional power," particularly in a hospital setting. The word *arts* in Arts in Medicine programs is not limited to traditional or typical concepts or products.

Primary functions of an AIM program are to enhance a hospital's physical environment with stationary arts products and performances and to humanize the hospital's social environment with interactive arts-related activities through contributions by community volunteers.

Alternative Names for AIM Programs and Related Issues

There are many program titles for arts contributions in hospitals. An excellent website for reviewing and finding references for examples of arts programs in hospitals and *other* health-related community agencies, such as hospice or shelters for homeless children, is http://www.nea.gov/news/news03/aihexamples.html. Table 4.1 provides a sample of the *hospital* programs in the list. All of these programs provide stationary or interactive arts contributions to hospital environments.

Table 4.1. Hospital Programs	
Program Name	**Facility**
Healing Arts Program	San Diego Children's Hospital
Cultural Services Program	Duke University
Museum on Rounds	Hasbro Children's Hospital, Rhode Island
Medical Humanities and the Arts in Health Care	University of Massachusetts Medical School
Gifts of Art	University of Michigan Health System
Cultural Enrichment Program	Vanderbilt University Medical Center
Arts in HealthCare Program	University of Kentucky Medical Center

Does it matter that similar programs are labeled differently? Regarding the services provided and benefits gained for patients, staff members, and families, the answer is "probably not." Enhancement and entertainment are appreciated in the moment by participants in all of the programs. Different labels can be somewhat problematic in other areas. For example, the variety of names makes communication with professional colleagues in other similar hospital programs difficult (e.g., "Yes, that program's a lot like ours, but we don't offer . . ."). The variety of names also causes problems when searching online for important research publications. The lack of uniformity of keywords can unintentionally result in excluding creative efforts that are excellent examples for a review of literature. Multiple program names are also consequential during efforts to define variables for replication of investigative research and submission of grant proposals. Equally important, the absence of a common title for a single approach (the arts) provided within a single agency (a hospital) definitely hampers public awareness and consumer demand for the service.

Although AIM and the other programs listed in Table 4.1 seem to fit a definition of "complementary medicine" provided by the National Center for Complementary and Alternative Medicine (NCCAM), that is, "non-mainstream approaches used *with* conventional medicine" (http://nccam.nih.gov/health/whatiscam), it is interesting to note that arts programs are excluded from the current National Institutes of Health's list of complementary medicine options. Perhaps the absence of a unified concept under a single title contributes to this exclusion. For the remainder of this chapter, *Arts in Medicine* (AIM) will be used as a global term that encompasses most arts programs that exist with different titles but provide stationary and interactive arts contributions to enhance the physical and social environment of a hospital.

In addition to facilitating public awareness and consumer demand for arts contributions in hospitals, the primary reason that it matters "what you call it" is related to the inherent confusion about the required training and credentialing for service providers in AIM programs compared to arts-therapy programs. Who delivers direct service to patients in AIM programs? What is the required training? Are credentials required? Some AIM programs are managed by a salaried full- or part-time hospital staff member, often a social worker or a child life specialist, whose qualifications and job descriptions are defined by the administration. There are no uniform qualifications required for AIM managers. The AIM manager's primary task is to develop and maintain connections to community artists in the local area to solicit art contributions and volunteers. Training and credentials for gathering stationary contributions (arts works, performances) may be minimal, particularly if the scope and size of the hospital are limited. For example, a knowledgeable arts consumer with excellent public relations skills could qualify to manage an AIM program and, in turn, recruit assistance from architectural and interior design volunteers to suggest placement and visual continuity for donated art works. Training and credentials for selecting, instructing, and monitoring volunteers who provide interactive direct services for patients seem more important. In some cases, artists who volunteer their services rely on on-site training by the AIM manager during brief weekend workshops, institutes, or certificate programs.

What are the qualifications for training volunteers for direct patient contact? After completing the hospital's clearance procedures including background checks, drug screening, and immunizations, most volunteers are eager and ready to entertain clients but have little or no experience in the hospital environment, including interacting with vulnerable patients. Their credentials, training, and resumes usually illuminate previous experiences with the arts. It is important to note that AIM service providers, and sometimes AIM managers, are community volunteers without specific prerequisite training or credentials related to medical services. Yet, training and providing protocols and guidelines for interactions with patients usually are part of the AIM manager's responsibilities. AIM volunteers have a common and noble desire to contribute their services to a hospital, but it is important to acknowledge there are no standard minimum training or credential requirements for directing or volunteering in an AIM program at the present time. Quality control of an AIM program and accountability to the hospital administration are left to the discretion of the AIM manager, who may or may not have a related arts therapy or health services degree. This is an important discrimination for public awareness regarding assumptions about qualifications of service providers in AIM programs, regardless of the differences in program names.

Resources

Table 4.2 provides a list of resources and publications for AIM programs and documents. Each source provides valuable information. Source #1 in the table is an excellent publication available online that describes several AIM programs and documents the absence of a uniform method for funding, staffing, and budgeting an AIM program. Mission statements and activities, however, are very similar. Another resource for exploring the diversity is the website for the Arts and Health Alliance (AHA), formerly the Society for Arts in Healthcare (Source #2). AHA is an active organization whose 1,400 members represent a variety of professional people and organizations that support AIM programs, e.g., (a) hospital administrators, (b) arts administrators, (c) physicians, (d) nurses, (e) artists, (f) child life specialists, (g) social workers, (h) hospitals, and (i) university medical schools. Conferences are held each year and a peer-reviewed journal, *Arts & Health: An International Journal for Research, Policy and Practice*, available in print and online (Source #3), is published three times a year. Links to AHA member organizations' websites are available online (Source #4) and include additional links to consulting firms, university colleges of medicine, hospitals, community programs, and state programs. AHA is the primary organization attempting to publicize all AIM concepts and programs.

A different example of a resource with a very specific AIM program for children's hospitals is Beads for Courage (Source #5). It lists children's hospitals in 34 states and 5 countries connected to Beads of Courage, Inc.: Providing Arts in Medicine for Children with Serious Illnesses, which began in 2007 and is currently a 501(c)(3) organization. There is wide-ranging support of the concept of AIM across professional disciplines and organizations as documented by the AHA's diversity of member organizations and the very specific Beads of Courage example.

For a list of all links in this chapter, see Appendix D.

Table 4.2. Resource Links	
Links	
1	http://www.thecreativecenter.org/tcc/publications__dvds/online_publications/Colloquium_White_Paper:en-us.pdf
2	http://www.thesah.org/template/index.cfm.
3	www.tandfonline.com
4	http://www1074.ssldomain.com/thesah/members/affiliate_list.cfm
5	http://www.beadsofcourage.org/pages/hospitals.htm.

These resources can be helpful for developers of AIM programs. There may be no limits to creativity. The diversity, however, makes it very difficult to determine any agreement on operational definitions and related standards for quality assurance across programs. This can be problematic for developers of AIM programs. There is no doubt that well-designed and organized AIM programs offer valuable contributions to hospitals. Continuation of efforts by dedicated professionals and volunteers will expedite, if not resolve, issues involving training standards, research specificity, funding efforts, and public awareness.

Three major differences between an AIM and an arts-therapy program in a hospital: (1) qualifications of persons providing direct services, (2) expected outcomes and documentation of interventions, and (3) funding.

Differences Between AIM and Arts-Therapy Programs in Hospitals

In addition to the confusion caused by the diversity of names for AIM programs, confusion between AIM and specific arts-therapy programs also occurs. It is important to note that there are at least three major differences between an AIM and an arts-therapy program in a hospital: *qualifications of persons providing direct services, expected outcomes and documentation of interventions, and funding.* The differences are interrelated, that is, it "costs" more to hire professionally trained arts therapists who are qualified to perform and document outcomes of interventions with patients referred by physicians for specific medical purposes than it does to hire directors of AIM programs who solicit, schedule, and supervise community artist volunteers who offer stationary and interactive arts-related contributions for hospitals. Both programs are valuable. One hospital's efforts to offer both programs, AIM and Medical Music Therapy (MMT), are described later in this chapter to further clarify differences that separate the two programs and facilitate discrimination of mutually exclusive operations.

The major difference between an AIM and an arts-therapy program, like MMT, is the professional qualifications of persons providing direct services. AIM service providers are volunteers who meet hospital clearance procedures for direct contact with patients; provide an arts-related service deemed appropriate and necessary by an AIM program director; and exhibit maturity, personal accountability, and interpersonal skills conducive to positive interactions with patients, family members, and hospital personnel. Volunteers receive on-site training and are accountable to and supervised by an AIM manager or contact person for volunteers. The AIM contact person or manager is often a child life specialist in a children's hospital or a social worker or volunteer coordinator in general hospitals. Successful track records of writing grant proposals or securing funds from private donors are often included in the resumes of some AIM program managers.

Professional qualifications for arts therapists are very different when compared to AIM service providers. Arts therapists and directors of arts-therapy programs have professional credentials in a specific arts area (e.g., MT-BC—board certified music therapist) and a college or university degree (e.g., BM or MM in Music Therapy), indicating successful completion of a 4year undergraduate or 2-year graduate arts-therapy academic program and related clinical internship. Their professions are supported by specific national organizations devoted to the promotion of the profession in hospitals and other health care agencies. Arts-therapy clinical training experiences often include interventions with several client populations, including (a) psychiatric, (b) medical, (c) geriatric, and (d) special education. Music therapy students, however, who know they want to eventually work in a medical setting, are encouraged by faculty members to select field experiences and practica in local hospital programs during early pre-professional courses and to continue with medical selections through upper-level professional courses and the full-time six-month clinical internship. These students enter the professional medical arena as graduates with diverse hands-on delivery of music therapy services in a hospital setting. In addition to providing direct services to patients using evidence-based protocols, they have also experienced working within the doctors' referral system, the units' staff accountability procedures, and the hospital's documentation system for accreditation and reimbursement purposes.

A second important difference between an AIM program and an arts-therapy program is related to the difference in professional qualifications and pertains to the expected outcomes and documentation methods of interventions. Expected outcomes of AIM programs are general and focus on the enhancement of the hospital's physical and social environment and the enhancements' indirect effect on the welfare of the patients and staff. Providing pleasing and attention-getting distractions and entertainment is a valuable addition in the hospital setting, but AIM service provider accountability and documentation of hospital enhancements vary across programs. The minimum requirement usually includes recording the time spent in the hospital units, number of patient contacts by volunteers, and types of activities implemented. Patient satisfaction surveys are sometimes used to gauge the general effect of AIM interactions or performances on patients' attitude, sense of well-being, and perceptions of the hospital. Brief interviews or written unit staff surveys are sometimes used to determine nurses' evaluation of volunteers on their unit and their perceptions of the effectiveness of AIM program activities. Suggestions for implementing additional AIM activities are often requested during these evaluations. Open communication among the nursing staff, volunteers, and the AIM program director is crucial for continual assessment of the effectiveness of an AIM program.

Expected outcomes of arts therapies (e.g., Medical Music Therapy–MMT) are very specific and individualized to meet a specific patient's needs based on a referral from medical personnel. Full documentation of any intervention by an arts therapist is required and must directly refer to specific objectives of the intervention as stated in the records of the referred patient by the referring physician. The documentation is recorded in a hospital's computer system for review by referring personnel and unit staff members. Arts therapists measure and report psychological or physiological results related to the expected outcome on an intervention for an individual patient. While documentation for AIM activities could be categorized as *program*-specific, documentation for arts-therapy interventions could be categorized as *patient*-specific.

A third difference between AIM and arts-therapy programs, also related to professional qualifications differences and operational differences, is financial support. Budgets for both programs depend on the size of the hospital and the scope of the proposal within a hospital. For example, will all units receive interactive services from AIM volunteers, or will performances in general waiting areas be the primary focus for the program? Will patients in all units be applicable for referrals for MMT services, or will specific units be targeted for specific interventions? Depending on the scope of the proposed program, a minimum budget for an AIM program in a small hospital could include hiring a part-time or full-time staff member to set standards, organize the program, and supervise community volunteers who maintain the patient contact schedule. A minimum budget for an arts-therapy program in a small hospital includes competitive full-time salaries and benefits for professionally credentialed therapists. Budgetary considerations for both programs include purchasing resources, equipment, and materials. There are major differences between an AIM and an arts-therapy program. The differences result in either-or propositions (e.g., it's either an AIM program or an arts-therapy program), even though there is a common element (e.g., the arts). Understanding the differences is consequential for everyone interested in supporting theoretically or financially either or both implementations of the arts in hospitals. Understanding the differences is also consequential for future patients and family members who request delivery of direct services. It is also important for professionals to respect the unique, distinctive, and valuable contributions each program adds to patients' daily hospital experiences, to clearly differentiate the *modus operandi* of providing entertaining distractions from that of implementing therapeutic interventions, and to separate research findings based on the purview of each program. Professionals, for example, agree that research findings "belong" to a community that includes any researcher focused on replicating a method or expanding or limiting a research question. The use of arts-therapy research findings by non-researchers to document and publicize effects of AIM programs not only obfuscates the inherent and valuable difference between AIM and arts-therapy programs, but misrepresents the benefits of AIM programs and prevents the development of AIM-specific research.

Do these differences suggest that it is an "either-or" proposition for hospitals? In other words, do hospital administrators have to decide between an AIM program and an arts-therapy program for their particular hospital? If one truly understands the value of both programs, the answer is an obvious and definite "no," and the next part of the chapter will eventually provide a description of a unified AIM and MMT program. This first section, however, provides recommendations for proposing, developing, and maintaining a "stand-alone" AIM program.

Developing an AIM Program

The following suggestions are practical but not necessarily sequential nor prioritized. Each hospital culture is unique and nothing actually takes the place of gathering information about current status and future goals of any specific hospital. That being said, if the possibility of finding financial and administrative support for implementing an AIM program seems imminent, there are several issues to consider while developing a proposal for an AIM program.

Determine the scope of an AIM program for the local hospital. Factors to consider are:

- the size of the hospital,

- the number of units,

- the diversity of patients,

- the existing volunteer program, and

- available funding options.

Find hospitals with AIM programs that are similar in size to the local hospital and gather examples of programs (see URL resources in Appendix D). Determine similar internal funding options (e.g., a local hospital's foundation) and external funding possibilities (e.g., grants from state and federal arts programs). Many AIM programs are funded exclusively by private donations. When looking for examples, carefully differentiate between hospital *arts-therapy programs* with credentialed trained professionals that include or do not include AIM volunteer programs, and hospitals with *AIM programs* that do not include arts-therapy professional staff members. This is important in determining the scope of the proposal.

Specify a basic job description for an AIM manager. A job description for a manager who wants to offer interactive humanizing, entertaining arts activities for patients is very different from a job description for a manager who wants to add stationary arts products and performances to the hospital environment. Most AIM programs include both approaches, but the job descriptions are separated here to assist in the determination of which job may be "phase one" for the proposal if both are not implemented at the same time.

Tasks for offering interactive humanizing and entertaining arts activities for patients include establishing and maintaining a schedule of activities. Table 4.3 provides some suggestions to consider when setting up interactive activities.

Table 4.3. Suggestions for Establishing Interactive AIM Activities		
Objective: **Establish an activities schedule**	**Objective:** **Recruit volunteers for** **probable arts activities**	**Objective:** **Maintain an** **AIM program schedule of activities**
Locate each hospital unit, determine nurse-patient ratio, and view space available for activities. Patients' rooms may be the primary venues for activities. Locate available space for supplies and equipment on units. Select units for AIM contacts based on probable patient engagement and determine a liaison nurse or unit staff person for communication. Be aware of supportive comments from individuals who may be willing to provide this role for the AIM program. Select "best times of the day" for arts activities by consulting with unit liaison. Mornings are often filled with scheduled procedures and doctors' visits. Meal times and visitation hours may be factors to consider when scheduling activities. If visitation is not limited consider activities that may include visitors, particularly in the pediatric units. Determine probable motor, communicative, and perceptual capabilities related to different types of illnesses or medical conditions of patients on a particular unit. Propose specific art activity options based on an active-passive continuum (e.g. patients in neurology units may be less active than patients in diabetes units, etc.)	Develop an eye-catching handout describing the purpose of AIM, possible activities, director's hospital contact information. Develop a web site or blog for communication with community arts coalitions. Contact/visit local high school music and arts teachers and classes, college or university music and arts programs, and local artists/performers coalitions to publicize the availability of volunteer experiences. Prepare a pre-service inventory to gather potential volunteers' contact information, previous hospital volunteering experience, specific talents, interests and personal preferences for volunteering, free time schedule and day/time preferences, and personal references. Communicate with the hospital's volunteer coordinator and personnel director re: standards and methods for assessing volunteers' maturity and interpersonal skills. Follow their lead in this respect and add specifics related to interactive contributions. Specify a priori reasons for accepting and rejecting volunteer applicants. Interview prospective volunteers and fill schedule with accepted recruits. Inform volunteers about hospital clearance procedures and assist them with completion.	Determine the administrative "chain of command" regarding documenting results of the AIM program. Establish communication with that person and office. Locate AIM program office space, a central storage space for supplies and materials, and group activity spaces on units or throughout the hospital. Develop an in-house website or blog to communicate with volunteers and unit liaisons. Prepare a manual that provides standards and protocol for patient contacts by volunteers including boundaries, dress code, and appropriate behavior. Include suggested activities and adaptations for different needs. Determine types of resources and materials needed for different types of art activities. Provide and maintain inventory of art materials for activities. Supervise volunteers as scheduled. Document volunteers' services with time cards, signed forms from units. Assess unit nurses'/ patients' satisfaction with AIM services Make changes based on assessments.

Include the scope and limitations of the program in the proposal and provide related job descriptions for AIM program staffing. Consider dividing the proposal into phases for initiating different options sequentially during a brief start-up period. Set goals and deadlines for implementation. Online links to similar programs can be added to the proposal. Search research topics like (a) quality of life, (b) patient well-being, (c) patient satisfaction, (d) family satisfaction, and (e) nurses' satisfaction. Limit research findings and references to AIM research only; do not include arts-therapy evidence-based research. Administrators know accreditation issues for qualifications of direct service providers. Stress the role of the AIM program for (a) enhancing the hospital environment for consumers, (b) developing community support for the hospital through volunteer services, (c) improving the quality of life for patients during their hospital stay, and (d) providing assistance to unit nurses for patient engagement and satisfaction. Additional tasks for adding works of art and scheduling live performances to enhance the hospital environment can be found in Table 4.4.

Table 4.4. Suggestions for Establishing Interactive AIM Activities		
Objective: **Survey the entire hospital**	**Objective:** **Recruit artists/ performers**	**Objective:** **Maintain art shows and performances**
Visit public areas, waiting rooms, procedural areas, and patient units for possible need and location of visual enhancements. Recruit interior design expert volunteers for suggested placement of art objects and paintings. Develop hospital layout drawing and rank priorities for potential placements. Locate hospital public areas for performances. Determine acoustic quality and potential noise distractions. Determine seating arrangements and the need for extra folding chairs. Determine "busiest" times in public waiting areas for live performances	Recruit community artists and performers from high schools, college and university programs, local museums and performance venues. Announce/recruit internally. Staff members may want to volunteer during their breaks or off-hours or provide potential contact info for potential volunteers. Advertise requests for art shows and performances. Provide contact information. Develop an inventory to record volunteers' contact info, expertise, preferred performance locations, and previous hospital volunteer experience. Determine minimum clearance procedure, dress code, and protocol for performers and provide handout.	Establish local media presence as a community showcase for local artists' temporary art shows and performances. Identify possible donors, benefactors, and other persons interested in supporting the arts. Maintain and update lists of community resources and philanthropic organizations for timely contacts. Establish media and TV schedule for publicity Announce acquisitions (financial/ art) internally and in local media. Publish annual recognition of contributions in hospital communications and local media.

A Unified AIM and MMT Program

In this section, a unique university AIM service learning course (AIMS) that provides volunteers for a local hospital's AIM program is described. The course was developed in conjunction with the establishment of a music therapy program in a hospital. In this particular case, the primary reason for the arrangement between the local university and the local hospital is related to the university's initial and continuing financial support for a music therapist faculty position at the hospital. Offering the AIMS course provides a way for students to register and receive academic credit for gaining practical experience working with patients. Offering an AIM program *and* an MMT program in a hospital expands the potential for informing students, the general public, and medical personnel of the beneficial and distinctive roles of each program.

The two programs—AIM and MMT—were established at the same time at the Tallahassee Memorial Healthcare (TMH), a general hospital in a city of approximately 187,000 people. The impetus for the development of the MMT program began after decades of music therapy research by music therapy faculty and students at Florida State University (FSU), also located in Tallahassee. They established a well-rounded database of published music therapy research during this time in (a) oncology, (b) radiology, (c) chemotherapy, (d) neonatal intensive care unit, (e) pediatrics, (f) emergency departments, (g) the cardiovascular unit, (h) outpatient surgery, (i) rehabilitation units, and (j) adult day services. The director of the FSU Music Therapy program consulted with the FSU administration regarding the establishment of a full-time MT faculty position at TMH to implement a medical music therapy program. In 1999, the FSU provost provided funds for a music therapist position at the hospital; implementation and expansion of the MMT program began immediately. The TMH MMT program continues to be associated with the FSU Music Therapy program.

Offering an elective AIM service learning course (AIMS) to all university students every semester was included in the proposal for the establishment of the hospital music therapist faculty position. When the TMH MT program began, the TMH music therapist collaborated with an FSU MT faculty member and together they developed the AIMS course. Additions to the TMH MT program have occurred since its establishment. The current TMH MT program personnel consists of (a) a full-time music therapy coordinator (MM, MT-BC) at the hospital funded by FSU and designated as an FSU faculty member, (b) a full-time music therapist (MM, MT-BC) funded by TMH, who primarily provides music therapy services while serving as the AIM contact person for FSU AIMS student volunteers, (c) two MT interns with stipends funded by the TMH Foundation, and (d) a one-quarter-time MT graduate assistant (10 hours/week) funded by FSU.

The AIM program at TMH is funded by the TMH Foundation. Personnel in the TMH Foundation office oversee the donation and placement of visual arts for the hospital and raise funds for and private donations for all hospital programs. A very small portion of the job description of the music therapist funded by TMH includes responsibilities for managing the AIM program of volunteers, communicating with the hospital staff about the TMH AIM program, and collaborating with FSU about the AIMS course.

AIMS Course Description

The AIMS course at FSU provides volunteers for the TMH AIM program each semester. It is offered to undergraduate and graduate students in all majors. It is a one-semester 15-week course that is repeatable and can be taken for 1, 2, or 3 academic credits. Students contract for 2 hours/week for each academic credit; that is, students receiving 1, 2, or 3 credits contract for 30, 60, or 90 hours of hospital contacts, respectively. The majority of students are undergraduates with majors in (a) pre-med and other health care studies, (b) child development, (c) psychology, and (d) music. The AIMS course is a 1-credit-hour requirement in the undergraduate music therapy curriculum and is usually completed by MT majors before their junior year.

An FSU music therapy faculty member and the TMH MT/AIM manager work together throughout the semester. Table 4.5 provides a list of duties for both the FSU faculty member and the on-site TMH AIM manager. Both the FSU faculty and staff member provide assistance to individual students throughout the semester. Appendix E provides a list of forms used with the course; this list can be viewed as a concise summary of the course requirements.

Table 4.5. Personnel Responsibilities	
Faculty Responsibilities	**On-site Manager Responsibilities**
Maintains the course web site and communicates with students each week	Administers the TMH on-site orientation session
Directs the on-campus orientation and final sessions	Provides materials and equipment for AIMS projects
Assists students with choices of projects and selection of units	Communicates with TMH service personnel about the AIMS course's expectations from volunteers.
Organizes and supervises group projects	
Evaluates student participation, weekly documentation and final essays	

Course Specifics

Initial enrollment in the AIMS course consisted primarily of relatively small groups of undergraduate music students, including music therapy majors, and has at different times included undergraduate students from 13 different departments across the university. When the course was initially offered, it was a very unique course at FSU and several recruitment alternatives were used to publicize it. Methods included:

- submitting an article for the campus newspaper;

- posting flyers on department bulletin boards;

- providing handouts at information tables set up at strategic places during days allotted for course advisement and registration;

- having conversations with advisors in specific programs;

- making presentations in related classes; and

- sending letters and flyers to academic advisors in several departments.

After two years of offering the course each semester, recruitment efforts were no longer needed to reach the proposed cap. Most students now report that they heard about the course offering from other students and from advisors. In addition to meeting their contracts for hospital contact hours, all students must complete assignments related to weekly contracts. Except for the group orientation sessions and final session, the course is totally community-based, self-directed, and managed with a Blackboard website. The course is described as experiential learning and is highly individualized according to students' (a) interests, (b) abilities, (c) project selection, (d) participation contracts, and (e) contact schedules.

A course website provides a common structure for communication between the instructor and students. It includes the following pages:

- Announcements;

- Staff Contact Information—FSU and TMH email links and phone numbers;

- Syllabus—explanation of course objectives, procedures, and grading policy;

- Assignments—includes course calendar and weekly updates;

- Forms—easy access to weekly documentation forms;

- Verification Chart—updated weekly to record receipt of students' assignments;

- Master Schedule—depicts each volunteer's hospital location by hours of the day in hospital units;

- Course Resource—links for the TMH clearance procedures, pre-contact training videos, and an online article differentiating the AIM from the MMT program.

Clearance, Orientation, and Scheduling

Students are notified three weeks before the semester begins to start the TMH clearance procedures, with instructions as to how to obtain their badge by the end of the second week of the semester. The clearance procedures include completing PPD skin tests, background checks, and drug screenings, and providing immunization records. Student liability insurance documentation was required when the course began but is no longer required for AIMS students. After completing the clearance procedures, students receive a TMH identification badge that allows entrance into hospital units. It must be worn during all hospital contacts.

The course does not have a specified meeting time or place in the registrar's list of courses. Before the semester begins students are notified to attend a mandatory on-campus orientation session Wednesday evening during the first week of classes and a mandatory TMH orientation session the following Thursday afternoon. The on-campus orientation session provides an opportunity for the instructor to cover a variety of essential course-related information. Occasionally former AIMS volunteers are invited to attend the on-campus orientation session to describe their experience and demonstrate AIMS projects. Likewise, the hospital orientation provides an introduction to pertinent hospital procedures and information. See Table 4.6 for detailed information. Appendices F and G provide example forms to assess student objectives/interests and hospital experience.

Table 4.6.Orientation Procedures for AIMs Courses	
On-Campus Orientation	**Hospital Orientation**
Meet Faculty Instructor	Meet Hospital on-site manager
Receive examples of AIMs projects	Learn hospital protocol for patient confidentiality, medical procedures, dress codes, and grooming standards,
Be introduced to the course's Blackboard website	Hear descriptions of available AIMS projects
Receive an explanation of course requirements	Participate in unit tour and AIMs space/material orientation
Complete inventories re: interests, objectives, previous hospital experience, and personal qualities	
Complete self-assessment of conversation & empathy skills	

During the second week of classes, students watch online video clips on the website. The clips provide probable scenarios that may occur in the hospital during interactions with patients. Suggestions are offered for handling a variety of predictable situations, such as (a) how to respond to patients' inappropriate questions, (b) how to converse with hesitant patients, and (c) how to respond to a disoriented patient. The students also read an online article that describes differences in (a) personnel, (b) objectives, and (c) procedures for the TMH AIM and MMT programs. They learn that music therapists, for example, are specified as clinically trained and credentialed hospital staff members with at least a bachelor's degree in music therapy and board certification, whose primary role is to interact with specific patients referred to music therapy by the medical staff to reach specific clinical objectives. Students learn to identify themselves with the AIM program as volunteers who serve as degree-seeking students contributing their time, skills, and talents to entertain and distract patients with arts activities and performances.

Students also read an online article and practice the role of an AIMS volunteer being referred to as a music therapist by hospital staff or patients by writing several hypothetical polite corrective answers to doctors, nurses, and patients. During the early years, this was an important exercise to help hospital personnel learn the difference between the AIM and MMT programs, because the programs began at the same time and were relatively unfamiliar services to the majority of staff members. Current observations suggest that the staff, for the most part, now know the difference, but occasionally a student will report they "got to" use their reading assignment's practice answers to help a staff member or a patient understand the difference between the two programs. The article also clarifies the *role of music* for AIMS volunteers, particularly for the musically experienced non-music majors, music majors, and music therapy majors. To minimize confusion about the role of music for the hospital personnel, the only music project option available to AIMS volunteers is performing in the atrium and other public venues. Only music therapists and music therapy interns receive music therapy referrals and interact with patients in their private rooms to provide indicated music therapy services.

After the first week of orientation and after receiving their TMH badge, students determine their individual schedules for weekly visits to specific units. Students maintain the same unit schedule each week for several reasons, the most important one being to develop rapport with a unit nurse who knows when to expect the volunteer on the unit. The student–nurse relationship facilitates the designation of patients for volunteers to contact during their hour on the unit, and the nurse's signature is required on the unit documentation form submitted by the student after each unit visit. Students are given a unit census upon arriving on a unit and are free to contact recommended patients for invitations to engage in AIM activities. A master schedule of possible contact hours is available online at the beginning of the semester, and students submit schedule requests after they receive their official TMH badge (see Appendix H). Requests are granted on a "first-come, first-served" basis. The child life specialist on the pediatric unit specifies the preferred week days and times for one or two AIMS volunteers to assist in the playroom and to make room visits. The nurses on the adult units usually specify afternoon and early evening hours on weekdays for preferred contacts. In most cases, only one AIMS volunteer is scheduled on an adult unit during an hour to make room visits.

The course website facilitates communication throughout the semester. Individual face-to-face conferences with instructors are offered to assist students who request appointments or who appear to have difficulty with some aspect of the course. One or two optional group projects are offered on campus to the students, and most students choose to participate to socialize with the other volunteers. One popular project is an activity-swap meet. Each student brings a new AIMS-appropriate activity and teaches it to the rest of the students. Examples of shared activities include (a) origami, (b) balloon animals, (c) magic tricks, (d) paper-cutting, and (e) poetry readings. Students are requested to try at least one of the newly learned activities at the hospital during their next contacts.

Another popular group project is a unit serenade, where AIMS singers and guitarists rehearse songs in the atrium before visiting hospital units to sing for the staff. Other projects have included:

- PR days in the atrium, with tables set up for arts and crafts participation led by students who also provide AIM pamphlets available for people who pass by;

- performances in the Cancer Center atrium, pediatric unit puppet shows;

- magic shows in the atrium presented by chemistry majors; and

- AIMS Nurse Appreciation Day, with cards and cookies provided on the units.

During the last week of the semester, students meet on campus to submit final essays and accountability logs, complete self-assessments and website evaluations, and share personally enlightening AIMS anecdotes. Figure 4.1 summarizes a basic timeline for the course.

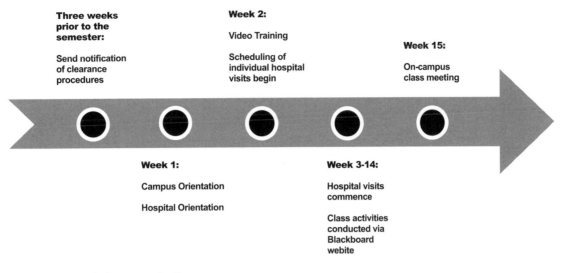

Figure 4.1. AIMS course basic semester timeline.

Documentation of Participation

Several documentation procedures are required throughout the semester. Every time students go to the hospital, they sign in and out on a typical TMH timecard that is maintained by the hospital. They record the date and units visited. Every time students visit a unit or perform at the hospital, they complete detailed documentation forms generated and maintained by the FSU faculty member. The forms are updated before Monday of each week with the current week's number and corresponding dates. They are uploaded to the course website for students to print each week before going to the hospital. Students print enough forms for each of the units and performances scheduled for a certain week and obtain signatures of a hospital staff member to verify their participation (see Appendices I and J for more information). These forms are collected at the end of the week and evaluated by the FSU faculty member. The academic assignments include submission of weekly reports and a final essay. Several items are requested for the weekly report (see Appendix K). Often a "question of the week" will be added to the weekly assignment and included in the evaluation. Students also maintain a cumulative log of AIMS activities and submit the log at the end of the semester (see Appendix L).

Grading includes timely completion of weekly scheduled hours, thorough documentation forms and weekly reports, and a reflective and extensive final essay (see Appendix M). At the beginning of the semester during the on-campus orientation, students receive a grade evaluation sheet detailing points for each week's participation and assignment submissions. They maintain the sheets and submit them with their final essays and cumulative logs at the end of the semester.

The final essay is structured around 15 open-ended questions requesting examples from experiences during the semester with references from previously submitted weekly reports (see Appendix M). Most of the questions are reflective in nature, for example, "What did you learn about yourself personally?" and "What, if any, impact did your experience have on your future plans?" The rest pertain to course evaluation questions, for example, "Do you have any recommendations for the course website?" The majority of responses to the first question, "What did you learn about yourself personally?" indicate that students experience an unsuspected ability to quickly or through time become comfortable interacting with unfamiliar people in new situations and/or in an environment initially perceived as stressful or sad. Other responses to this question pertain to a variety of topics, such as:

- enjoying working with a particular age group,
- learning how to be patient,
- recognizing false preconceptions and stereotypical thinking, and
- learning the value of effective communication.

Responses to the "impact on future plans" question usually reinforce current degree choices or provided assistance in deciding to pursue a service profession degree. Most final essay responses validate the AIMS course as a service learning course.

At the final class meeting, students submit written evaluations of the website and their suggestions, usually minor, are implemented for the next semester. Student input when the course was initiated and in its pilot phase was helpful. At this point, the course has become relatively standardized and ratings are consistently high and comments are positive. Once a year, a brief paper-and-pencil survey is given to nurses on the AIMS units (see Appendix N). Staff ratings are usually very high and specific comments provide feedback for any suggested changes or additions to the AIMS course and the AIM program. Establishing the AIMS course in conjunction with funding a hospital's MMT program with university financial support is considered to be a unique and helpful model for other MT academic programs establishing medical music therapy programs in local hospitals.

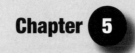

Chapter 5

Grant Writing for Music Therapy
Darcy DeLoach, PhD, MT-BC, and Andrea Cevasco-Trotter, PhD, MT-BC

Funding needs are at the top of the list for most agencies providing therapeutic services. With grant opportunities available through federal and state government entities, as well as private foundations and charities, it is common for individuals to avoid the grant-writing process due to the overwhelming requirements that differ from each granting body. The intent of this chapter is to shed some light on the grant-writing process for those considering pursuit of a funding source. The information discussed includes competition sources, purposes of various granting agencies, common differences in proposal length requirements and submission processes, research team qualifications, and types of evaluators.

Identifying a Funding Source

The most common red flag for any agency reviewing a funding proposal is a project that seems tailored to the request for proposals (RFP). It is a risk for funders to award money for a project that is created solely in response to a RFP and does not already have proven systems in place. Many funding agencies are looking for a well-established program that has a high chance of success in carrying out the proposed project. There are start-up and new program development funding opportunities, which commonly require very detailed previous work accomplishments and rationale for the new venture. However, the majority of funding opportunities assume the applicant can demonstrate how the proposed project is a natural extension of ongoing services that will utilize previously demonstrated staff expertise.

When looking for a funding source, it is common to search through many funding opportunity announcements before finding the right fit for a proposed project or program. Therefore, this process does not necessitate a rushed and hectic grant submission, but rather a carefully thought out and intentional proposal, as most agencies post RFPs on a recurring basis. Additionally, communication with the granting agency from the very beginning will help elucidate whether the proposed project may be a good fit for both parties.

Looking through past proposals that were awarded funding is also a good idea. Even if there is not a history of funding your type of project, seeing which projects did garner the support of the funding agency will tell you a lot about the interest areas of the agency. The previously funded projects may or may not align with the stated funding areas for the agency. This information will also aid in the decision-making process to submit or not submit your project proposal. Understanding the funding priorities of the foundation, charity, or government agency is imperative in making the decision to move forward with a funding proposal.

The Request for Proposals

When submitting a grant, whether a (a) federal, (b) corporate, (c) professional, or (d) university-related grant, thoroughly read the RFP and priorities for funding. Address the priorities within the proposal. Evidence-based outcomes are necessary.

Many RFPs provide the areas of evaluation for the proposed project (background or literature review, significance of the problem, methodology, data analysis, evaluation plan/metric for success, research team, budget, etc.). Each evaluated/scored area must be succinctly but thoroughly addressed within the grant application. Thus, make sure that you do not spend most of the time on the review of literature and have an underdeveloped budget or criteria/metric for success. Similarly, be sure to include research studies that are pertinent to your proposal; leaving studies out of the proposal is often considered conspicuous, and failure to do so results in negative evaluations.

Regardless of funding source, every review group is unique. Most people do not know what music therapy is and what it involves. Thus, a brief explanation of music therapy might be helpful, but it is more important to have a theoretical framework to support the significance and reasoning of the therapeutic technique/intervention. Explain or define terminology so the reviewers can understand and advocate for your proposal. Within the proposal, diagrams, figures and tables, and bullets help the reviewers understand complex information. The use of headings provides clarity.

Gain reviewers' attention and interest in your proposal by discussing the potential impact this research has on the public. Define how the project addresses important problems or barriers within the area, as well as how it will change treatment and services within the profession; make sure this aligns with the mission/purpose of the funding mechanism. Also, delineate the aims/goals/objectives of the project.

Be realistic regarding time and what can be accomplished given the timeframe and research team's areas of expertise. Government funding sources prefer that you have a thorough research team and past experience on a research team receiving federal funding. It is recommended that an individual qualified to analyze the type of research design used in the proposed study be included on the research team. Also, providing too many outcomes from the proposed project is also viewed negatively.

The amount of time necessary to prepare a grant proposal will differ drastically depending on the funding source. Government grants typically take 6 to 9 months to write completely and be reviewed by colleagues for recommended edits. Federal grant applications are lengthy and have very specific instructions on the myriad of requirements to be completed before submission. If your university or agency has a grant specialist, it is highly recommended to reach out for assistance when submitting a federal grant. Private grant agencies have a range of application requirements. Some will take only a few hours to complete, while others choose to follow the federal submission format. Ensuring that every submission requirement is met is crucial.

Proofread the entire grant proposal for (a) grammar, (b) spelling, (c) content, and (d) flow/ continuity. Have other individuals read it for grammar, but also for content. If a family member understands your proposal, it is likely that a board member of a corporation or a peer within the university will also understand it.

The Review Process

NIH Funding

Once a proposal has been electronically submitted, a Scientific Review Officer (SRO) determines who will be needed to review the application. The SRO recruits qualified reviewers based on knowledge in their scientific field and ability to provide quality, fair, and objective reviews. The SRO assigns applications to be reviewed, and each application has a first reviewer, second reviewer, and third reviewer. Reviewers cannot have any conflicts of interest; specific guidelines exist. The reviewers have a 6-week time period to evaluate and provide a written summary for approximately six applications. Each reviewer prepares a critique and assigns individual criterion scores. The SRO organizes a meeting to discuss the applications following the review process.

A 1- to 2-day meeting takes place, where approximately 30 individuals are gathered together, representing various expertise areas. The chair of the meeting is a moderator for the discussion of the scientific and technical merit of the reviewed applications and is also a reviewer. Proposals with high scores are discussed at the meeting. Everyone provides a final score of the proposal based on the three reviewers' comments and the discussion of the application. Some applications receive a Not Discussed (ND) status. These applications are considered to be less competitive and are usually scored in the bottom half of the applications. Comments from the three assigned reviewers are provided to the applicants.

A second level of review occurs in which an advisory council or board performs a second review. This board consists of scientists from the extramural research community and a public representative. They examine the applications, the overall impact scores, percentile rankings, and their summary statements and examine these areas against the NIH Institute/Center's (IC) needs. The IC director decides final funding based on the advice of the staff and advisory council/board.

Scoring. Every area within NIH requires an overall impact score; this score indicates the probability that the project will make an important scientific contribution to the research field. Most grants for Parent Announcements involve five scored review criteria, although some may involve more than five. Typical criteria include (a) the significance of the proposal, (b) the investigator(s), (c) innovation, (d) approach, and (e) environment. Other additional criteria, not scored individually but considered within the impact score, typically involve protections for human subjects; inclusion of women, minorities, and children; and other considerations.

The aforementioned areas and the impact score are based on a 9-point scale. All ratings are whole numbers only, and typically scores of 1 and 9 are uncommon; 5 is considered an average score, is considered good, and has a medium-impact. The strengths and weaknesses are evaluated for each criterion. Scores of 1, 2, and 3 are considered "high" impact applications. (A score of 1 is exceptional, 2 outstanding, and 3 excellent.) Applications that receive a score of 4 (very good), 5 (good), and 6 (satisfactory) are considered to have a medium impact. Scores of 7, 8, and 9 are low impact applications and indicate fair, marginal, or poor applications.

Sometimes a moderate score is assigned to some of the criterion but the proposal receives a high impact score because one review criterion is very important and scored highly. Similarly, the opposite could happen, in which there are high criterion ratings but the overall impact score is low due to one criterion that was not rated highly.

Overall, the process of submitting a NIH grant is lengthy, and the preparation should take place across a number of months. The application should include:

- the significance of the problem;

- facilities and resources (with supporting documentation from the agencies);

- equipment;

- biographical sketches of key personnel;

- complete budget and justification;

- research plan (including the aims, significance, innovation, approach, outcomes, strategy, human subjects); and

- other research plans (such as letters of support, etc.).

Reviewers are extremely diverse and many of them have been evaluating grant proposals for years. Within the proposal, the aims should be evaluated through psychometrically valid and reliable measurements (include the properties of the evaluation tools within the proposal) and, as appropriate, a mixed-methods model for evaluating the outcomes. Focus groups are often used to gain information and solidify protocols prior to the implementation of a study. The investigators should include individuals (collaborators and consultants) who are experts within their area. Letters of support from collaborators and consultants as well as permission to conduct the study from agencies/facilities are necessary.

Terms used by NIH include:

- Funding Opportunity Announcement (FOA)

- Institute/Center (IC)

- Parent Announcement (PA)

- Scientific Review Officer (SRO)

Private Foundation/Corporate Funding

Corporations support nonprofits through private foundations and/or public charities. There are company-sponsored foundations and corporate direct-giving programs, and both provide funding closely related to the corporation's interests, often to communities where the company is located. Foundation grants often fund education, human services, health, arts/culture, public/society benefit, science/technology, etc. Thus, grant seekers must determine the corporation's goals and mission; this sometimes involves capital or program support rather than research. Geographical preferences must be taken into consideration. Sometimes grants are restricted to specific regions, states, and communities. If this is the case, it is very unusual for a foundation to make an exception to the specifications listed as to who receives funding. If a foundation states that it does not accept unsolicited requests for funding, it is inappropriate to submit a proposal without first discussing with the board your funding need and receiving a request for submission.

Letters of Intent (LOIs) are the initial form of contact. Because LOIs are often limited to one or two pages, the proposal must be succinct. The review process might involve staff and peer reviewers, although oftentimes the board reviews the proposal. Depending on the agency, LOIs might be accepted on a rolling basis year-round and are reviewed on perhaps a monthly schedule; others have limited time periods for LOIs before they close the window and move to the full application process.

Professional Grants (from AMTA)

As of early 2014, the American Music Therapy Association (AMTA) provides two types of funding for research.

Clinician-Based Grant Program. The Clinician-Based Grant Program exists to encourage and assist clinician-based applied research. Currently five funding priorities exist, and all types of research (qualitative, quantitative, and mixed methods) are eligible. Preferred research includes (a) research that contributes to evidence-based practice; (b) pilot projects that examine evidence-based interventions or protocols in clinical settings; (c) research that examines cost-effectiveness; and (d) projects that disseminate research results to providers, payers, and/or consumers is preferred. Other important considerations include collaborating with an academic partner for the proposed project. The research proposal is limited to two pages; the detailed budget is one page.

The Arthur Flagler Fultz Research Fund. The Arthur Flagler Fultz Research Fund encourages and promotes research, especially novel music therapy treatment within clinical and health services research. Seven funding priorities exist, and there is a preference for research that addresses at least one funding priority and includes collaborative efforts between music therapy clinicians and experienced researchers. The proposal should be no longer than 15 pages, with no more than 4 pages for the review of literature. The budget is limited to two pages, not including the explanation and justification.

The reviewers for these funding initiatives are typically music therapists. The Clinician-Based Grant Program is reviewed by members of the Research Committee. The Arthur Flagler Fultz Research Fund consists of three blind reviewers, followed by approval from the AMTA Board of Directors. Strict guidelines exist regarding conflicts of interest.

AMTA grant reviewers understand music therapy and do not need extensive information regarding what music therapy is. On the other hand, a theoretical framework and a comprehensive but succinct overview of the related research literature are necessary. Create a case for the relevance and significance of the proposal; relate all information back to the funding priorities. Give careful attention to the other requirements for the proposal, including the methodology; plan of operations; data analysis, assessment, and evaluation plan; as well as the budget and budget justification. Too often grant seekers start with strong applications for the first two areas of the proposal, and then the later sections, listed in the preceding sentence, contain minimal information or do not provide a thorough explanation. Make sure that the methodology, including the procedures, relates to the listed items on the budget (such as time involved in the implementation of the protocol/intervention by music therapist). Reviewers appreciate greater detail and transparency.

University-wide Grants

The process of receiving "internal" funding, or grants within your university or organization, will vary according to each institution and even within different departments in the institution. Oftentimes research universities provide "seed" funding for a pilot project in hopes that the individual will be able to use the results from the pilot project to obtain external funding outside the university.

Examine the mission and goals of the internal funding source. Some internal grants are for assistant professors; others encourage interdisciplinary work. Sometimes summer salary is considered; other times funding priorities emphasize opportunities for undergraduate student involvement in the research proposal. Be sure to address as many of the considerations/priorities for funding as possible within the proposal.

Typically, the university posts previous awardees on their webpage, including the (a) name of the professor, (b) department, (c) title, (d) abstract, and (e) amount of the award. Examine this page to gain an idea of funding amounts and what types of topics they seem to fund. It may be beneficial for you to contact one or two previous grant awardees within your university and ask if they would share their proposals.

Address the audience, which might include individuals whose research covers the entire continuum from the hard sciences to those who are in theatre and dance. Regardless, the reviewers for internal funding within a university want to read a clearly devised plan and know that the research could not be done without the funding. This is probably the most important aspect of your proposal. For example, reviewers do not believe paying a graduate research assistant to enter data is necessary for completing a project.

Be sure to use language that non-specialists can understand. Avoid jargon and multiple acronyms, which tend to be confusing for the reviewer. For proposals that have a limit of five total pages, it is imperative to explain why this is an extremely important project for the population you are serving and why funding must be in place to complete the proposed project. Make sure to have a clear plan of action. Most grant proposals ask for the criteria for success of the project. Be sure to clearly delineate this information, but also examine and set realistic goals for the project for the duration of the funding.

After Being Funded or Declined

After receiving funding, there is still paperwork to be done for the funding source. The amount of communication during the grant period will vary depending on the funding source. Some agencies will require quarterly communication on specified forms. Others will only require communication of results and outcomes of the grant-funded project. If a situation arises where the timeframe of the proposed project needs to be extended to meet the stated goals of the project, it is possible to ask for an extension of the grant period from some funders. This does not typically mean the funder will provide additional monies to complete the project; rather, submission of the results of the project can be delayed to allow the project goals to be met. To do so typically requires financial support from the grant recipient's employer to finish out the grant project.

It is very common to not receive grant funding for proposals submitted. This does not mean you should abandon all hope of ever receiving funding. Rather, the feedback given when grants proposals are not funded can be invaluable in moving forward and either revising or submitting a new proposal. Depending on the fiscal health of the government, the level of federal grant support allocated, and the number of submissions received, the federal grant funding success rate has ranged from 5% to 20% in any given year (http://report.nih.gov). Private agencies do not commonly report proposal funding success rates but may share that information if requested. Most funding sources are very specific with feedback about why a proposal was not funded and encourage future submission or revisions if the proposal appears to have the potential for being a good fit.

Conclusion

The grant-writing process is time-consuming and there is no certain outcome. Support from your employer or resources allocated for the time spent on grant development calls for consideration and discussion. Spending a significant amount of time and attention at the beginning of the process in choosing and communicating with a funding source is highly recommended. Identifying a call for proposals or request for proposals that aligns with your agency's mission and work is imperative. Careful attention must be paid to proposal submission guidelines as well as inclusion of qualified research or project team members. Grant writing can be an enjoyable experience when planned out and approached in a systematic fashion. Utilizing the many tips and recommendations on funders' websites can be extremely helpful. Table 5.1 summarizes considerations for grant funding.

Table 5. 1. Summary of Considerations for Grant Funding				
	NIH	**Corporate**	**Professional**	**University**
Competition	Competing with researchers in differing disciplines.	Competing with various service organizations and differing agendas, including philanthropic support for service initiatives, including sponsorships.	Competing with other professional board-certified music therapists. Judges should understand the language/ terminology.	Competing with other disciplines in the university/institution.
Purpose	To support research that has the possibility of providing a convincing and influential impact on the research field.	To support the corporation's goals and mission; this sometimes involves service initiatives rather than research. Oftentimes considered to be charitable giving.	To further research in music therapy or related areas.	To provide opportunities for faculty to achieve excellence in research. (Probably varies at each institution, but often the intent is to lead to larger funding sources and enhance scholarly work.)
Length of proposal	Varies according to type of grant program. For an R03, research strategy should be limited to 6 pages; however, additional and supporting paperwork make the application length around 30 or more pages.	LOI is usually one to two pages. Agency decides, based on LOI, whether you are eligible to submit a full application. Oftentimes, it will contact you to submit a full application after reviewing the LOI.	Arthur Flagler Fultz – research proposal limited to 15 pages; however, supporting paperwork results in longer length. Clinician Grant is limited to a 2-page research proposal.	Typically, but not always, limited to shorter lengths, such as 5 pages.
Process to submit	Work with your university or corporation's Office of Sponsored Research. Must file paperwork within this office.	Work with your university or corporation's Office of Sponsored Research (or Programs) as they will help prepare your tax information and verify your nonprofit status.	Submit as directed, although the university's Office of Sponsored Research will probably want to have that information processed within their office as part of their accountability of what grant funding was sought during each fiscal year.	Submit as directed.
Research team qualifications	Will want a solid research team consisting of qualified individuals from various disciplines (i.e., quantitative, mixed-methods, nurse/medical staff, or technology expert)	Some do not have as much interest in this area. Read call for proposal to determine whether this needs to be addressed.	MT-BC and member of AMTA. Arthur Flagler Fultz encourages collaboration between clinicians and researchers. Clinician-Based Grant requires collaboration between clinician and experienced researcher.	Sometimes grants are delineated for new/junior faculty, and others might be for any full-time faculty member or tenured faculty members who are starting a new line of research.
Who evaluates	Peer review process and a second level of review by advisory council/board.	Evaluation takes place by board members.	Several individuals selected by the professional organization. Reviewers receive proposals, evaluate individually, and submit written response to the organization.	Most likely individuals from varying disciplines. Most likely no one in music therapy, possibly someone in psychology or a similar related area to music therapy. Sometimes evaluations are done by committees for various disciplines (humanities and fine arts, social sciences, and mathematics and natural sciences).

Chapter 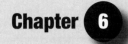 6

Staff Interactions and Ethical Considerations

Darcy DeLoach, PhD, MT-BC, and Jennifer Jarred Peyton, MM, MT-BC

When working in a hospital environment, a music therapist has the opportunity to interact with a variety of health care professionals. Commonly, music therapists are responsible for providing intervention services throughout multiple units and therefore interact with many health care staff. While nurses are likely the most frequent health care workers music therapists encounter, there are several others included in the medical team and hospital environment. Clinical staff includes, but is not limited to:

- physicians,

- nurse practitioners,

- registered nurses,

- licensed practical nurses,

- certified nursing assistants,

- physical therapists,

- occupational therapists,

- speech-language pathologists,

- recreational therapists,

- therapy assistants,

- child life specialists,

- social workers,

- case managers (usually a nurse or social worker),

- chaplains,

- pharmacists,

- phlebotomists,

- patient transporters,

- sonographers,

- radiology technicians, and

- medical assistants.

Some administrators are also considered clinical staff, such as the director of nursing, chief nursing officer, and unit directors. Non-clinical administrative staff may include the chief executive officer, chief operating officer, chief financial officer, and ethics officer. There are several non-clinical staff members a music therapist must know, including, but not limited to: (a) information technology personnel, (b) human resources, (c) clerical staff, (d) hospitality team, (e) security, (f) educators, (g) environmental services, (h) maintenance, and (i) volunteers. Such a list of relevant staff might be somewhat intimidating to a music therapist entering a new medical setting, but with moderate effort, one can quickly become acquainted with the team members pertinent to the success of a music therapy program. Of primary importance are those professionals who make decisions regarding funding and program implementation, leadership positions, or referral sources, as well as anyone who makes the music therapist's job possible.

While the music therapy field is progressively growing and becoming more integrated in the medical community, not all medical staff (clinical and non-clinical) know what music therapy is. Staff familiarity with music therapy effectiveness, purposes, and anticipated outcomes will vary greatly and is one of the most challenging aspects of integrating services in health care environments. Several factors contribute to the initial response health care staff will have about music therapy services as part of the multidisciplinary team. Previous exposure to music therapy services, personal responses to music, and a holistic versus traditional medical mindset all impact staff perceptions of music therapy.

Previous Exposure to Music Therapy Services

With the multitude of therapeutic approaches existing in the field of music therapy (Darrow, 2004), it is possible for health care staff to be exposed to music therapy patient care that is significantly different in approaches or outcomes, especially when interacting with different therapists or health care systems. When this occurs, a health care professional's framework of music therapy outcomes can be limited in scope. Initial responses to expanding music therapy services may be affected by what staff members anticipate an outcome to be. For example, if staff has been exposed only to a wellness model of music therapy that primarily addresses stress reduction and coping with life change, it may be difficult for that staff member to support expansion into pediatric rehabilitative services without in-service education. Similarly, varying intervention approaches within a patient population can cause confusion for staff members as well. For example, there are very specific approaches to Autism Spectrum Disorders (ASD) intervention services implemented by professionals outside of the field of music therapy. A multidisciplinary center for ASD services that primarily employs Applied Behavior Analysis (ABA) discrete trial intervention may not support inclusion of developmental music therapy services, and vice versa. A developmental ASD center would most likely not support inclusion of music therapists who implement an ABA intervention approach.

This can be further applied to the various specializations music therapists are able to pursue and incorporate into patient care. Protocol-driven service provision from a behavioral framework looks very different to some health care staff than humanistic or psychodynamic approaches utilized by music therapists. The high employee turnover rate in health care facilities necessitates ongoing staff education about what the music therapy department is providing, along with the anticipated outcomes. It is helpful to know if previous exposure to music therapy exists for staff who will receive education about music therapy services.

Health care professionals who have had positive past experiences with music therapy or music therapists will be excited to see the addition of a music therapy program within their hospital. One ultrasound technician at a regional medical center, who was accustomed to music therapy assisted procedures for pediatric patients, interviewed for a position at a children's hospital in another city.

Upon her return to work, she informed the music therapist that she didn't take the job because that hospital didn't utilize music therapy in the area she would be working. Her exposure to music therapy was so positive and impactful on her own job satisfaction that she will likely be a lifelong supporter of the field.

Unfortunately, there are health care workers who have had negative past exposure to music therapy, either by inexperienced students, sub-par music therapists, or music therapists with an approach viewed as strange by the staff. This is a difficult obstacle for the current music therapist who is battling projected perceptions from the naysayers. As is commonly known, it is much harder to convince someone that music therapy is good if they have already determined it is not. These negative past experiences with music therapy can significantly hinder the success of a program. Not only will the music therapist not receive referrals from that source, but that source has the potential to negatively impact other staff's view of music therapy.

There are also staff members who have been exposed to music therapy in previous settings, but are being introduced to a new style or approach in their current employment. In one situation, a nurse who had moved and changed hospital systems found it shocking that music therapists required a referral for services and documented outcomes, instead of rounding for all patients and providing no written documentation of outcomes. While her view of music therapy was positive, she had never imagined music therapy serving specific patient needs. Her perception of music therapy was clearly a result of positive experiences, but a lack of education from the music therapy department in her previous setting. Health care team members who have had no previous exposure to music therapy are blank slates, and their initial perception will likely be based upon their personal experiences with and responses to music.

Personal Responses to Music

It would be hard to find someone who has not had a personal interaction with or response to music at some point in life. There is a wide range of personal music experiences and expertise that people possess. Even those who do not play any instruments or consider themselves singers can still have very strong opinions about how music affects people. Those who love music and have primarily very positive associations with music are often delighted to see music introduced into the medical environment. Their previous experiences allow them to easily see that music therapy will be "good for the patients," even if they do not fully understand what music therapy is at first. These staff members are often amazed when they observe their first session and quickly become cheerleaders for the music therapy department.

There are also staff members who, although they like music, are reluctant to see its value in such a delicate and sterile environment. These professionals, as well as those who have negative past music experiences or none at all, may require more education, evidence-based data, and clinical observation before they believe in music therapy's vast benefits. The health care worker who has had limited exposure to music experiences can be just as skeptical as the one who dislikes music or anything "artsy." This puts music therapists in a very interesting situation when engaging staff in conversations about "What is music therapy?" When considering the previous involvement each person has had with music, it becomes easier to understand why there are so many preconceived ideas and misconceptions about what music can or cannot do in a health care environment. Music therapists frequently encounter statements from health care professionals that warrant education about what music therapy actually is and the purpose it serves for those receiving it.

Common Staff Statements and Misconceptions

"Music always makes me feel better when I'm stressed out."

Passive music listening is a very common coping tool in our society. Escaping into a favorite song to divert attention away from stressors is a quick and easy way to momentarily forget about life's troubles. Music for self-care in health care workers has been written about anecdotally (Bates, 2008; Harrison, 2004; Servodidio, 2007) as well as researched with positive findings (Cooke, Holzhauser, Jones, Davis, & Finucane, 2007; Lai, Liap, Huang, Chen, & Peng, 2013), which may contribute to the commonly held belief that music is most effective for stress reduction. Without staff education about music therapy interventions and outcomes, it is natural for a staff member to arrive at this conclusion.

A music therapist walks into a patient room in an intensive care unit when an RN, who is unfamiliar with the reason for the patient referral, looks at the music therapist and says something to the effect of "Oh good! I know music is going to make him feel better today . . . Mr. X has been under a lot of stress." At that moment, the music therapist has a choice: either stop and share the reason for the referral with the RN and the anticipated evidenced-based outcomes, or smile and make a comment in agreement that yes, music therapy will make a positive impact on the patient. Many factors will impact which direction the music therapist takes, including patient load, time-sensitive needs of the patient, and the level of familiarity with the staff member.

The underlying concern about this type of experience is that a health care professional is not aware of the specific reason for referral or the varying benefits of music therapy for patients. If staff members are exposed to music therapy only for stress reduction and do not see other therapeutic goals being addressed, the misconception may be perpetuated that music therapy is beneficial only to patients experiencing stress.

"Classical music should make him less agitated."

The first problem with this statement is that those who say it sometimes use the term *classical* interchangeably with *relaxing* in reference to music. It is not uncommon for non-musicians to believe that classical music makes one smarter and is innately relaxing. Most musicians would disagree, citing that the classical music genre is characteristically complex in nature and often more stimulating than calming. The second issue is the assumption that one type of music should have the same effect on everyone. There is a plethora of CDs and albums in the "relaxation music" category available for people to use when they need to calm down or relax. Depending on staff members' previous use of or exposure to calming and relaxation music, there may be preconceived ideas about the appropriate music to use when a patient is agitated. The fact is, there is no prescriptive music; no one style of music functions the same for every individual. Even if "classical" really meant "relaxing," it still wouldn't necessarily be appropriate for every agitated patient.

Music therapists commonly utilize the iso-principle when working with agitated patients. This approach starts with matching the intensity of the music to the mood and/or behavior state of the patient (Altshuler, 2001; Davis, 2003). When using the iso-principle with an extremely agitated patient, a song is chosen that is within the patient's preferred music genre, has high rhythmic complexity, and is played at a loud volume to match the intensity of agitation. Nurses who witness the start of this technique have made initial comments such as, "Well, that is just going to make it worse!" or "How is he supposed to calm down with music like that?" When framing the situation from a health care worker's perspective and personal context of music for relaxation, it is easy to understand why there may be confusion. Music therapists in this situation are put in a delicate position because the needs of the patient come first, but at the same time, damaging a staff relationship could be detrimental to the music therapy program. Inviting the staff member to stay and watch the process of the iso-principle at work, or making a plan to discuss the patient's outcome after the session or later that day, may help the staff understand. It might even increase the number of future referrals for agitated patients from that staff member.

It is counterintuitive for some people to think that music matched to a behavior can be a catalyst for change. Many think that matching music to a negative mood or behavior state will make it worse or perpetuate a negative experience or emotional state. Music therapists who frequently use the iso-principle are usually able to verbally explain how the technique works, but until someone sees the effects, it can be a difficult concept to understand. It is often helpful to suggest that a staff member return in 30 minutes to see how the patient is responding to the treatment process. When the staff member does return, the response is typically positive and has a lasting impact.

"Heavy metal is the only kind of music that anyone will be able to hear over the sound of the MRI."

This remains an all-time favorite statement made about procedural-support music therapy because it makes so much sense. Anyone who has heard the sounds a Magnetic Resonance Imaging (MRI) machine produces would nod in agreement that, yes, in fact, heavy metal music really is all a patient would be able to hear during the procedure. Without an in-depth understanding about how music affects cognition and expectations, it is hard to explain why music of any genre would be effective as a supportive service for patients undergoing a variety of medical procedures. The fact that live music therapy using patient preferred genres (compared to recorded music of preferred genres) is able to increase the positive perception of MRI procedures, decrease the time for procedures, and decrease the number of breaks requested by patients supports the existence of cognitive and expectation elements of patient experiences within music therapy (Walworth, 2010). For MRI assisted interventions, the music therapist matches the rhythmic qualities of the songs played to the sounds the MRI machine produced. Although the MRI sounds change frequently, the meter construct of the sound does not drastically shift. This enables the songs played by the music therapist to mask the MRI sounds and gives the listener a framework for processing the MRI machine sounds. Walworth's (2010) study revealed that even though no one was told about the synchronization of songs to the MRI scan, adult patients were able to predict when a scan was going to end based on the song played by the music therapist. The music therapist made this possible by watching the time left on a scan and repeating verses or creating tags for songs to synchronize the song ending with the conclusion of each scan. Patient familiarity with each song played is crucial for this process to work. Many patients report singing along in their head to the songs the music therapist plays and report knowing they can request songs in between scans. Giving a patient an element of control in an otherwise uncontrollable situation may contribute to the positive perception of the experience. Music therapy-assisted procedures may be another setting where observing the patient experience makes it easier for health care staff to understand the effectiveness than hearing or reading about the process. After witnessing many adult patients undergoing music therapy-assisted MRI scans, the MRI technologists were able to explain to other staff both how and why music therapy impacted the patient experience positively.

"Church music always lifts me up."

As with some of the previously discussed preconceptions about music effectiveness, it is common to hear staff make suggestions concerning what music to use with patients based on their own personal music experiences. Some of these personal musical experiences may occur in religious settings. Most religious groups incorporate music into their corporate meeting times. When one listens to a soloist or sings with a group, the musical experience is commonly uplifting or reflective. Upon hospital admission, many patients will identify whether they have a religious affiliation. It is natural for a staff member to conclude that a patient with a certain religious affiliation may benefit from hearing songs from their faith base while receiving hospital care. Religious music can have a positive impact on patients' spiritual well-being (Wlodarczyk, 2003). Previous positive associations with religious music can be very strong for certain patients, which can aid in the therapeutic process. Acceptance, personal goal-setting, security, determination, encouragement, and optimism are among the feelings that can be accessed through religious music.

Interestingly though, sometimes patients who state they have a strong faith base may not want to hear religious music during their hospitalization. In these situations, patients may be struggling with questions of "why" or "what next" that are interrelated with their faith. Hearing church music may also be an unwanted reminder that they are unable to attend church while in the hospital. For patients who are unable to communicate and do not have family present to identify music preferences, religious music is not typically chosen by music therapists for intervention use due to the complexity of possible responses. The structural elements of music are able to facilitate many music therapy interventions, making it possible to have effective outcomes regardless of the music genre chosen for sessions.

If health care staff suggest any music for a patient (religious or not), it is recommended to simply ask if it is specifically what the patient or family requested. If not, then delicately inform the team member that music therapy will be most effective if the patient's preferred music is used. Some well-meaning family members may also push religious music onto a patient who would prefer something else. If the patient is able to communicate his or her preferences, that is always a good starting place. If not, treat all music requests from others with judicious caution. Those who know the patient best will typically be able to adequately convey the best music selection.

"Happy music will make her forget why she is depressed."

When a patient is experiencing feelings of depression or sadness, distracting the patient from those feelings may not be the most appropriate intervention approach. Some staff may voice concern about a patient being exposed to "sad" music when experiencing depressed mood states for fear of intensifying the negativity. The iso-principle technique is commonly used by music therapists to elevate mood state by matching the musical and lyrical qualities to the patient's mood state at the beginning of the session. After the patient's mood state has been reflected by the music, the musical and lyrical qualities can be progressively altered to improve the patient's mood. This process is effective, non-intrusive, and is patient-led. Rarely will a patient move from a depressed mood state to dancing and laughing within a single session. If a patient is not emotionally ready to shift his or her mood state, the shift in musical elements cannot force a change. However, if a patient is emotionally ready to move toward positive change, the musical and lyrical elements of songs offer a supportive structure to help the patient experience an improved mood state. Staff members who are able to observe this change within a session are usually amazed at the progress patients make, especially when verbal counseling has not resulted in change or growth. If staff members are not able to observe, a report of progress from the music therapist after the session may leave the staff member equally impressed with the technique.

"Oh, good—the entertainment is here!"

This statement has the potential to make a music therapist want to explain how much time, money, and effort has gone into his or her education and training, including credentials and specialized certifications. While some music therapists greatly enjoy entertaining audiences with their talent, few appreciate being called the "e word" while working in a medical setting. Before damaging professional relationships with health care staff by showing you are offended, consider their frame of reference. If most of their previous exposure to live music has been in the context of entertainment, it is natural for one to assume that the musician entering a hospital unit is there to cheer up the patients with a performance. After all, music therapists are professional musicians. Even health care professionals who have observed music-filled music therapy sessions may not be aware of all the therapeutic elements and considerations specifically calculated and tailored by the music therapist for each individual patient. Some music therapy sessions can look like entertainment to an observer who is unfamiliar with evidence-based outcomes.

It becomes the responsibility of the music therapist to educate the staff about music therapy and its clinical benefits. When being referred to as an entertainer, music man/lady, troubadour, strolling minstrel, or songstress, music therapists can choose to smile and nod, or stop and say something. First, consider if the nickname is a term of endearment or a misconception before making that decision. Then determine if education is needed immediately for only that staff member, or later for the unit or the entire hospital.

Educating Staff

Orientation to Evidence-Based Practices

For some health care workers, evidence-based practices are the deciding factor for music therapy service inclusion. Without data to support anticipated outcomes, there will be no support given. This viewpoint is often seen in the medical attending staff at teaching hospitals. Meta-analyses on various topics can be distributed or presentations at monthly physician meetings can be given to summarize the research base supporting specific music therapy protocols and treatment areas. For other hospital staff, meaningful patient outcome examples are pivotal for service inclusion. Videos or pictures demonstrating what music therapy inclusion would actually look like on a unit is helpful for these health care professionals. Patient examples and music therapy stories can be recounted from past clinical work, clinical case study examples in the literature, or colleague experiences. Knowing what speaks to each staff member is an important part of assessing staff communication needs. One can typically assess when his or her audience is motivated or compelled by research data, numbers and statistics, or anecdotal patient stories that pull on heart strings.

In-Service Presentations

The most common form of education in health care settings is the in-service presentation. Every clinical unit typically offers in-services to the staff on a regular basis to provide the information they need to most effectively do their jobs. These presentations can include hospital protocol, patient satisfaction reports, new clinical techniques, documentation recommendations, patient care guidelines, and a variety of other pertinent topics. As live demonstrations or videos are typically the most compelling way to educate others about music therapy, the in-service presentation is the most accessible and beneficial education platform. In-services can vary in duration from 15 minutes to 2 hours, and the music therapist may have only a portion of that time. The challenge, then, is to deliver as much relevant information as possible in the amount of time given, in a way that will leave a lasting impact until the next presentation opportunity.

The first consideration in preparing for an in-service is to know the audience. As discussed earlier, staff members connect with information in various forms. While some are moved by heart-warming success stories, others require hard scientific data to be convinced of an intervention's validity. Information provided in the form the audience finds most compelling yields a more effective presentation with enduring results. Typically, physicians respond to research statistics, administrators respond to financial data and patient satisfaction, and clinical staff appreciate anecdotal stories. However, the wide variance within these groups of health care professionals warrants the recommendation to include both data and stories in presentations. Live demonstrations or video of specific techniques aid staff in understanding concepts and interventions with which they likely have no experience or exposure. As is commonly said, "A picture is worth a thousand words." A music therapist can talk about music therapy for hours, but until someone sees it in action, it is likely too abstract or not understood.

While in-service presentations are very efficacious in educating staff, just one is not sufficient. When starting a new music therapy program or expanding services to units/areas not previously served, the music therapist may need to provide in-services to multiple units and shifts. For example, even though the NICU staff working the night shift may never see the music therapist at work, they may make as many referrals as the day shift, and therefore need to receive the same in-service presentation as the day shift staff.

The most successful presenters are those who actively engage their audience and effectively deliver information that remains with the attendees long after the presentation concludes. Figuratively placing oneself in the staff's shoes to gain perspective on best educational techniques is always recommended. Most people do not respond well or attend to boring lectures in which information is read to them or provided in only one format. A presenter who offers no more to the audience than simply reading a handout or PowerPoint presentation misses an opportunity to make the information "come alive," as is so easy to do with music. Even a verse or two of an original song can connect the dots for those who learn aurally or who simply need an example to understand a concept. Providing evidence-based data, current research findings, and references is especially beneficial when presenting to physicians, administrators, and funding sources.

Printed Material

It is common practice to provide handouts when giving a presentation, as they are a great way to give more information than can be covered in the timeframe allotted. They also function as a printed reminder of goals, outcomes, and referral protocols when staff leave an in-service. Many hospitals post printed protocol pathways at nurses' stations, staff lounges, and even restrooms. It is not uncommon for the music therapist to hear staff say that they had "the perfect patient for music therapy the other day" but they weren't sure how to make a referral. This problem is easily remedied by placing printed material in an accessible location. If a nurse knows to go the green binder above the copier for instructions or protocols on making a physical therapy or chaplain referral, then the music therapy referral process should be included in that same binder and should be easy to find. As most health care providers are moving toward electronic information storage, it is becoming more common to have paperless units. Depending on the department in which music therapy is housed within the hospital, staff should be able to find music therapy policies and procedures in the same location or in the same fashion as all other referrals and orders.

Badge cards or pocket cards are another way to educate health care staff. Several hospitals provide staff with small laminated cards that attach to staff name badges that contain pertinent information like code keys, acronyms for fire safety, and hospital mission statements or patient care tips. Discriminating badge cards that highlight the most important information about music therapy and referral process offer an effective tool, as they are worn daily by staff and therefore are always at their fingertips. Likewise, small cards that can be placed in lab coats and scrub pockets can be useful to staff. These pocket cards can contain symptoms music therapy can address, therapeutic goals, desired outcomes, referral process, contact information, and any other information deemed necessary. Music therapists can carry pocket cards in a guitar bag, lab coat, or pocket and can hand them out daily to staff who are unfamiliar with music therapy or who need a reminder.

The One-on-One Approach

Sometimes the best education takes less than 5 minutes and is given to just one staff member during his or her shift. Because employee turnover is high in medical settings, staff members come and go frequently, often missing in-service presentations and interactions with music therapists. Whether requesting referrals on the unit or eating lunch in the cafeteria, music therapists can educate a fellow health care professional about the benefits of music therapy with just a few minutes of one-on-one time.

When seeking referrals on any particular unit, music therapists commonly find a nurse and ask if any patients are appropriate candidates for music therapy. If the nurse is unfamiliar with who qualifies as an appropriate candidate, the music therapist has an opportunity to briefly explain and provide a pocket card, if available. For example, a music therapist visits the oncology unit without any specific referrals and finds one or two nurses charting at the nurses' station. The music therapist asks if any of their patients are currently depressed, having trouble coping, in pain, or terminally restless/agitated. Simply by suggesting a few of the issues music therapy can address, the music therapist prompts the nurses to think about which patients would benefit most. The nurses have an opportunity to ask questions, and the music therapist can take a few minutes to give the explanation needed to help them understand why the music therapist is there. If they have time to join the session or even observe for a few minutes, then they can see firsthand how effective even one session of music therapy can be. This impression will likely last long enough for the nurses to think of music therapy the next time they encounter a patient with similar needs. If the staff members are unable to observe, a quick summary of the session or relevant patient responses following the session can reinforce the appropriateness of the referral and encourage the staff to remember that music therapy services are available.

Unit Rounds

In hospitals where the music therapist makes unit rounds with the multidisciplinary team, education opportunities are abundant, but very short. Rounds are typically fast-paced and only pertinent information is discussed. If and when the music therapist identifies a patient who would be a good candidate for services during rounds, a simple "Music therapy can assist with pain management" or "Would music therapy be appropriate for this patient?" may be all that is needed to obtain a referral. Team members who are unfamiliar with music therapy may take several rounds to catch on, but they will likely detect trends in the types of patients the music therapist requests to see or patient needs music therapy can address. Unit rounds that are slower paced lend themselves to more information from the music therapist and the opportunity for staff to ask questions. Even if none of the patients on any given rounding is appropriate for music therapy at that time, the music therapist's presence at the unit rounds is important for staff to see. It reminds them of music therapy's availability and that the music therapist is a part of the multidisciplinary team.

Considerations for Starting and Maintaining a Program

Staff Mindset of Holistic Versus Traditional Medical Approaches

With the continued movement toward holistic health and care for many patient consumers, health care environments are becoming more inclusive of supportive services. From an administrative perspective, the ability of an institution to financially support adjunctive or supportive therapies is the first determination. Health care systems with a whole health mission will most likely have donor funding sources that are interested in supporting the addition or expansion of music therapy services. Many people in our culture have positive experiences with music and believe music is beneficial for whole health, even if they are not aware of the music therapy profession or its beneficial outcomes for patients. For health care systems with a more traditional medical approach, there may not be awareness of the cost savings available for music therapy interventions and protocols (Walworth, 2005, 2010). The inclusion of cost savings data into proposals for music therapy service initiation or expansion is very helpful for administrators.

Once funding has been secured, the next step is deciding where within the hospital to offer supportive services such as music therapy. Factors that determine where services are offered range from the decision makers' previous exposure to music therapy services to their personal views of holistic versus traditional medical care. When considering the various units offering music therapy services across health care systems, it becomes apparent that there is not a typical pathway for service inclusion. Examples of where music therapists in health care systems are housed include, but are not limited to:

- pastoral care departments,

- child life departments,

- rehabilitation departments,

- neuroscience centers,

- cancer centers,

- recreation therapy departments,

- allied health departments, and

- arts in medicine departments.

If commonality existed in health care environments for music therapy service delivery, there would not be such a wide range of departments overseeing music therapy services.

A music therapist's specialization may determine in which unit administrators decide to first include services. A grant written specifically for music therapy service provision could be the determining factor. A personal interest in music therapy from a service line coordinator can also play an integral role. At Tallahassee Memorial Healthcare, the administration decided to offer music therapy services throughout the institution and asked the service line coordinators if any of them were interested in overseeing the music therapist being hired. The director who volunteered to oversee the music therapy department had a whole health approach to wellness and care and believed strongly in the supportive services provided by music therapists in all units of the health care system. For this reason, the music therapy department was housed in the Neuroscience Center, and then moved to being housed within the Cancer Center when the Neuroscience Center director changed positions to become the Cancer Services Coordinator. Remaining under the leadership of the Cancer Center Coordinator was requested by the director to ensure the music therapy department had complete support and a voice in funding decisions.

Music Therapy Advocates, Finding a Champion

Many music therapists are able to quickly identify a "champion" who understands, values, and advocates for music therapy service inclusion throughout the health care environment. These advocates can be anyone in the health care system, and they play an integral role in the health and growth of a music therapy department. In health care environments where music therapists serve multiple units and interact with many different staff, these advocates are vital to the continued support and understanding of music therapy services. When employee turnover occurs on units, it is not unusual for staff to educate new hires about music therapy services/goals/outcomes for their patients before the music therapist has a chance to even meet the new staff hire. When this happens, the groundwork is laid for continued staff support. Nurses and CNAs who work on multiple units will have the possibility of interacting with music therapists at a higher frequency than those who are assigned to a single unit. Many times these nurses will be the advocates for music therapists across units and will have interactions with multiple administrators.

Out of Sight, Out of Mind

Despite all the education provided to staff through in-services, printed material, unit rounds, and personal one-on-one contact, maintaining a visual presence is essential to maintaining a successful music therapy program. The old saying "out of sight, out of mind" proves itself true in this field that is mostly viewed as non-essential or supplementary. Even health care professionals who have had a profound experience with music therapy can sometimes forget about it if they are not frequently reminded of its availability. Medical music therapists are often surprised how quickly referrals can escalate or diminish depending on how much time they spend on a particular unit. After a MRSA outbreak in the ICU of one hospital, all non-essential staff were not allowed to enter while the ICU was thoroughly cleaned and renovated, which took a few months to complete. Once the music therapist was permitted to enter, it took another few months to regain the number of referrals typically held in that unit. Some staff admitted, "Oh, I forgot all about you," when the music therapist made rounds.

It is a particular challenge to maintain presence in areas not frequently served by the music therapy department. Because every program is different and every hospital's needs vary, music therapists must be aware where services are being provided and how often. It is also crucial to be seen periodically (if not frequently) by administrators, directors, donors, and decision makers. This is why many music therapists join certain committees or attend specific meetings within the hospital, to constantly remind those who may not see music therapy daily of the program's role in clinical services.

Staff Services

It is common for music therapists to provide stress reduction services, using live or recorded music, for health care workers. This can be a beneficial service for health care workers who work extremely long shifts with responsibility loads that are very high. Guided relaxation or brief live music sung together by unit staff allow personal experiences with music therapy that can help build collegial relationships. In settings where music therapy staff services are not routinely offered, assessing staff stress levels may lead to the addition of supportive services as needed. It is not uncommon to hear nursing staff say that they could use some music, when the music therapist walks by the nurses' station. If providing nursing supportive services fits within the mission of the hospital, stopping and playing requested songs for the nursing staff can lead to decreased stress levels and increased unit morale.

Some music therapy departments incorporate weekly scheduled music for the staff in various units. In this situation, any staff members with a couple of minutes to spare are invited to sing, play instruments, or simply listen to one or more requested or preselected live songs provided by the music therapist each week. In one hospital, the Neuro ICU nurse manager routinely requested "Ain't No Mountain High Enough" during the weekly staff "morale booster" music therapy time. She felt it gave the staff the needed "lift" during the middle of the week and always requested that the music therapist arrive in the middle of the shift.

Comments from staff often indicate that music therapy sessions for patients are nearly as beneficial to the health care workers in the room as they are for the patients. In one hospital, the wound care nurse frequently requested music therapy to co-treat patients with exceptionally long wound dressing changes, or those with severe pain or anxiety associated with the dressing changes. This nurse almost always reported that music therapy not only decreased the amount of time it took to complete the procedure, but also kept both the patient's and her stress level to a minimum. NICU nurses also often comment that music therapy for the infants has a positive effect on the staff members who are able to hear the music. They frequently report that the music is calming to them, lowering their blood pressure, and they will even request specific songs. Even though the music is directed toward the patients, the staff often listen and benefit in various ways.

Changing Procedure

Instances may arise that require a music therapist to examine and reevaluate procedures, policies, and protocols in the medical setting. While music therapy is generally viewed as an overall positive service to the patients, staff can be inadvertently negatively affected by it. One example occurred in a NICU several years ago, when the only music used for multimodal stimulation was Brahms' Lullaby, hummed repeatedly. After years of listening to music therapists humming the same song over and over, the NICU staff's perception of music therapy declined; they started calling the music therapy staff "the hummers," and referrals decreased. This situation warranted a change in the music being provided, not only to keep the staff happy, but also to maintain referrals in a unit where music therapy is significantly beneficial to patients and families. Data were collected on various types of music to determine the appropriateness for infants hearing the music (Standley et al., 2005). Although this situation was initially a negative one, the implemented changes resulted in a restored professional relationship with the NICU staff, an expanded repertoire of songs found to be appropriate for premature infants, and an increased number of referrals for services.

When referrals decrease in a particular unit or area of the hospital, the music therapist must analyze the situation to determine the cause(s) and create a solution. There are several reasons why referrals decline, and most are tied to the staff's perception of services. If the staff doesn't care for a particular music therapist and his or her music skills, they may discontinue music therapy requests. Likewise, if a staff member has a negative music therapy experience, he or she will be less inclined to enlist further services. It is common for the staff to stop making referrals (or never start) if the referral process is too difficult, complicated, or time-consuming. It may be appropriate or beneficial to have different referral processes for different units if there is not a standard protocol hospital-wide. For example, the outpatient procedure unit may be accustomed to calling for services, while the rehabilitation therapy department inputs orders into the computer system. The ICU waits for the music therapist to make rounds, while the pediatric charge nurse highlights patients' names on a census when the music therapist visits on Tuesdays and Thursdays. As long as the music therapist is willing to receive orders/referrals in various forms, maintaining consistency within a department or unit is likely to keep that department/unit's staff happy and generate referrals the way they do for all other services.

Non-Musical Gestures (Cookies)

There are plenty of times when it is entirely appropriate to "butter up" staff members with gestures that have nothing to do with music. The holidays are filled with food baskets delivered to various units by administrators, directors, physicians, and families to show their appreciation to the staff. Health care workers are often overworked and commonly fueled by coffee and sugar. A plate of cookies, brownies, or other tasty treats can have a surprising and tremendous impact on the staff's attitude and morale. It is also a good way to remind the staff about music therapy if printed material/ education is included.

A happy staff results in a positive work environment, and anything the music therapist can do to make the staff's work easier or more enjoyable will yield more positive perceptions of the music therapy program.

Ethical Issues

Assessment of Patient Need for Services

An assessment is necessary when deciding if a patient is appropriate for music therapy services. In health care settings, there are possibilities for rounding to determine the patients appropriate for treatment at a given time. Health care environments that use musicians to improve the environmental aesthetics and the patient experience should have a process to determine who should receive interaction with a musician. Rounding allows the music therapist to determine which patients would be appropriate for volunteer or paid musicians in health care versus music therapy interventions. In cases where rounding is not used for patient referrals, other health care staff (who are well informed about music therapy) may be able to determine who would be appropriate to interact with a musician, listen to a performance, or receive music therapy services.

It is imperative to differentiate who is appropriate to receive music therapy services and who is not, in order to remain within the assessment guidelines of the CBMT Scope of Practice (CBMT, 2010). One aspect of concern is how music can potentially harm patients in the health care environment. It stands to reason that if music can be beneficial for patient outcomes, it also has the ability to do harm. This possibility is most evident in the fragile patient populations. Premature infants and critically ill children and adults in intensive care units are all in a survival state where music therapy may or may not be beneficial for patient outcomes. Without documented research evidence to support the inclusion of music therapy services with fragile populations, it is unethical to provide services based on intervention models with other patient groups. The systematic inquiry concerning patient outcomes in fragile populations will support which treatment interventions are appropriate for use to ensure no harm is done. For example, there is no body of research providing evidence for how premature infants cognitively process sound. To make the assumption that premature infants will respond positively to womb-like sounds is unfounded and questionable, given that many premature infants have had little to no exposure to the sounds of the womb before entering the NICU. All major structures of the ear are not in place until 23 to 25 weeks gestation, and infants are not able to react to auditory information until approximately 26 weeks gestation (McMahon, Wintermark, & Lahav, 2012). Pediatricians with Brigham and Women's Hospital, Montreal Children's Hospital, Mass General Hospital, and Harvard Medical School who investigated premature infant hearing development concluded that the evidence-based recommendation for inclusion of sound in the NICU is to use only vocal music (McMahon et al., 2012). Evidence-based practices provide ethical inclusion of services for fragile populations.

The assessment of patients will also yield what treatment plan is appropriate for intervention services. For music therapists who view patient assessment as a unique and informal process, it is imperative to document the ethical justification for service provision. Using a formalized assessment tool provides reliability and validity of the resulting treatment plan recommendation. For example, when working with children with Autism Spectrum Disorders (ASD) in outpatient rehabilitation settings, the SCERTS tool is available for multidisciplinary assessment and treatment intervention recommendations. The SCERTS tool is appropriate for use by music therapists and generates very specific and achievable goals, objectives, and subobjectives to address communication needs (Walworth, Register, & Engel, 2009). The tool is designed to be implemented every 3 months to capture gains made and re-evaluate for new treatment goals (Walworth, 2007). Using a validated assessment tool increases the ease of communicating intervention targets and aims with other therapeutic staff through the use of common language between disciplines.

Reassessment for Termination of Services

Once services have been implemented, reassessing for termination of services is required. The presence of a goal to be working toward in a therapeutic environment assumes that there is the possibility of the goal being achieved. It is unethical to provide treatment services on a continual basis in a medical environment with no clear therapeutic direction. If a goal/objective or subobjective is not met by a patient, the conclusion can be drawn that the goal/objective/subobjective was not appropriate for the patient to be working on. This becomes crucial in audit situations, where therapeutic services need to reflect a congruent and similar patient status between disciplines providing services. Without the ability to re-assess and show completion/meeting of stated goals, there is no ability to terminate services. In short-term hospital stays, this issue is not as prevalent due to the patient meeting discharge criteria. However, it still is possible for a patient to meet the stated music therapy goals before their discharge date is determined. Patients who are admitted for longer stays are more likely to receive services that require more time for completion of goals. Having a reassessment plan is recommended to ensure that all service provisions are necessary and ethical. For example, if a patient is receiving music therapy services for improved mood state, it is important to assess for mood state at regular intervals to ensure that services are terminated or new goals are identified once mood is improved.

Multidisciplinary Rounds

The topic of attending rounds was addressed briefly in relation to determining appropriateness of service provision. When attending rounds, it is very possible for health care staff to make a recommendation for a music therapist to see a patient. Clarifying that the patient will be assessed for appropriateness of music therapy interventions is commonly needed, unless the entire staff attending rounds is already educated about the assessment process within music therapy. When patient treatment needs are identified by staff while rounding, it is appropriate for music therapists to suggest a patient be assessed for inclusion of music therapy services. In this situation, a music therapist has an opportunity to increase the staff awareness about what treatment options are available from music therapists providing intervention services. It is ethical for music therapists to suggest a patient be assessed for intervention needs. However, the occurrence of rounding and providing services to patients who state they would like to receive music therapy services should be approached with caution. Without the ability to identify a measurable objective through an assessment, the argument can be made that there is no difference between a volunteer musician and a music therapist seeing the patients.

Standing Orders and Staff Referrals

Another avenue for identifying patients for services is through referrals from health care staff. Some hospital systems use standing referrals for any patients admitted who are identified within a certain pathway. For example, upon admission, all patients with symptoms that place them at risk for stroke are flagged for stroke pathway interventions. All health care staff who address stroke recovery are simultaneously referred to assess these patients. This decreases the time spent by health care staff in determining which patients should be referred for music therapy services. However, in this referral pathway, the music therapist must create an assessment system that allows for the ethical decision of who receives treatment first. Issues related to triaging patient caseloads are discussed below.

Music therapists providing reimbursable services are commonly required to first obtain a physician referral. This process can be time-intensive, and therefore the option for standing physician referrals for patients meeting certain criteria may be preferable. Ethically, all patients who receive physician referrals must receive the services ordered. If a music therapy staff member is not able to meet the patient demand for services, the standing order referral pathway is not recommended. The ability to discharge a patient based on an inappropriate standing referral is possible, but not typically done. A standing referral is typically initiated only in situations where common patient symptoms necessitate music therapy interventions.

Non-reimbursable services may be handled differently. Staff referrals can be made verbally, can be written, or can be entered into patient tracking software. Verbal referrals are most often received at nurses' stations, or in the hallway when passing a staff member. Ethical considerations of patient confidentiality are paramount when receiving a verbal order. It is common for family members or visitors to be standing at nurses' stations to receive updates about patients, and hearing another patient's name would be a violation of patient confidentiality. With a written referral, a violation of patient confidentiality is also possible. Any identifiable information is considered protected health information (PHI) under the Health Insurance Portability and Accountability Act (HIPAA) (Health Resources and Services Administration [HRSA], 2013). This includes patient names, medical record numbers, financial numbers, and date of birth. These identifiers are commonly listed on patient census sheets, which are printed and used by therapeutic staff when creating daily caseloads. Any paper containing identifiers must be discarded in a secure fashion, such as confidential paper shredding services. Shredding with an in-office store-bought shredder is not considered secure and should be avoided. This relates to research practices as well. Any researcher completing a research ethics or HIPAA training should be aware of the security issues surrounding storage of PHI patient data for analysis.

Triaging Patients for Order of Visits

Some health care systems prefer to enter all non-reimbursable requests for intervention services to track the ability of various departments to provide services. This can be beneficial when determining staffing increase needs or division of time needs. This situation also requires the ethical decision regarding who receives services first. In a triage system, the most critical patients receive intervention services first. When a music therapist provides intervention services across patient units, it can be difficult to determine who first requires the services, and what should be the order of administration of patient services. Within music therapy interventions, the most critical patients may not be the patients located in the intensive care units (ICUs). A patient who is making a breakthrough with an emotional coping goal may be the most critical patient to receive services on any particular day. Or, a terminally ill patient who has family visiting and is in need of assistance in communicating final wishes may be placed higher in a triage list than a comatose patient in the ICU who is in need of sensory stimulation. The decision of triaging patient caseloads is complex and also involves the hospital mission and value statements. Music therapy departments that are funded to increase patient satisfaction scores and ratings will most likely not triage patients the same way as a music therapy department that is funded by a research grant.

Documentation

The need to document changes in patient status is crucial for accreditation and reimbursement practices. The movement toward interdisciplinary provision of care necessitates that all health care staff communicate about patient status, progress, and decline. In situations where staff members are not seeing similar progress, plateau, or decline for the same patient, accountability requires documentation as to why the patient is presenting differently within different treatment settings. This accountability exists to improve patient care services. Disciplines that do not clearly communicate outcomes are at risk of being eliminated from treatment teams who receive reimbursement services. Ethically, the provision of services must be terminated if no progress is being made. Without a clear documentation of patient status over the course of a treatment session, it is impossible to document change over time. In medical settings, this includes the presenting symptoms that may not be directly related to the purpose of the session. For example, a patient with congestive heart failure (CHF) may be receiving music therapy services to decrease pain, increase comfort, and improve coping skills. A music therapist in this situation is required to document the physical presenting symptoms related to pain and comfort such as a grimace face, clenched hands, and shifting in bed, as well as coping-related behaviors such as negative verbalizations and stated absence of hope. Additionally, the documentation note must include the physical presenting symptoms related to CHF such as swollen extremities, secretions, or inflammation, so that changes in admitting diagnosis can be confirmed across disciplines.

Co-Treating and Scope of Practice Interaction

It is common for music therapists to co-treat with related professionals. In this situation, the clear delineation of service provisions provided within each staff member's scope of practice is essential. It is unethical for a music therapist for provide a service outside of the CBMT Scope of Practice (SOP) (CBMT, 2010). There may be situations when another staff member requests a service from a music therapist that is not within the SOP, simply because the staff member is not familiar with the SOP. Having a copy of the SOP to distribute to staff members is helpful.

Gifts and Gratuity

While music therapists strive to educate staff, patients, and families that music therapy is not entertainment, some still perceive it that way. It is not uncommon for family members to slip money into a music therapist's hand at the end of a session with words of sincere gratitude for the beautiful music. Their perspective is that a nice smiling lady/gentleman came to their loved one's hospital room, played some of their favorite songs, took them on a trip down memory lane, and simply "made their day." As most people's experiences with live musicians are in the context of entertainment, it seems natural to them to give a tip for exceptional service or performance. Most health care facilities have policies that restrict employees from accepting gratuity, tips, or gifts from patients and families, as does the AMTA Code of Ethics, as stated in 9.3 and 9.4 (AMTA, 2013).

While it is usually deemed appropriate for an entire unit or department that cared for a particular patient to accept a gift, muffin basket, or pizzas given by a family member, gifts to one staff member are typically not allowed (unless the gift is under a specified monetary value determined by the facility). Gifts of varying forms and amounts are common, and sometimes simply arrive in the mail. One patient sent an entire anthology of The Beatles sheet music in a box addressed to a specific music therapist who, during a session, had admitted them as her favorite band. Because the gift far exceeded the $25 value set by the hospital, the music therapy supervisor consulted the department director overseeing the music therapy department. It was determined that the department as a whole would accept the gift (as it was specifically music and not appropriate to return) and a letter of gratitude from the director was sent to the patient.

Patients' families are usually not aware of these rules regarding gifts and, if they are, occasionally disregard them. When music therapists are faced with the awkward situation of being offered a tip, the most appropriate response is to graciously decline, explaining that hospital employees are not allowed to accept gifts for doing their jobs. If and when the family insists and refuses to take the money back, the music therapist can then suggest that the family make a donation to the hospital in appreciation of the music therapy services they received. This option is actually preferred because the administration is then made aware of the family's wonderful experience with music therapy, which likely enhanced patient satisfaction scores. If the family member offering the tip prefers not to go through the process of making a donation and insists that the music therapist "just take the money," the music therapist can inform the family that the money will be given to the department director as a donation and ask if the family prefers to be recognized or remain anonymous. With either decision, a thank you note on facility letterhead should be sent to the family as soon as possible.

Conclusion

While not exhaustive, the information presented in this chapter concerns commonly experienced staff interactions as well as ethical considerations for music therapists working in health care environments. As the field of music therapy advances and grows within health care settings, the need to communicate effectively and educate health care staff about music therapy efficacy becomes of paramount importance.

References

Altshuler, I. (2001). A psychiatrist's experience with music as a therapeutic agent. *Nordic Journal of Music Therapy, 10*, 69–76.

AMTA. (2013). *Code of ethics.* Retrieved from http://www.musictherapy.org/about/ethics/

Bates, J. (2008). Sing for sanity. *Nursing Standard, 22*(19), 27.

CBMT. (2010). *CBMT Scope of Practice.* Retrieved from http://cbmt.org/

Cooke, M., Holzhauser, K., Jones, M., Davis, C., & Finucane, J. (2007). The effect of aromatherapy massage with music on the stress and anxiety levels of emergency nurses: Comparison between summer and winter. *Journal of Clinical Nursing, 16*(9), 1695–1703.

Darrow, A. A. (2004). *Introduction to approaches in music therapy.* Silver Spring, MD: American Music Therapy Association.

Davis, W. (2003). Ira Maximilian Altshuler: Psychiatrist and pioneer music therapist. *Journal of Music Therapy, 40*, 247–263.

Harrison, S. (2004). Music reduces stress levels among staff and patients. *Nursing Standard, 18*(30), 4.

Health Resources and Services Administration (HRSA). (2013). What is "protected health information" (PHI) and "electronic protected health information" (ePHI) under HIPAA? Retrieved from the HRSA website: http://www.hrsa.gov/healthit/toolbox/HealthITAdoptiontoolbox/PrivacyandSecurity/underhipaa.html

Lai, H.-L., Liap, K.-W., Huang, C.-Y., Chen, P.-W., & Peng, T.-C. (2013). Effects of music on immunity and physiological responses in healthcare workers: A randomized controlled trial. *Stress and Health, 29*, 91–98.

McMahon, E., Wintermark, P., & Lahav, A. (2012). Auditory brain development in premature infants: The importance of early experience. *Annals of the New York Academy of Sciences, 1252*, 17–24.

Servodidio, C. (2007). Nurses provide care and comfort to patients while also remembering themselves. *ONS Connect, 22*(2), 21.

Standley, J. M., Gregory, D., Whipple, J., Walworth, D., Nguyen, J., Jarred, J., ... Cevasco, A. (2005). *Medical music therapy: A model program for clinical practice, education, training, and research.* Silver Spring, MD: American Music Therapy Association.

Walworth, D. (2010). Effect of live music therapy on anxiety, perception of procedure, repeating procedure, and time for completion for patients undergoing magnetic resonance imaging. *Journal of Music Therapy, 47*, 335–350.

Walworth, D., Register, D., & Engel, J. N. (2009). Using the SCERTS model assessment tool to identify music therapy goals for clients with Autism Spectrum Disorder. *Journal of Music Therapy, 46*, 204–216.

Walworth, D. D. (2005). Procedural support music therapy in the healthcare setting: A cost and effectiveness analysis. *Journal of Pediatric Nursing, 20*, 276–284.

Walworth, D. D. (2007). The use of music therapy within the SCERTS model for children with Autism Spectrum Disorder. *Journal of Music Therapy, 44*, 2–22.

Wlodarczyk, N. (2007). The effect of music therapy on the spirituality of persons in an in-patient hospice unit as measured by self-report. *Journal of Music Therapy, 44*, 113–122.

Section 3: Evidence-Based Clinical Applications

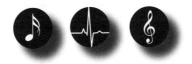

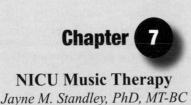

Chapter 7

NICU Music Therapy
Jayne M. Standley, PhD, MT-BC

The NICU-MT program is a research-based music therapy treatment for premature infants to improve medical outcomes and to promote growth and development. Clinically, it integrates identification of individual patient problems (medical, social, and developmental) with knowledge of neurologic maturation and patterns of premature infant growth. The premature infant is not just a small baby, but one whose development was interrupted and whose remaining months of gestational growth will occur, not in the buffered womb, but in the NICU amid stressors of (a) noise, (b) light, (c) touch, and (d) painful/irritating medical treatments. Music therapy can (a) nurture, (b) soothe, (c) promote developmental milestones, and (d) facilitate earlier discharge for the infant.

Problems of Premature Birth and Development

Premature birth is defined as less than 37 weeks gestation, while *low birth weight* (LBW) is less than 2500 g (5 lbs., 8 oz.). With contemporary medical intervention, very premature infants born as early as 24 weeks gestation have a 56% probability of surviving in the U.S., while those born at 32.5 weeks have over a 95% survival rate (Centers for Disease Control [CDC], 1999).

Prematurity and LBW are the second leading cause of infant mortality, and children born LBW will often have medical and developmental long-term problems. LBW children are twice as likely to be hospitalized during early childhood and will spend longer in the hospital. The average cost for infants hospitalized in the NICU is $41,610 versus $2,830 for a term infant, and the average costs for health care through the first year of life for preterm infants is $32,000 as compared to $3,000 for full-term infants (Kornhauser, 2010). When they attain school age, LBW children are 50% more likely to be enrolled in special education. The most common neurological problem is cerebral palsy with incidence increasing as birth weight decreases. Other problems are (a) hyperactivity, (b) specific learning disability, or (c) learning disorders. The most common medical problems are (a) asthma, (b) upper and lower respiratory infections, (c) ear infections, and (d) organ immaturity (heart, lungs, kidneys, or bowels). Medical treatment can cause stress that disrupts neurologic development, leading to future problems. Additionally, the provision of oxygen can cause retrolental fibroplasia (visual impairment), while some necessary treatment drugs can cause hearing loss.

During fetal development, the right side of the brain grows faster and will usually favor the more primitive human attributes. Further along in gestation during the third trimester, the left side of the brain starts growing and will eventually perform those human behaviors acquired later in evolution, such as language (Chiron et al., 1997; Kotulak, 1993). In the third trimester while the premature infant is in the NICU, he or she is adding 250,000 neurons per minute in the developing brain. During this period, 100 billion neurons will form, all a human will get throughout a lifetime. These neural cells compete with each other, connecting across tiny spaces called synapses to link up with a specific neurological function (Fischer & Rose, 1994) and stop dividing during periods of stress and overstimulation. Thus, the premature infant who will complete the third trimester of fetal development in the NICU is vulnerable to neurologic damage but in need of cause/effect learning opportunities. Nurturing can offset some of this damage while promoting improved growth and development.

Music Therapy Intervention

The premature infant is hypersensitive to stimuli, and stimulation across senses is cumulative; therefore, stimuli (sound, light, touch, smell, and taste) for the least mature infants must be restricted and controlled. Overstimulation disrupts neurological development and should be avoided as much as possible. Hearing develops as early as 18 gestational weeks, and the fetus responds to music during the third trimester of development (Lecanuet et al., 2000). The addition of music to the premature infant's environment must be done with great care and according to neurologic "readiness" or tolerance.

According to APA, ambient noise levels should be kept below 45 dBA

High ambient noise levels in the NICU (a) raise stress levels, (b) disrupt sleep cycles, (c) cause startle responses reflected in highly variable physiological measures, and (d) reduce growth and development of premature infants (Perlman, 2001). As a result, the American Academy of Pediatrics (APA) formed a Sound Study Group and called for reductions in sound levels. Specifically, they suggest that sound levels be maintained below an hourly loudness equivalent of 50 db, an hourly L10 (sound level exceeded 10% of the time) of 55 dB and a 1-second maximum of 70 dB using the A-weighted, slow response scale (American Academy of Pediatrics, 1997; Krueger, Wall, Parker & Nealis, 2005).

Research with music in the NICU has shown that premature babies thrive when provided with musical auditory stimuli, whether recorded or live (Loewy et al., 2013; Standley, 2012). Physiologic measures such as heart rate and respiration rate stabilize and oxygen saturation levels increase (Cassidy & Standley, 1995; Coleman et al., 1997; Standley & Moore, 1995). Music infants gain weight and are discharged sooner than those not receiving such stimulation (Caine, 1991). The majority of these studies have provided music to individual infants with tape players or speakers placed directly in the incubator to avoid sound pollution of the entire NICU environment (Cassidy & Ditty, 1998).

The speed with which an infant can adjust or habituate to stimuli is an indication of neurologic maturation. Conversely, interruption of neurological development decreases habituation ability of tolerance. Tolerance to multiple stimuli can be promoted by using music for soothing and homeostasis and then systematically increasing other stimuli without interrupting homeostasis. Stroking promotes breathing in the neonate; therefore, massage and kangaroo care are excellent therapies as is music combined with touch when the infant is developmentally ready for this complexity. This is usually around 32 gestational weeks.

Between 24 and 33 gestational weeks, the brain is too immature to support oral feeding. The suck–swallow–breathe coordinated response develops at 34 weeks. At this time, the infant must be taught to suck if he or she was tube fed for an extended period. Music can be used to reinforce non-nutritive sucking, which helps with this transition and leads to earlier acquisition of independent oral feeding.

Language development is faster if the language is directed to the infant in "parentese" (song-like qualities). Live lullabies are highly effective therapy for soothing and for promoting language development. Singing directly to the infant and adapting the interaction according to the child's responses is important in furthering neurologic development and initiating social interaction and attachment.

Kemper et al. (2004) surveyed NICU physicians and nurses about their expectations for music provision in the NICU. The majority (68%) agreed that they would like to have music played throughout the NICU and that their preference was for recorded rather than live music. One study examined the effect of recorded music played free field at 62 dB (Scale C) throughout the entire NICU environment (Standley, 2003). In this 7-week study, speakers were placed at each end near the ceiling of the NICU. Decibel levels were measured in the room under no music and recorded music conditions across 7 weeks. It was determined that overall dB levels in the room dropped as a result of staff speaking more quietly with each other and as a result of infants crying less. However, control of auditory stimuli (appropriate selections, duration, dB levels) across 24 hours/day, 365 days/ year was difficult since NICU-MTs were not available throughout the extended days and weeks. Additionally, the diverse individual needs of each child according to gestational age, gender, and/ or medical complications could not be controlled. Therefore, music played throughout the NICU is generally less effective than individually selected music placed within each infant's incubator or crib.

Male and female infants develop differently in the NICU. Female infants thrive more robustly and learn developmental skills more quickly. Male infants are bigger at birth, are more active, and are more easily overstimulated. They often do not thrive as readily and may stay longer in the NICU before discharge. Female infants respond more effectively to NICU-MT than male infants, though both groups receive benefit (Standley, 2012).

Reasons for Referral and Expected Outcomes

A meta-analysis or research summary of the NICU MT literature (Standley, 2012) and analysis of clinical NICU-MT programs (Standley & Swedberg, 2011) document a variety of expected outcomes that can be used to determine appropriate reasons for referral. Table 7.1 highlights patient benefits and expected outcomes of music therapy in the NICU setting.

Table 7.1. Benefits of Music Therapy with Premature Infants		
Intervention	**Appropriate Starting Age**	**Benefits/Expected Outcomes**
Music listening to live singing or recorded lullaby music in the isolette	28 weeks AGA	• Improves oxygen saturation levels (Moore, Gladstone & Standley, 1994) • Stabilizes physiologic measures of pulse and respiration (Lorch et al., 1994) • Increases weight gain • Shortens hospital stay • Reduces crying • Improves sleep (Loewy et al., 2013)
Live singing and progressive multimodal stimulation	31–32 weeks AGA	• Shortens hospital stay • Increases tolerance for stimulation • Speeds extubation and decreases time on the ventilator (Standley, 1998; Walworth et al., 2012)
Parent training in the multimodal stimulation program	31–32 weeks AGA	• Reduces overstimulation (Whipple, 2000) • Increases visitation time in the NICU • Empowers parents and promotes bonding
The PAL© (Pacifier-Activated-Lullaby system):	34 weeks AGA	• Reinforces non-nutritive sucking (as early as 34 weeks) (Standley, 2000) • Increases feeding rate of poor feeders at 34–36 weeks (Standley, 2003; Standley & Walworth, 2010) • Soothes infants more quickly following painful stimuli (Whipple, 2008)

Evidence-Based Techniques

Music Listening

Music listening has been shown to be safe with low birth weight infants (Cassidy & Standley, 1995), providing positive benefits like reduction in inconsolable crying, improved physiological measures, and deeper sleep (Arnon et al., 2006; Cassidy & Standley, 1995; Keith, Russell, & Weaver, 2009). Some data indicate parents and/or caregivers (nurses, physicians) prefer the use of recorded music (Polkki, Korhonen, & Laukkala, 2012; Tarja, Korhonen, Timo, Outi, & Helena, 2012), but other data show that parents believe that live music, in the form of singing or humming, is most suitable (Tarja et al., 2012). Furthermore, research shows that live music leads to greater reductions in heart rate and deeper sleep in stable preterm infants (Arnon et al., 2006). Precautions should be taken to ensure that music listening is implemented properly with infants in the NICU setting. Table 7.2 provides an overview of evidence-based music listening protocols.

Table 7. 2. Music Listening Protocols (Live or Recorded)		
Referral Characteristics	**Music Listening Procedures**	**Contraindications**
• Can begin around 28 weeks • Infant is medically stable	• Daily approval of the nurse providing care to the infant should be obtained for provision of music stimulation • Maximum time/day for continuously playing music 4 hours. Preferred method is alternating ½ hr. on and ½ hr. off across 1.5 hrs. • Speakers should be placed binaurally	• Musical or sound generating toys and mobiles should be prohibited as they are usually repetitive and the volume can seldom be controlled
Musical Characteristics		

• Selection of Lullabies: Sounds in the NICU should be soothing, constant, stable, and relatively unchanging to reduce alerting responses. Lullabies promote language development with emphasis on vowels, rising/falling phrases, and the recognition of soothing sounds and should be provided in the native language of the infant's family when possible. The least alerting lullabies would have these characteristics:
  ✓ Voice alone or only 1 accompanying instrument
  ✓ Light rhythmic emphasis, constant rhythm, slow tempo
  ✓ Constant quiet volume. Music volume should remain in the 50–55 dB range on Scale C. Note: male hearing acuity is less developed than female acuity and may require slightly greater dB level (Cassidy & Ditty, 2001)
  ✓ Melodies in the higher vocal ranges, which infants hear best and prefer
  ✓ Use of female vocalists since normally developing fetuses hear this in the womb and develop a preference for women's voices
  ✓ Use of children's voices since infants attend to and learn from other children
  ✓ Use of lullabies in the child's native language
• Live singing is excellent when it is steady, constant, quiet, soothing, higher pitched, at slower tempi, and infant directed.
• At very early gestational ages (prior to 32 weeks) social interaction is too overwhelming for the immature neurologic system and should be avoided. This is more critical for males than for females. To obtain the most calming influence on heart rate, the music should be hummed in lullaby style in a major key with the fewest chord changes possible.		

Use of PAL© to Reinforce Non-Nutritive Sucking

Before the premature infant can be discharged from the hospital, he or she must learn to coordinate the suck, swallow, and breathe responses while feeding. The infant must also independently take in enough nutrition during oral feeding to gain weight consistently and grow across time. Research shows that non-nutritive sucking (NNS) is an excellent activity since it stimulates the brain to release hormones that benefit physiological measures and improve behavior states while preparing the infants for oral feeding. The PAL© is an FDA-approved medical device that reinforces non-nutritive sucking with a short period of recorded music. Sustained sucking causes sustained music. Research has shown that the PAL© (a) increases sucking endurance, (b) increases feeding rate, and (c) develops sucking bursts of 10 to 12 sucks before pause, which is well suited to oral feeding skill. According to Standley et al. (2010), PAL© trials significantly reduced gavage feeding length for infants at 34 weeks (AGA), with three trials superior to one trial. Female infants also learned to nipple feed significantly faster than male infants. See Table 7.3 for PAL© protocols.

Table 7.3. Use of PAL© to Reinforce Non-Nutritive Sucking		
Referral Characteristics	**PAL©Procedures**	**Contraindications**
• Medically stable • Has begun gavage feeding • Demonstrates apnea during nipple feeding • Evinces early fatigue and frantic short bursts followed by fatigue (PAL© is used to lengthen sucking pattern.) • Still receiving gavage feedings at 34 weeks GA or greater. • Medically able to receive a pacifier following painful procedures (PAL© is used to teach NNS for pain relief.)	• Consult nursing for daily approval of PAL© use. • Duration of use is 10–15 minutes once or twice a day. PAL© should be stopped when infant experiences overstimulation or ceases to suck for 1-minute duration despite stimulation of pacifier in mouth • Initial use settings include lowest level pressure criteria, music reinforcement of 10 seconds, and suck criterion of 1. • Insert pacifier into infant's mouth from side with nipple on top of the tongue. If infant does not suck immediately move pacifier in and out of mouth or stroke cheek to stimulate sucking. • If the infant is sucking consistently and demonstrating progress, then increase PAL© criteria for music reinforcement by gradually increasing sucking pressure and the sucking criteria to desired burst level of 10–12 sucks. • Continue PAL© opportunities until infant completes 10–15 minutes of NNS and demonstrates improvements in feeding.	• PAL© is not recommended for infants under 34 weeks GA.
Musical Characteristics		
• Volume levels should be set at approximately 60–65 dB (Scale C) or 1 bar line on the PAL© read out. • Select pacifying music (usually lullabies are selected due to the constant rhythm and volume level as well as for language development)		

Use of Music to Teach Neurologic Tolerance/Habituation to Stimulation

During the cautious stimulation phase ($\geq$ 30 weeks), music can be used to increase tolerance to stimulation. This is primarily accomplished through multimodal stimulation, an adaptation of the White-Traut and Tubeszewski auditory, tactile, vestibular, visual protocol by Standley (1998). Multimodal stimulation is not appropriate for infants younger than 30 weeks and should be carefully monitored for signs of overstimulation when administered (Gooding, 2010). See Table 7.4 for an overview of the use of music to teach neurologic tolerance/habituation to stimulation.

Table 7.4. Use of Music to Teach Neurologic Tolerance/Habituation to Stimulation		
Referral Characteristics	**Music Listening Procedures**	**Contraindications**

• Adjusted gestational age of 30–32 weeks
• Medically stable
• Overresponsive to stimuli
	• Get approval of the nurse providing care to the individual infant for appropriateness of this procedure for this day/time.
	• Swaddle the infant and sit silently, unmoving in a rocking chair while holding him/her. Begin quietly humming a lullaby to the infant without touch or other movement. Assure that the infant is totally relaxed (homeostasis) which usually takes 30–60 seconds.
	• Continuing humming and implement stimulation sequence listed below. Note that stroking should be slow, repetitious, and firm since light touch is hyper-alerting to the premature infant.
	• Begin slow stroking, then light massage in the following order:
	  ✓ Scalp-linear
	  ✓ Back-linear
	  ✓ Throat-liner
	  ✓ Arms-linear or circular
	  ✓ Abdomen-linear
	  ✓ Linea alba (abdomen/vertical midline)-linear
	  ✓ Legs-linear
	  ✓ Checks-linear
	  ✓ Forehead-linear
	  ✓ Nose to ears-linear
	• If infant stays in homeostasis during sequence above, then maintain auditory, add slow rocking, and repeat tactile steps looking for engagement cues of eye contact and finger contact. Note any of the following infant responses and reinforce: head orientation, smiling, eye contact, vocalization, snuggling
		• **Notice and respond to any adverse physiologic reactions that occur at any point in the procedure, including:** oxygen saturation drops below 86%; heart rate increases to <100, >200, or >20% over baseline; respiratory rate increases >20 over baseline; apnea/bradycardia occur.
		Response: If any of the above occurs, **pause 15 seconds.** Then if HR/RR is within normal limits, continue. If the HR/RR does not go to normal limits or accelerates when stroking begins again, **stop** all music therapy stimulation for the day.
		• **Notice and respond to any subtle disengagement cues, including:** hiccoughs, grimace, clinched eyes, eyes averted, tongue protrusion, finger splay, struggling movement.
		Response: When any of these occur, pause singing and touching for 15 seconds. If cue abates, continue stimulation as before.
		• **Notice and respond to any potent disengagement cues, including:** crying, whining, fussing, cry face, spitting/ vomiting, hand in halt position, reaching out/stretching.
		Response: If any of these occur pause 15 seconds. When cue abates, continue. If cue does not abate or reoccurs in the presence of music and touching, discontinue the procedure for that day

Musical Characteristics		
• Quiet singing or humming is recommended. • Simple guitar accompaniment may be used with female infants.		

Additional Interventions

Parent training. Parents who wish more opportunities to be involved in their child's therapy or who have been observed to overstimulate their child may be trained in the use of music to teach neurologic tolerance/habituation to stimulation procedure. Research shows that they will effectively use the procedure and will visit more often in the NICU (Whipple, 2000). Parents can also be trained in ways to use music for soothing/bonding and developmental stimulation. Examples include the use of music for soothing (e.g., singing lullabies) or the use of music for developmental play (e.g., use of play songs like *Itsy Bitsy Spider*) (Trehub & Trainor, 1998; Trehub, Hill, & Kamenetsky, 1997). Data suggest that NICU staff believe that music can also be beneficial for the parents by decreasing stress and focusing/enhancing performance of required tasks, and that the use of music in the NICU could improve parent mood and increase overall comfort in the unit (Tarja et al., 2012).

Recommendations for Clinical Practice

We conducted a 1-year analysis of the impact of our NICU-MT program. Using applications pioneered in research studies, we found that clinical results were identical to researched outcomes for infants born 28 to 35 gestational weeks (Standley & Swedberg, 2011). Those applications are summarized in this chapter with complete clinical applications of all NICU-MT procedures given in the second edition of *Music Therapy for Premature Infants* (Standley & Walworth, 2010), and the total clinical program with infants and families has been described (Hillmer, Swedberg, & Standley, 2011).

There are anecdotal reports of volunteer musicians petitioning NICUs to perform live, calming music for premature infants. Premature infant responses to stimuli are so volatile that untrained musicians who may be naive about appropriate (a) repertoire, (b) style, or (c) signs of infant distress should not be allowed to play in this location. Similarly, toys and mobiles placed by child life or parents should be monitored. Professional training and ongoing data collection are crucial to understanding the most medically appropriate and therapeutic musical selections. The NICU music therapist should serve as an advocate for the child and use his or her expertise to ensure the safety of these vulnerable infants.

Music Recommendations:

- *Humming and a cappella maintain HR/RR*
- *Accompaniment, when added, should be simple*
- *Major keys decrease HR more than minor keys*

It is our value that lullabies in the child's native language are the most soothing and beneficial NICU music when the child reaches approximately 28 gestational weeks. Term infants enter the world with a great deal of language knowledge gained from third trimester womb eavesdropping on their mothers talking. The premature infant is born before this benefit ensues and is, therefore, language deprived. Lullabies of all cultures carry a preponderance of beginning language sounds and are capable of soothing while conveying highly effective language input. Therefore, lullabies with language content are considered more beneficial than purely instrumental music selections.

Lullabies with language content are considered more beneficial than purely instrumental selections.

NICU Recommended Song Lists

It is known that premature infants at the earliest gestational ages and those who are more seriously ill are affected by minimal changes in the music presented. Our research has shown that humming maintained and calmed HR/RR more than did singing, and that singing a cappella was slightly more calming than singing with guitar accompaniment (Standley et al., 2003). Simple accompaniment (three chords or less with unchanging arpeggio or strumming style) had the most calming influence on the infant. Songs in a major key produced a slightly greater decrease in heart rate than did those in a minor key.

Songs should be performed a cappella or with the simplest accompaniment possible and with as few chord changes as possible. If the NICU infant is critically sick, greater care should be taken in song selection according to results documented previously. Avoid all simulated, low-quality recordings, as these will not provide the desired benefits.

Least Alerting Songs recommended for the most critical infants. These songs are considered to be "least alerting songs" for the most fragile, sickest, most premature infants for the following reasons: three chords or less, major chords, and lullaby style (repetitious, no separate melody for a chorus or bridge). All should be played slowly and softly.

Other acceptable NICU songs. Acceptable songs for more medically stable infants or for those at later gestational ages incorporate the following components: (a) songs in a major key, (b) all chords are major or minor (no diminished or augmented), and (c) no more than four chords within a lyrical phrase. Again, all should be played slowly and softly. See Table 7.5 for a list of appropriate songs.

Table 7. 5. Least Alerting and Other Acceptable Songs	
Least Alerting Songs	**Other Acceptable Songs**
A-Hunting We Will Go Alphabet Song Are You Sleeping Baby Bumble Bee Barney Song The Bear Went Over the Mountain Bingo Blowin' in the Wind Boom Boom (Ain't It Great to Be Crazy) Cold, Cold Heart Down by the Bay Down in the Valley Farmer in the Dell Five Green and Speckled Frogs God Bless America Going Over the Sea Head, Shoulders, Knees, and Toes He's Got the Whole World Hush, Little Baby I Fall to Pieces I Know an Old Lady Who Swallowed a Fly If All the Raindrops If You're Happy and You Know It I'm a Little Teapot Itsy, Bitsy Spider London Bridge Looby Loo Mary Had a Little Lamb The More We Get Together The Muffin Man Old MacDonald's Farm On Top of Old Smokey Peace Like a River Red River Valley Row, Row, Row Your Boat Shake My Sillies Out Sing a Song of Sixpence Sing, Sing a Song Singing in the Rain Six Little Ducks Skidda-ma Rinky Dinky Skip to My Lou This Old Man Twinkle, Twinkle Little Star Wheels on the Bus Willoughby Wallaby You Are My Sunshine Zip-a-dee-doo-dah	Accentuate the Positive America the Beautiful Annie's Song (You Fill Up My Senses) Baby Mine Beautiful Dreamer Blue Moon Blueberry Hill Brahms Lullaby Candle on the Water Can't Help Falling in Love Could I Have This Dance Country Roads The Dance Dream, Dream, Dream A Dream Is a Wish Your Heart Makes Edelweiss From This Moment On Getting to Know You Have You Ever Seen the Rain Hey, Jude Home on the Range I Can See Clearly Now I Hope You Dance I Will I'm Forever Blowing Bubbles In the Still of the Night Kiss the Girl Lean on Me Leaving on a Jet Plane Let It Be Let Me Call You Sweetheart Love Me Tender Moon River My Heart Will Go On Oh, What a Beautiful Morning Old Folks at Home (Swanee River) Over the Rainbow Peaceful Easy Feeling The River The Rose Shenandoah Simple Gifts Simple Man Stand by Me Try to Remember Unchained Melody Under the Boardwalk What a Wonderful World When You Wish Upon a Star Wonderful Tonight

Conclusion

Premature infants are among the most medically and developmentally fragile populations served by music therapy. The possibility of harm to these fragile, neurologically immature infants exists, and their unique needs must be recognized. Without specialized training, there is little precedent for guiding early intervention music therapy strategies for premature infants in the NICU. Because NICU research focused on developmental therapies for premature infants usually does not include music or the addition of auditory stimuli, NICU-MTs must follow evidence-based medical protocols and abstain from innovative creativity in treatment until research can document benefits for new methodology.

It is important to know that premature infants pass through phases of development that affect neurologic and adaptive responses (survival, withdrawal, and social/interactive); therefore, music therapy treatment must be developmentally appropriate as per each gestational week of development. Early in gestation the infant should remain in the most relaxed state for effective growth and neurologic development, that is, with arms and legs folded in the fetal position. The immature brain is easily overwhelmed. This is evidenced by the infant startling or extending arms or legs. When either is observed, it is an indication of potential harm since brain cells quit dividing during this response to stimulation. Music that is too loud or too interactive can cause harm. Music therapy procedures seeking or stimulating interaction prior to 32 gestational weeks are usually contraindicated.

Protection of the infant is paramount. The location and criticality of the problem dictate a medical model for service provision. In accordance with a medical model, NICU-MT should adhere to a biomedical/evidence-based approach for treatment and research. Research should (a) meet medical standards for design and methodology, (b) employ evidence-based protocols, and (c) use of dependent variables that measure medical and developmental parameters such as

- heart rate,

- respiration rate,

- behavior state,

- length of NICU stay, and

- gestational developmental milestones.

Presentation of results should carefully and correctly label gestational age of subjects at the time of interaction and provide medical or developmental reasons for the procedure. Interpretation of interpersonal interactions with a severely premature infant based on a theoretical model does not meet these guidelines.

Before working with preemies, music therapists should have expertise in premature (a) infant physiology, (b) NICU medicine, and (c) fetal development. This training is currently available and literature has been widely disseminated. A recent survey found that NICU-MT training offers perceived benefits of higher quality of care and somewhat higher salaries for therapists (Peczeniuk-Hoffman, 2012). We hope that the profession will continue to recognize the benefits and need for training as the field expands its contribution to the well-being, growth, and development of premature infants.

References

American Academy of Pediatrics. Committee on Environmental Health. (1997). Noise: A hazard for the fetus and newborn. *Pediatrics, 100*, 724–727.

Arnon, S., Shapsa, A., Forman, L., Regev, R., Bauer, S., Litmanovitz, I., & Dolfin, T. (2006). Live music is beneficial to preterm infants in the neonatal intensive care unit environment. *Birth, 33*, 131–136.

Caine, J. (1991). The effects of music on the selected stress behaviors, weight, caloric and formula intake, and length of hospital stay of premature and low birth weight neonates in a newborn intensive care unit. *Journal of Music Therapy, 28*, 180–192.

Cassidy, J., & Ditty, K. (2001). Gender differences among newborns on a transient otoacoustic emissions test for hearing. *Journal of Music Therapy, 38*, 28–35.

Cassidy, J. W., & Ditty, K. M. (1998). Presentation of aural stimuli to newborns and premature infants: An audiological perspective. *Journal of Music Therapy, 35*, 70–87.

Cassidy, J. W., & Standley, J. M. (1995). The effect of music listening on physiological responses of premature infants in the NICU. *Journal of Music Therapy, 32*, 208–227.

Centers for Disease Control. (1999, April 29). *National Vital Statistics Report, 47*(18).

Chiron, C., Jambaque, I., Nabbout, R., Lounes, R., Syrota, A., & Dulac, O. (1997). The right brain hemisphere is dominant in human infants. *Brain, 120*, 1057–1065.

Coleman, J. M., Pratt, R. R., Stoddard, R. A., Gerstmann, D. R., & Abel, H.H. (1997). The effects of the male and female singing and speaking voices on selected physiological and behavioral measures of premature infants in the intensive care unit. *International Journal of Arts Medicine, 5*(2), 4–11.

Fischer, K. W., & Rose, S. T. (1994). Dynamic development of coordination of components in brain and behavior: A framework for theory and research. In G. Dawson & K. W. Fischer (Eds.), *Human behavior and the developing brain* (pp. 3–66). New York: Guilford Press.

Gooding, L. F. (2010). Using music therapy protocols in the treatment of premature infants: An introduction to current practices. *The Arts in Psychotherapy, 37*, 211–214.

Hillmer, M., Swedberg, O., & Standley, J. (2011). Medical music therapy with premature infants: Family-centered services. In A. Meadows (Ed.), *Developments in music therapy practice: Case study perspectives* (pp. 49–69). Gilsum, NH: Barcelona.

Keith, D., Russell, K., & Weaver, B. (2009). The effects of music listening on inconsolable crying in premature infants. *Journal of Music Therapy, 46*, 191–203.

Kemper, K., Martin, K., Block, S., Shoaf, R., & Woods, C. (2004). Attitudes and expectations about music therapy for premature infants among staff in a neonatal intensive care unit. *Alternative Therapies in Health & Medicine, 10*(2), 50–54.

Kornhauser, M. (2010, January). How plans can improve outcomes and cut costs for preterm infant care. Retrieved from the Managed Care website: http://www.managedcaremag.com/archives/1001/1001.preterm.html

Kotulak, R. (1993, April 11). Unlocking the mind: A prize-winning series from the *Chicago Tribune*. *Chicago Tribune*, p. 1.

Kreuger, C., Wall, S., Parker, L., & Nealis, R. (2005). Elevated sound levels within a busy NICU. *Neonatal Network, 24*, 33–37.

Lecanuet, J., Graniere-Deferre, C., Jacquet, A., & DeCasper, A. (2000). Fetal discrimination of low-pitched musical notes. *Developmental Psychobiology, 36,* 29–39.

Loewy, J., Stewart, K., Dassler, A., Telsey, A., & Homel, P. (2013). The effects of music therapy on vital signs, feeding, and sleep in premature infants. *Pediatrics, 131*(5), 1–17.

Lorch, C., Lorch, V., Diefendorf, A., & Earl, P. (1994). Effect of stimulative and sedative music on systolic blood pressure, heart rate, and respiratory rate in premature infants. *Journal of Music Therapy, 31*, 105–118.

Moore, R., Gladstone, I., & Standley, J. (1994). *Effects of music, maternal voice, intrauterine sounds and white noise on the oxygen saturation levels of premature infants.* Paper presented at the National Conference of the National Association for Music Therapy, Orlando, FL.

Peczeniuk-Hoffman, S. (2012). *Music therapy in the NICU: Interventions and techniques in current practice and a survey of experience and designation implications* (Unpublished master's thesis). Western Michigan University, Kalamazoo.

Perlman, J. (2001). Neurobehavioral deficits in premature graduates of intensive care—Potential medical and neonatal environmental risk factors. *Pediatrics, 108*, 1339–1348.

Polkki, T., Korhonen, A., & Laukkala, H. (2012). Expectations associated with the use of music in neonatal intensive care: A survey from the viewpoint of parents. *Pediatric Nursing, 17,* 321–328.

Standley, J. (2012). Music therapy research in the NICU: An updated meta-analysis. *Neonatal Network: The Journal of Neonatal Nursing, 31*(5), 311–316.

Standley, J., Cassidy, J., Grant, R., Cevasco, A., Szuch, C., Nguyen, J., … Adams, K. (2010). The effect of music reinforcement for non-nutritive sucking via the PAL (Pacifier-Activated Lullabies apparatus) on achievement of oral feeding by premature infants in the NICU. *Pediatric Nursing, 36*(3), 138–145.

Standley, J, Gregory, D., Whipple, J., Walworth, D., Nguyen, J., Jarred, J., … Cevasco, A. (2003). *Medical music therapy: A model program for clinical practice, education, training, and research.* Silver Spring, MD: American Music Therapy Association.

Standley, J., & Swedberg, O. (2011). NICU music therapy: Post hoc analysis of an early intervention clinical program. *Arts in Psychotherapy, 38*, 36–40.

Standley, J., & Walworth, D. (2010). *Music therapy with premature infants: Research and developmental interventions.* Silver Spring, MD: American Music Therapy Association.

Standley, J. M. (1998). The effect of music and multimodal stimulation on physiological and developmental responses of premature infants in neonatal intensive care. *Pediatric Nursing, 24*, 532–539.

Standley, J. M. (2000). The effect of contingent music to increase non-nutritive sucking of premature infants. *Pediatric Nursing, 26*, 493–499.

Standley, J. M. (2003). The effect of music-reinforced non-nutritive sucking on feeding rate of premature infants. *Journal of Pediatric Nursing, 18*, 169–173.

Standley, J. M., & Moore, R. S. (1995). Therapeutic effects of music and mother's voice on premature infants. *Pediatric Nursing, 21*, 509–512, 574.

Tarja, P., Korhonen, A., Timo, S., Outi, P., & Helena, L. (2012). Are there differences between the expectations of parents, nurses and physicians when using music in the NICU? *Open Journal of Nursing, 2,* 215–221.

Trehub, S., Hill, D. S., & Kamenetsky, S. B. (1997). Parents' sung performances for infants. *Canadian Journal of Experimental Psychology, 51*, 385–396.

Trehub, S. E., & Trainor, L. (1998). Singing to infants: Lullabies and play songs. In C. Rovee-Collier, L. P. Lipsitt, & H. Hayne (Eds.), *Advances in Infancy Research* (Vol. 12; pp. 43–77). Stanford, CT: Alex.

Walworth, D., Standley, J., Robertson, A., Smith, A., Swedberg, O., & Peyton, J. J. (2012). Effects of neurodevelopmental stimulation on premature infants in neonatal intensive care: Randomized controlled trial. *Neonatal Network: The Journal of Neonatal Nursing, 18*, 210–216.

Whipple, J. (2000). The effect of parent training in music and multimodal stimulation on parent-neonate interactions in the Neonatal Intensive Care Unit. *Journal of Music Therapy, 37*, 250–268.

Whipple, J. (2008). The effect of music-reinforced nonnutritive sucking on state of preterm, low birthweight infants experiencing heelstick. *Journal of Music Therapy, 45*, 227–272.

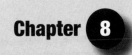

Chapter 8

Pediatric Medical Music Therapy

Jayne M. Standley, PhD, MT-BC, Lori F. Gooding, PhD, MT-BC, and Olivia Swedberg Yinger, PhD, MT-BC

By the 1980s, pediatric hospital medicine increasingly began to focus on patients with higher acuity and complexity (Fisher, 2012). Today, infants, children, and adolescents ranging in age from newborns (post initial discharge) to 18 years treated in the hospital setting often have serious, long-term, or even terminal illnesses. Children undergoing extensive treatment related to serious illness and their families often require counseling or structured family interactions to deal with illness symptoms, treatment side effects, and related psychosocial needs.

Pediatric medical treatment may be painful, unfamiliar, or uncomfortable. In particular, younger children often do not understand medical treatment and may even be traumatized by it. This can lead to developmental regression and/or lifelong fear/avoidance of medical treatment (Pate, Blount, Cohen, & Smith, 1996). Increasingly, hospitals are looking for ways to help pediatric patients and their families cope with the challenges of illness and hospitalization. Music therapy has been used in pediatric services for many years and is more and more recognized as a viable treatment option. A meta-analysis of pediatric music therapy research showed that, in all studies, music benefitted medical outcomes and patient welfare (Standley & Whipple, 2003). The data further suggest that music therapy can be a cost-effective intervention, decreasing the need for sedation during medical procedures, reducing procedural times, and decreasing staffing needs (Walworth, 2005). Music therapy is used throughout pediatric treatment to address issues as diverse as (a) anxiety, (b) trauma, (c) pain, and (d) end-of-life care. Additionally, neurologic music activities are used to address deficits in motor functioning. A recent survey identified over 200 board-certified music therapists (MT-BCs) who currently provide pediatric MT services in the U.S. (Tabinowski, 2013). The following information highlights some of the aspects for consideration when establishing a pediatric music therapy program.

Reasons for Referral

According to a 2008 study by Mathur, Duda, and Kamat, pediatric practitioners referred patients to music therapy services for (a) socialization, (b) emotional expression/communication, (c) premature infant care, (d) motor skills/gait training/rehabilitation, and (e) perioperative care. Additionally, patients in intensive care, patients with anxiety attacks, and patients undergoing burn care were also referred for music therapy services. These data suggest that music therapy services are referred to address a variety of needs, and, as a result, it is important to establish a cohesive system to ensure effective patient care. The establishment of referral-based pediatric medical music therapy services is dependent on (a) medical staff approval, (b) physician referrals, (c) open communication between interdisciplinary staff members and the music therapist, and (d) identification of appropriate reasons for referral and related music therapy protocols. Negotiation with the business office for appropriate documentation conducive to the hospital's reimbursement policies and contracts may also be important if pursuing reimbursement. However, given the ongoing changes in health care reform and the current use of the per diem and DRG (diagnosis-related groups) pay structures, it should be noted that reimbursement for music therapy services in an inpatient setting may not always be possible. (For a concise overview of hospital billing, see http://economix.blogs.nytimes.com/2009/01/23/how-do-hospitals-get-paid-a-primer/?_r=1.)

Referral processes vary from unit to unit due to the (a) mission, (b) patient needs, (c) staff leadership, and (d) communication differences of each area. Referrals for music therapy should be specific and relevant to (a) diagnosis, (b) treatment, and (c) discharge timeline (Standley, 2000). One possible approach may involve targeting music therapy services toward patients with higher acuity and complicated situations. This can not only improve the patient experience, but can also improve patient outcomes and reimbursement potentials. In fact, patient satisfaction has been shown to improve when music therapy services are present (Swedberg & Standley, 2011). Additionally, it can help solidify the value of music therapy services in pediatric inpatient care.

Educating medical staff through (a) in-services, (b) presentations, (c) demonstrations, and (d) interdisciplinary team input is necessary to generate and coordinate referrals. Fact sheets or referral algorithms may also be beneficial for medical providers. Identifying colleagues who support music therapy services and can encourage other staff members to try new techniques in patient care is invaluable to setting up a new program. Finding the optimal fit within the existing communication network in each unit is also essential. Music therapists may be notified of patient referrals and scheduled procedures by fax, pager, email, or telephone. Once a new program is in place, the MT-BC should be visible in the area where referrals are desired. The more exposure music therapy receives, the greater the probability of future referrals.

Evidence-Based Techniques

A thorough literature review reveals a number of techniques generally used in pediatric music therapy (Colwell, Edwards, Hernandez, & Brees, 2013; Gooding, 2012; Robb, 2003; Standley & Whipple, 2003; Wolfe & Waldon, 2009). The techniques listed in Table 8.1 have been shown to be effective in addressing a myriad of needs in pediatric patients in the hospital setting.

Table 8.1. Common Pediatric Music Therapy Techniques	
Techniques	**Objectives/Purpose**
Music for distraction	Distraction; reduce distress/anxiety
Music-assisted relaxation and/or music to induce sleep	Induce sleep and/or decrease distress
Music-based psychoeducation and procedural education	Cooperation during medical treatment; anxiety reduction
Active music participation (movement, instrument playing, singing, etc.)	Normalization; Improve family interactions
Music combined with counseling techniques (common interventions include lyric analysis, song writing, video production, etc.)	Coping skills development
Developmental music activities	Achieve/maintain developmental milestones
Neurologic music therapy techniques (including melodic intonation therapy)	Rehabilitation of physical or communication deficits (often co-treating with speech of physical therapy)
Orff-based music interventions	Improved psychosocial objectives
Improvisation	Improved mood and well-being

Recommendations for Clinical Practice

Research shows that all music interventions are significantly better than no music in pediatric medical treatment and the benefits are very large (Standley & Whipple, 2003). Research also shows that children respond to medical treatment differentially by age range (Standley & Whipple, 2003).

Active music involvement is better than passive listening, and live music is better than recorded. Though patient-preferred music is generally recommended (Standley, 1986, 2000), with children it does not matter who selects the music content (patient vs. MT vs. medical personnel)—outcomes will be similar (Standley & Whipple, 2003). It is also important to remember that success of the music intervention is enhanced by the therapists' ability to assess and to incorporate patient (a) musical preferences when appropriate, (b) perceptions of musical properties, (c) familiarity with the music, (d) cultural context, and (e) previous experiences (Stouffer, Shirk, & Polomano, 2007). Likewise, the music therapist must consider the child's developmental level and functioning when designing appropriate interventions.

Research shows that children fear unfamiliar medical treatments and cannot differentiate a minor versus major procedure. Music therapy functions better for non-invasive and major invasive procedures than for minor invasive procedures. By age, adolescents show the greatest benefits, compared to infants. Least beneficial effects occur for children aged 4–12 years who show more fear due to understanding the painful implications of proposed treatment, while being too immature developmentally to accept the short-term discomfort for long-term gain. Research with children in music therapy does not show differentiated effects by gender (Standley, 2000).

- *Music is better than no music.*
- *Adolescents and infants show the greatest benefit.*
- *Active engagement is more effective than passive listening.*
- *Live music is better than recorded music.*
- *Music therapy should start prior to the onset of painful procedures.*

All methods for documenting benefits show positive results, meaning music therapy is equally effective whether assessed by (a) patient or parent self-report, (b) monitored physiologic measures, or (c) observation of patient behavior and affect. Behavioral observation of pain and distress reveal modest effects in comparison to physiological and self- report measures, which are somewhat more inflated. Research shows that when music therapy is used for distraction from painful invasive procedures, it should start before the painful stimulus (Standley, 2000). Table 8.2 highlights some of the goals/objectives and related techniques available in the music therapy literature.

Table 8.2. Evidence-Based MT Outcomes and Techniques		
Goal/Objective	**Applicable Procedures and/or Treatment Settings**	**MT Techniques**
Pain reduction/ management during or following invasive procedures [1-3]	• Surgical and post-operative care [4-7] • Debridement and dressing changes for burns [8-11] • Bone marrow aspirations [12] • Lumbar punctures [13] • Venipunctures and hypodermics [14-17] • Immunizations [18-20] • Sutures [21] • Cardiac catheterization [22-24] • Cancer treatment [25-29] • Emergency department assessment and treatment [30]	• Active music participation to live music with choices exercised by the patient [31] • Music-assisted relaxation • Background, recorded music with passive listening (least effective)
Anxiety reduction [32-34]	• Pre-operative anxiety [35-38] • Pre-treatment or repetitive, painful, invasive procedures; trauma [39] • Pre labor and delivery [40] • Procedures such as roentgenography [41] • Nausea and vomiting [42]	• Active music participation to live music with choices exercised by the patient • Music- assisted relaxation • Song writing and video production about illness [43-45] • Focused music listening
Infant pacification in the newborn nursery	• Healthy newborns [46-49] • Colic-related crying [50]	• Recorded lullabies or live singing of lullabies • Lullabies paired with touch for layering multi-modal stimulation
Decreased respiratory distress [51-53]	• Children with mechanical respiratory assistance	• Passive listening to recorded background music with tempo for desired RR
Increased enjoyment of physiotherapy [54]	• Children receiving chest physiotherapy for cystic fibrosis	• Recorded music paired with physiotherapy
Maintenance of developmental milestones [55-56]	• Pediatric patients	• MT developmental activities (cognitive, motor, social)
Expression of feeling, communication skills [44, 57-58]	• Hospitalized children	• Lyric analysis, song writing, counseling
Improved hospital satisfaction [59]	• Pediatric patients	• Various techniques

[1] Clinton, 1984; [2] Loewy, 1997; [3] Loewy 1999; [4] Aldridge, 1993; [5] Bradt, 2001; [6] Siegel, 1983; [7] Steinke, 1991; [8] Rudenberg & Royka, 1989; [9] Schieffelin, 1988; [10] Schneider, 1982; [11] Whitehead-Peaux, Baryza, & Sheridan, 2006; [12] Pfaff, Smith & Gowan, 1989; [13] Rasco, 1992; Schur, 1986; [14] Arts et al., 1994; [15] Fowler-Kerry & Lander, 1987; [16] Hua, 1997; [17] Malone, 1996; [18] Megel, Houser & Gleaves, 1998; [19] Noguchi, 2006; [20] Yinger, 2012; [21] Lutz, 1997; [22] Claire & Erickson, 1986; [23] Gettel, 1985; [24] Micci, 1984; [25] Bailey, 1984; [26] Barrera, Kykov & Doyle, 2002; [27] Brodsky, 1989; [28] Slivka & Magill, 1986; [29] Standley & Hanser, 1995; [30] Barton, 2008; [31] Robb, 2003; [32] Edwards, 1999; [33] Fagen, 1982; [34] Lane, 1991; [35] Chetta, 1981; [36] Ogenfuss, 2001; [37] Robb et al., 1995; [38] Scheve, 2002; [39] McDonnell, 1984; [40] Liebman & MacLaren, 1991; [41] Hanamoto & Kajiyama, 1974; [42] Keller, 1995; [43] Robb, 1996; [44] Robb 2000; [45] Robb & Ebberts, 2003; [46] Kaminski & Hall, 1996; [47] Lininger, 1987; [48] Marley, 1984; [49] Owens, 1979; [50] Larson & Ayllon, 1990; [51] Ammon, 1968; [52] Behrens, 1982; [53] Wade, 2002; [54] Grasso, et al., 2000; [55] Barrickman, 1989; [56] Goforth, 2008; [57] Froehlich, 1984; [58] Monro & Mount, 1978; [59] Swedberg & Standley, 2011

Targeting Specific Diagnoses and Objectives

Music Therapy and Cancer Care

Music therapy in pediatric hematology/oncology can play a vital role in supportive care for pediatric patients and their families. Music therapy interventions can help pediatric cancer patients and their families cope as well as stay connected with "normal" life (O'Callaghan, Baron, Barry, & Dun, 2011). Music therapists who work with pediatric cancer patients frequently use music therapy techniques to (a) reduce anxiety and pain reduction, (b) promote tension release/relaxation, (c) provide opportunities for control and normalization, (d) improve quality of life, (e) improve interpersonal relationships, (f) facilitate emotional expression, and (g) enhance self-esteem (Bailey, 1984; Hilliard, 2006; Standley & Hanser, 1995). Music therapists in pediatric oncology also address patients' palliative and hospice care needs. Common objectives targeted include (a) pain and nausea, (b) comfort, (c) communication problems, (d) psychosocial needs, (e) anticipatory grief, and (f) family conflict (Daveson & Kennelly, 2000; Hilliard, 2003).

Counseling and Coping Skills

Serious or prolonged illnesses with multiple hospitalizations, such as cancer or burn treatment, may include repeated painful, invasive, or debilitating treatments. Patient and parent stress may be cumulative, increasing with time. Seriously ill children often perceive the threat to their mortality and wish to discuss it. They may have to cope with the loss of friends—fellow patients met in treatment settings. Contextual support counseling within a process of song writing, lyric analysis, and/or video production can be very valuable (Robb, 2000).

Normalizing Activities for Play and Socialization

Hospitalized children need opportunities to play and socialize with other children. Group music activities are an excellent means for accomplishing this. Children who are stable enough to leave their rooms and those who are not contagious can gather in a waiting area for group music therapy. Parents can be encouraged to participate, and research shows that active involvement by parents or caregivers during music therapy can decrease child stress behaviors and increase appropriate parent/caregiver interactions (Whipple, 2000; Yinger, 2012). Likewise, staff, other therapists, and volunteers can all be invited for group participation. The group activities can be designed to include all ages, with each person participating at his or her level of capability.

A child's quality of play often diminishes in the hospital, and this can lead to disruptions in normal development (Kennelly, 2000). As a result, children in sterile isolation need a great deal of stimulation. Hospitals with internal broadcasting capabilities can allow children confined to their rooms to watch and join in group activities by phoning in responses. One-to-one music therapy sessions can utilize many creative resources to develop and maintain children's interests. Facilitating use of the Internet as a support in the therapeutic process is also important.

Music Therapy and Outpatient Rehabilitation Services

The term *rehabilitation* typically denotes a return to a previous level of functioning, whereas the term *habilitation* refers to the process of developing a previously unlearned skill in order to maximize one's abilities to function more effectively in the environment. In practice, the term *pediatric rehabilitation* is used in reference to both rehabilitative and habilitative processes. Pediatric rehabilitation services are medical, therapeutic, and educational interventions provided by an interdisciplinary team to children with either acquired injuries/illness (such as a traumatic brain injury or a tumor) or congenital disorders (such as cerebral palsy, spina bifida, or developmental delay) (Shulman, Kathirithamby, Rosenberg, & Stern, 2009). Outpatient pediatric rehabilitation services commonly include occupational, physical, and speech therapy. The inclusion of music therapy within pediatric rehabilitation has become more common and is an area in which there is a need for additional research.

Kennelly and Brien-Elliott (2001), in an article on the role of music therapy in pediatric rehabilitation, suggest that music therapy fulfills three primary needs in pediatric rehabilitation: promoting adaptive coping, reducing pain and distress, and promoting developmentally appropriate skills. Specifically, goals in pediatric rehabilitation fall into four main categories: psychosocial care, motor skills, behavioral/cognitive skills, and speech/language/communication skills. The authors emphasize the importance of working closely with the interdisciplinary team to deliver pediatric rehabilitation treatment. Examples of music therapy interventions in pediatric rehabilitation include:

- using song writing to address the emotional needs of children or adolescents who have experienced trauma or illness;

- using singing and vocal exercises to improve rate of speech and verbal intelligibility;

- co-treating with occupational or physical therapists, using music as motivation to complete exercise routines.

Procedural Support in the Hospital Setting

Pediatric Sedation

When fear of medical treatment does lead to noncompliance, sedation is often used to ensure treatment compliance. Because sedation is associated with serious risks, the American Academy of Pediatrics and the American Academy of Pediatric Dentistry (2006) developed guidelines to ensure safe administration. These guidelines, adopted by The Joint Commission, require the presence of "at least one person whose only responsibility is to constantly observe the patient" (p. 2594). This can place a serious strain on precious medical resources (RNs, etc.) that are in short supply nationally by requiring increased staffing and resulting in increased costs (Perry, Hooper, & Masiongale, 2012). The use of sedation is especially common in children under age 6 and individuals with developmental delays (Walworth, 2005). Sometimes a pediatric patient will have an adverse reaction to the sedation and can become extremely irritable or dangerously ill. Obviously, too much sedation is risky and harmful for children. Moderate or conscious sedation is defined "as a drug induced depression of consciousness. The patient maintains the ability to respond purposely to verbal direction or verbal direction either alone or accompanied by light tactile stimulation. Interventions are not required to maintain the patient's airway" (American College of Emergency Physicians, 2013).

Because sedation-to-anesthesia is a continuum, it is not always possible to predict how an individual patient receiving medication intended to achieve moderate or deep sedation will respond. Chloral hydrate and midazolam (Versed) are the most common sedatives used with children in the U.S. (National Institute for Health and Care Excellence, 2010). Common side effects associated with oral sedation are nausea, vomiting, stomach pain, mild respiratory depression, irritability, and hyperactivity (Greenberg, Faerber, Aspinall, & Adams., 1993; Sifton, 1998). More adverse outcomes include seizures, respiratory failure requiring bag ventilation, laryngospasm, significant increases in middle ear pressure, oxygen desaturation/ hypoxemia, sinus arrhythmia, and/or death (Abdul-Baqi, 1991; Biban, Baraldi, Pettenazzo, Filippone, & Zacchello, 1993; Cote, Alderfer, Notterman, & Fanta, 1995; Munoz et al. 1997; Polaner et al. 2001; Sing, Erickson, Amitai, & Hryhorczuk, 1996).

Pediatric Procedural Support

Procedural support is the use of music within a therapeutic relationship to promote healthy coping, decrease distress, and decrease pain perception during and after a procedure (Ghetti, 2012). In pediatrics, procedural support is provided during medical treatment to facilitate its accomplishment with the child's cooperation and with the least amount of trauma. Procedural support involves live music interventions provided by a music therapist to eliminate the need for sedation and/or reduce anxiety. Techniques for completion of this goal vary according to the procedure and each patient. Common procedures include (a) CT scans, (b) echocardiograms, (c) electroencephalograms (EEGs), (d) X-rays, (e) intravenous (IV) starts, and (f) ventilator extubation trials. Procedural support functions as a distraction to lower anxiety or to induce sleep in young patients needing to remain still for an extended period. Procedural support (a) saves the hospital money; (b) releases RNs for other duties; (c) increases the probability of a successful procedure; and (d) reduces parental, child, and staff trauma (Walworth, 2005).

Procedural support involves live music interventions provided by a music therapist to eliminate the need for sedation and/or reduce anxiety.

Procedural Support Protocols

In our practice, MT procedural support protocols are an approved policy document for medical staff reference and standard practice guidelines that include how soon the MT will begin before the procedure. Sample protocols for common procedures follow.

CT scan. For a CT scan, the patient is required to lie completely still for an image to be captured successfully. In pediatric patients, this generally requires the patient to be asleep. In an unfamiliar, noisy, and brightly lit environment, a pediatric patient usually has difficulty going to sleep, even after sleep deprivation. The music therapy staff member acts as the patient advocate in this situation, assessing all variables causing increased patient anxiety, which interferes with the patient falling asleep. Variables for assessment are listed in Table 8.3.

Table 8.3 Procedural Variables for Consideration		
Environmental Variables	**Emotional Variables**	**Physiological Variables**
● Number of people in waiting room ● Activity/noise level in room and hallway	● Previous negative medical procedures ● Quality of family support	● Age of child ● Amount of sleep deprivation, if any

When a patient requires an IV for the CT scan, the increased anxiety due to perception of pain also becomes a factor for the music therapist to consider. Since no two patients are the same when combining all of the previously mentioned variables, fine-tuned assessment skills are a necessity. Figure 8.1 provides specific protocols for various CT scan implementation procedures.

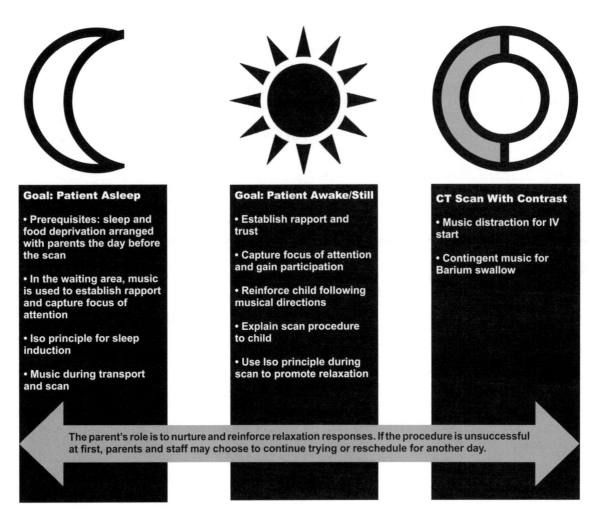

Figure 8.1. CT scan protocols.

Echocardiogram. An echocardiogram is a sonogram/ultrasound of the heart. Pictures are captured at different angles with the same type of device used for pregnant women. Emergency center services can include any of the discussed procedures and can differ in the amount of time before notification of the procedural support needed and the baseline level of patient anxiety prior to procedure.

Echocardiograms, X-rays, IV starts, and ventilator extubation trials all require distraction from patient anxiety to successfully complete the procedure. Each of these procedures is completed while the patient is awake and fully conscious, and therefore the patient can attend to whatever live music stimulus is present. All live music played is each patient's preferred genre or song. Due to the same patient and environmental variables discussed earlier (Table 8.3), every session varies as it progresses and as the music therapist assesses each situation. See Figure 8.2 for specific protocol information.

Electroencephalogram (EEG). Electroencephalogram (EEG) patients are often required to be sleeping for administration of the test. Pediatric patients receiving this test also experience increased anxiety due to the leads placed on the patient's head to transmit data as well as the other variables mentioned above. Some patients completing this procedure may be given a mild sedative with music therapy services used to lower the amount of sedation needed for the patient to fall asleep. See Figure 8.2 for specific protocol information.

Extubation. Extubation is removal of a ventilator tube from the mouth or nose, which can create great anxiety and agitation in patients. During ventilator assistance, sedation may be reduced daily for a neurologic assessment. This awakening from sedated sleep may be disconcerting to children. There may also be extubation trial periods for weaning of ventilator assistance. Children may be frightened by these processes and resist extubation. The MT-BC is usually enlisted to reduce agitation and anxiety. See Figure 8.2 for specific protocol information.

Burn debridement. Burn debridement is a medical treatment involving daily immersion in sterile solution with scrubbing of burned tissue. It is extremely painful and analgesia may not completely mask the pain. Music can be effective in helping burn patients tolerate this very painful procedure. See Figure 8.2 for specific protocol information.

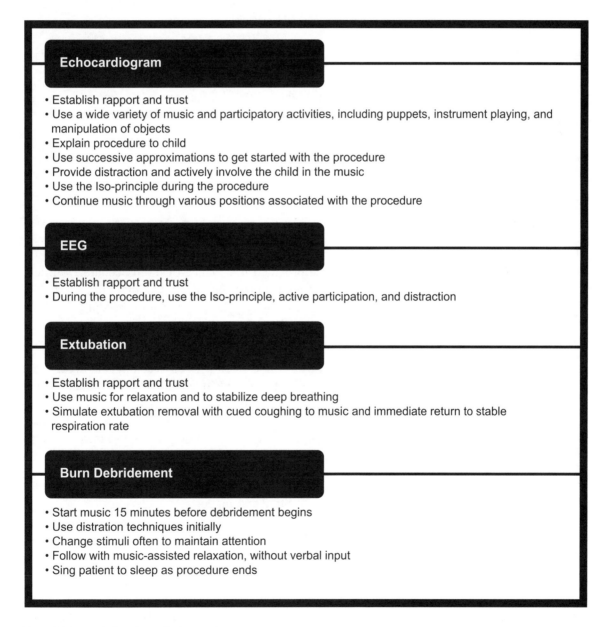

Echocardiogram

- Establish rapport and trust
- Use a wide variety of music and participatory activities, including puppets, instrument playing, and manipulation of objects
- Explain procedure to child
- Use successive approximations to get started with the procedure
- Provide distraction and actively involve the child in the music
- Use the Iso-principle during the procedure
- Continue music through various positions associated with the procedure

EEG

- Establish rapport and trust
- During the procedure, use the Iso-principle, active participation, and distraction

Extubation

- Establish rapport and trust
- Use music for relaxation and to stabilize deep breathing
- Simulate extubation removal with cued coughing to music and immediate return to stable respiration rate

Burn Debridement

- Start music 15 minutes before debridement begins
- Use distraction techniques initially
- Change stimuli often to maintain attention
- Follow with music-assisted relaxation, without verbal input
- Sing patient to sleep as procedure ends

Figure 8.2. Protocols for other pediatric procedures.

In addition to procedural support, music therapy can also be extended to provide pre-procedural support by facilitating procedural education in pediatric patients. For example, Mondarao (2008) used music therapy interventions to improve patient understanding and awareness in patients with Epilepsy. Chetta (1981) effectively used music as part of a preoperative teaching session designed to provide information to pediatric patients about their upcoming surgical procedures. When providing procedural education, there are several factors that must be considered. Jaaniste, Hayes, and von Baeyer (2007) suggest that providers consider the following factors:

- Information presented must be consistent with the child's developmental state. Music therapists should also recognize that children who are anxious may be functioning at a lower cognitive level than they typically would.

- Information presented must be timely and appropriate.

- Information should be accurate and specific. Include what the child will see, hear, smell, taste and feel.

- Information presented must be understandable by the child, clear, and engaging. Language used should be appropriate for the child's cognitive-developmental level.

- Information presented should include procedural aspects (a description of what will happen) as well as sensory aspects (description of what the child will experience).

- Allow children to ask questions or share concerns.

- Provide accompanying illustrations along with procedural education in order to improve understanding.

- Procedural education ideally should be provided in advance of the procedure, with less new information given just before or during the procedure itself. Optimal timing (i.e., just how far in advance) will vary based on the child's age and the type of procedure.

- Children should be prompted to use coping strategies just before or during a procedure.

- Providers should consider using a variety of elements when teaching children about procedures. Possibilities applicable to music therapy include medical play, modeling, and oral or written summaries. All of these elements could be easily incorporated into song writing, music paired with books, or active music engagement. For example, a music therapist and patient could act out a song about a specific procedure or use instruments to provide sound effects for a story about a procedure.

- Individual characteristics like temperament and coping style must also be considered for each child when providing procedural education and support.

Conclusion

Descriptions of existing pediatric music therapy clinical programs and procedures are readily available in existing literature (Cohen, 1984; Froehlich, 1996; Marley, 1984; Robb, 2003; Wolfe & Waldon, 2009). In a new setting, the many possible contributions of music therapy will have to be matched to the hospital's mission and priorities. Then, evidence-based protocols, documentation, and reimbursement codes for each approved service will have to be negotiated with medical personnel, interdisciplinary therapy staff, and the billing office. In some cases, it may be important to demonstrate clinically the procedures being proposed on paper. The benefits of MT are so dramatic that few medical staff, therapists, or parents will fail to be swayed by the effects. In clinical practice, it is important to participate in interdisciplinary team meetings to elicit referrals and to educate other staff about music therapy functions. Outcomes of clinical music therapy should be documented in the medical chart and can provide the data for an annual summary of music therapy benefits to patients and families. A cost/benefit analysis is an effective method for such a summary and can contribute to program expansion since it usually shows great benefit at low cost to the agency. Medical music therapy for pediatric patients facilitates medical assessment and treatment, reduces pain and trauma, and teaches children to cope and cooperate with the distressing reality of modern medicine. It is a growing and important service for children and their families.

References

Abdul-Baqi, K. J. (1991). Chloral hydrate and middle ear pressure. *Journal of Laryngol Otolaryngology, 105*, 421–423.

Aldridge, K. (1993). The use of music to relieve pre-operational anxiety in children attending day surgery. *The Australian Journal of Music Therapy, 4*, 19–35.

American Academy of Pediatrics, & American Academy of Pediatric Dentistry. (2006). Guidelines for monitoring and management of pediatric patients during and after sedation for diagnostic and therapeutic procedures: An update. *Pediatrics, 118,* 2587–2602.

American College of Emergency Physicians. (2013). Moderate (conscious) sedation FAQ. Retrieved from http://www.acep.org/Legislation-and-Advocacy/Practice-Management-Issues/Physician-Payment-Reform/Moderate-(Conscious)-Sedation-FAQ/

Ammon, K .J. (1968). The effects of music on children in respiratory distress. *American Nurses' Association Clinical Sessions*, 127–133.

Arts, S. E., Abu-Saad, H. H., Champion, G. D., Crawford, M. R., Fisher, R. J., Juniper, K. H., & Ziegler, J. B. (1994). Age-related response to Lidocaine-Prilocaine (EMLA) emulsion and effect of music distraction on the pain of intravenous cannulation. *Pediatrics, 93*, 797–801.

Bailey, L. M. (1984). The use of songs in music therapy with cancer patients and their families. *Music Therapy, 4*, 5–17.

Barrera, M. E., Kykov, M. H., & Doyle, S. L. (2002). The effects of interactive music therapy on hospitalized children with cancer: A pilot study. *Psycho-Oncology, 11*, 379–388.

Barrickman, J. (1989). A developmental music therapy approach for preschool hospitalized children. *Music Therapy Perspectives, 7*, 10–16.

Barton, S. (2008). *The effect of music on pediatric anxiety and pain during medical procedures in the main hospital or the emergency department* (Unpublished master's thesis). Florida State University, Tallahassee.

Behrens, G. A. (1982). *The use of music activities to improve the capacity, inhalation, and exhalation capabilities of handicapped children's respiration* (Unpublished master's thesis). Kent State University, Kent, OH.

Biban, P., Baraldi, E., Pettenazzo, A., Filippone, M., & Zacchello, F. (1993). Adverse effect of chloral hydrate in two young children with obstructive sleep apnea. *Pediatrics, 92,* 461–463.

Bradt, J. (2001). *The effects of music entrainment on postoperative pain perception in pediatric patients* (Unpublished doctoral dissertation). Temple University, Philadelphia, PA.

Brodsky, W. (1989). Music therapy as an intervention for children with cancer in isolation rooms. *Music Therapy, 8*, 17–34.

Chetta, H.D. (1981). The effect of music and desensitization on pre-operative anxiety in children. *Journal of Music Therapy, 18*, 74–87.

Claire, J. B., & Erickson, S. (1986). Reducing distress in pediatrics patients undergoing cardiac catheterization. *Children's Health Care, 14*, 146–152.

Clinton, P. K. (1984). *Music as a nursing intervention for children during painful procedures* (Unpublished master's thesis). The University of Iowa, Iowa City.

Cohen, Z. N. (1984). *The development and implementation of a pediatric music therapy program in a short-term medical facility* (Unpublished master's thesis). New York University, New York, NY.

Colwell, C. M., Edwards, R., Hernandez, E., & Brees, K. (2013). Impact of music therapy interventions (listening, composition, Orff-based) on the physiological and psychosocial behaviors of hospitalized children: A feasibility study. *Journal of Pediatric Nursing, 28*, 249–257.

Cote, C. J., Alderfer, R. J., Notterman, D. A., & Fanta, K. B. (1995). Sedation disasters: Adverse drug reports in pediatrics—FDA, USP, and others. *Anesthesiology, 83*(3A), 1183.

Daveson, B. A., & Kennelly, J. (2000). Music therapy in palliative care for hospitalized children and adolescents. *Journal of Palliative Care, 16*, 35–38.

Edwards, J. (1999). Anxiety management in pediatric music therapy. In C. Dileo (Ed.), *Music therapy and medicine: Theoretical and clinical applications* (pp. 69–76). Silver Spring, MD: American Music Therapy Association.

Fagen, T. S. (1982). *Music therapy as a tool for the assessment and treatment of fear and anxiety in pediatric cancer patients* (Unpublished master's thesis). New York University, New York, NY.

Fisher, E. S. (2012). Pediatric hospital medicine: Historical perspectives, inspired future. *Current Problems in Pediatric and Adolescent Health Care, 42*, 107–112.

Fowler-Kerry, S., & Lander, J. R. (1987). Management of injection pain in children. *Pain, 30*, 169–175.

Froehlich, M. R. (1984). A comparison of the effect of music therapy and medical play therapy on the verbalization behavior of pediatric patients. *Journal of Music Therapy, 21*, 2–15.

Froehlich, M. R. (Ed.). (1996). *Music therapy with hospitalized children.* Cherry Hill, NJ: Jeffery Books.

Gettel, M. K. (1985). *The effect of music on anxiety in children undergoing cardiac catheterization* (Unpublished master's thesis). Hahnemann University, Philadelphia, PA.

Ghetti, C. (2012). Music therapy as procedural support for invasive medical procedures: Toward the development of music therapy theory. *Nordic Journal of Music Therapy, 21*, 3–35.

Goforth, K. (2008). *Collaborating goals and interventions to effectively promote psychosocial development of pediatric patients during hospitalization: A survey of music therapists and child life specialists* (Unpublished master's thesis). Florida State University, Tallahassee.

Gooding, L. F. (2012). Music therapy in pediatric oncology treatment: Clinical practice guidelines from the research literature. In L. E. Schraer-Joiner (Ed.), *Proceedings of the 18th International Seminar of the Commission on Music in Special Education, Music Therapy, and Music Medicine.* Nedlands, WA: International Society for Music Education.

Gorman, A. (2013, July 20). Healthcare overhaul leads hospitals to focus on patient satisfaction. *Los Angeles Times.* Retrieved from http://articles.latimes.com/2013/jul/20/local/la-me- patient-satisfaction-20130721

Grasso, M. C., Button, B. M., Allison, D. J., & Sawyer, S. M. (2000). Benefits of music therapy as an adjunct to chest physiotherapy in infants and toddlers with cystic fibrosis. *Pediatric Pulmonology, 29,* 371–381.

Greenberg, S. B., Faerber, E. N., Aspinall, C. L., & Adams, R. C. (1993). High-dose chloral hydrate sedation for children undergoing MR imaging: Safety and efficacy in relation to age. *American Journal of Roentgenology, 161,* 639–641.

Hanamoto, J., & Kajiyama, T. (1974). Some experiences in use of environmental music in pediatric roentgenography. *Radiologia Diagnostica, 15,* 787–794.

Hilliard, R. E. (2003). Music therapy in pediatric palliative care: Complementing the interdisciplinary approach. *Journal of Palliative Care, 19,* 127–132.

Hilliard, R. E. (2006). Music therapy in pediatric oncology: A review of the literature. *Journal of the Society for Integrated Oncology, 4,* 75–78.

Hua, X. (1997). The effects of music in relieving pain for children receiving intramuscular injection. *Journal of Nursing Science, 12,* 135.

Jaaniste, T., Hayes, B., & von Baeyer, C. L. (2007). Providing children with information about forthcoming medical procedures: A review and synthesis. *Clinical Psychology: Science and Practice, 14,* 124-143.

Kaminski, J., & Hall, W. (1996). The effect of soothing music on neonatal behavioral states in the hospital newborn nursery. *Neonatal Network, 15,* 45–54.

Keller, V. E. (1995). Management of nausea and vomiting in children. *Journal of Pediatric Nursing, 10*(5), 280–286.

Kennelly, J. (2000). The specialist role of the music therapist in developmental programs for hospitalized children. *Journal of Pediatric Health Care, 14,* 56–59.

Kennelly, J., & Brien-Elliott, K. (2001). The role of music therapy in paediatric rehabilitation. *Pediatric Rehabilitation, 4,* 137–143.

Kreuger, C., Wall, S., Parker, L., & Nealis, R. (2005). Elevated sound levels within a busy NICU. *Neonatal Network, 24,* 33–37.

Lane, D. L. (1991). *The effect of a single music therapy session on hospitalized children as measured by salivary Immunoglobulin A, speech pause time, and a patient opinion Likert scale* (Unpublished doctoral dissertation). Case Western Reserve University, Cleveland, OH. (UMI No. 9137062)

Larson, K., & Ayllon, T. (1990). The effects of contingent music and differential reinforcement on infantile colic. *Behavior Research and Therapy, 28*, 119–125.

Liebman, S. S., & MacLaren, A. (1991). The effects of music and relaxation on third trimester anxiety in adolescent pregnancy. *Journal of Music Therapy, 28*, 89–100.

Lininger, L.W. (1987). *The effects of instrumental and vocal lullabies on the crying behavior of newborn infants* (Unpublished master's thesis). Southern Methodist University, Dallas, TX.

Loewy, J. (1999). The use of music psychotherapy in the treatment of pediatric pain. In C. Dileo (Ed.), *Music therapy and medicine: Theoretical and clinical applications* (pp. 189–206). Silver Spring, MD: American Music Therapy Association.

Loewy, J. V. (Ed.). (1997). *Music therapy and pediatric pain.* Cherry Hill, NJ: Jeffrey Books.

Lutz, W. G. (1997). *The effect of music distraction on children's pain, fear, and behavior during laceration repairs* (Unpublished master's thesis). The University of Texas at Arlington.

Malone, A. B. (1996). The effects of live music on the distress of pediatric patients receiving intravenous starts, venipunctures, injections, and heel sticks. *Journal of Music Therapy, 33*, 19–33.

Marley, L. S. (1984). The use of music with hospitalized infants and toddlers: A descriptive study. *Journal of Music Therapy, 21*, 126–132.

Mathur, A., Duda, L., & Kamat, D. M. (2008). Knowledge and use of music therapy among pediatric practitioners in Michigan. *Clinical Pediatrics, 47,* 155–159.

McDonnell, L. (1984). Music therapy with trauma patients and their families on a pediatric service. *Music Therapy, 4*, 55–63.

Megel, M. E., Houser, C. W., & Gleaves, L. S. (1998). Children's responses to immunizations: Lullabies as a distraction. *Issues in Comprehensive Pediatric Nursing, 21*, 129–145.

Micci, N. O. (1984). The use of music therapy with pediatric patients undergoing cardiac catheterization. *The Arts in Psychotherapy, 11*, 261–266.

Mondanaro, J. F. (2008). Music therapy in the psychosocial care of pediatric patients with Epilepsy. *Music Therapy Perspectives, 26*, 102-109.

Munoz, M., Gomez, A., Soult, J. A., Marquez, C., Lopez-Castilla, J. D., Cervera, A., et al. (1997). Seizures caused by chloral hydrate sedative doses (letter). *Journal of Pediatrics, 131*(5), 787–788.

Munro, S., & Mount, B. (1978). Music therapy in palliative care. *Canadian Medical Association Journal, 119*, 1029–1034.

National Institute for Health and Care Excellence. (2010). Sedation in children and young people: Sedation for diagnostic and therapeutic procedures in children and young people. Retrieved from http://egap.evidence.nhs.uk/CG112

Noguchi, L. (2006). The effect of music versus nonmusic on behavioural signs of distress and self-report of pain in pediatric injection patients. *Journal of Music Therapy, 43,* 16–38.

O'Callaghan, C., Baron, A., Barry, P., & Dun, B. (2011). Music's relevance for pediatric cancer patients: A constructivist and mosaic research approach. *Supportive Care in Cancer, 19,* 779–788.

Ogenfuss, J. W. (2001). *Pediatric surgery and patient anxiety: Can music therapy effectively reduce stress and anxiety levels while waiting to go to surgery?* (Unpublished master's thesis). Florida State University, Tallahassee.

Owens, L.D. (1979). The effects of music on the weight loss, crying, and physical movement of newborns. *Journal of Music Therapy, 1,* 83–90.

Pate, J., Blount, R., Cohen, L., & Smith, A. (1996). Childhood medical experience and temperament as predictors of adult functioning in medical situations. *Children's Health Care, 25,* 281–298.

Perry, J. N., Hooper, V. D., & Masiongale, J. (2012). Reduction of preoperative anxiety in pediatric surgery patients using age-appropriate teaching interventions. *Journal of PeriAnesthesia Nursing, 27,* 69–81.

Pfaff, V., Smith, K., & Gowan, D. (1989). The effects of music-assisted relaxation on the distress of pediatric cancer patients undergoing bone marrow aspirations. *Children's Health Care, 18,* 232–236.

Polaner, D. M., Houck, C. S., Rockoff, M. A., Mancuso, T. J., Finley, G. A., Maxwell, L. G., et al. (2001). Sedation, risk, and safety: do we really have data at last? *Pediatrics, 108,* 1006–1008.

Rasco, C. (1992). Using music therapy as distraction during lumbar punctures. *Journal of Pediatric Oncology Nursing, 9,* 33–34.

Robb, S. (2003). *Music therapy in pediatric healthcare.* Silver Spring, MD: American Music Therapy Association.

Robb, S. L. (1996). Techniques in song writing: Restoring emotional and physical wellbeing in adolescents who have been traumatically injured. *Music Therapy Perspectives, 14,* 30–37.

Robb, S. L. (2000). The effect of therapeutic music interventions on the behavior of hospitalized children in isolation: Developing a contextual support model of music therapy. *Journal of Music Therapy, 37,* 118–146.

Robb, S. L., & Ebberts, A. G. (2003). Songwriting and digital video production interventions for pediatric patients undergoing bone marrow transplantation part I: An analysis of depression and anxiety levels according to phase of treatment. *Journal of Pediatric Oncology Nursing, 20,* 1–14.

Robb, S. L., Nichols, R. J., Rutan, R. L., Bishop, B. L., & Parker, J. C. (1995). The effects of music assisted relaxation on preoperative anxiety. *Journal of Music Therapy, 32,* 2–21.

Rudenberg, M. T., & Royka, A. M. (1989). Promoting psychosocial adjustment in pediatric burn patients through music therapy and child life therapy. *Music Therapy Perspectives, 7,* 40–43.

Scheve, A. M. (2002). *The effect of music therapy intervention on pre-operative anxiety of pediatric patients as measured by self-report* (Unpublished master's thesis). Florida State University, Tallahassee.

Schieffelin, C. (1988, April). *A case study: Stevens-Johnson Syndrome.* Paper presented at the Annual Conference of the Southeastern Conference of the National Association for Music Therapy, Tallahassee, FL.

Schneider, F. A. (1982). *Assessment and evaluation of audio-analgesic effects on the pain experience of acutely burned children during dressing changes* (Unpublished doctoral dissertation). University of Cincinnati, Cincinnati, OH.

Schur, J. M. (1986). *Alleviating behavioral distress with music or Lamaze pant-blow breathing in children undergoing bone marrow aspirations and lumbar punctures* (Unpublished doctoral dissertation). The University of Texas Health Science Center at Dallas.

Shulman, L., Kathirithamby, D. R., Rosenberg, M. D., & Stern, E. L. (2009). Pediatric rehabilitation. In T. K. McInerny (Ed.) *American Academy of Pediatrics textbook of pediatric care.* Washington, DC: American Academy of Pediatrics.

Siegel, S. L. (1983). *The use of music as treatment in pain perception with post-surgical patients in a pediatric setting* (Unpublished master's thesis). University of Miami, Coral Gables, FL.

Sifton, D. W. (Ed.). (1998). *PDR® Generics™.* Montvale, NJ: Medical Economics.

Sing, K., Erickson, T., Amitai, Y., & Hryhorczuk, D. (1996). Chloral hydrate toxicity from oral and intravenous administration. *Clinical Toxicology, 34,* 101–106.

Slivka, H. H., & Magill, L. (1986). The conjoint use of social work and music therapy in working with children of cancer patients, *Music Therapy, 6A*(1), 30–40.

Standley, J., & Whipple, J. (2003). Music therapy with pediatric patients: A meta-analysis. In S. L. Robb (Ed.), *Music therapy in pediatric healthcare research and evidence-based practice* (pp. 1–18). Silver Spring, MD: American Music Therapy Association.

Standley, J. M. (1986). Music research in medical/dental treatment: Meta-analysis and clinical applications. *Journal of Music Therapy, 23,* 56-122.

Standley, J. M. (2000). Music research in medical treatment. In AMTA (Ed.), *Effectiveness of music therapy procedures: Documentation of research and clinical practice* (3rd ed., pp. 1–64). Silver Spring, MD: American Music Therapy Association.

Standley, J. M., & Hanser, S. B. (1995). Music therapy research and applications in pediatric oncology treatment. *Journal of Pediatric Oncology Nursing, 12,* 3–8.

Steinke, W. R. (1991). The use of music, relaxation, and imagery in the management of postsurgical pain for scoliosis. In C. Maranto (Ed.), *Applications of music in medicine* (pp. 141–162). Washington, DC: National Association for Music Therapy.

Stouffer, J. W., Shirk, B. J., & Polomano, R. C. (2007). Practice guidelines for music interventions with hospitalized pediatric patients. *Journal of Pediatric Nursing, 22,* 448–456.

Swedberg, O., & Standley, J. (2011). The effects of medical music therapy on patient satisfaction as measured by the Press Ganey Inpatient Survey. *Music Therapy Perspectives, 29,* 149–156.

Tabinowski, K. (2013*). A survey of current music therapy practices in pediatric hospitals and units* (Unpublished master's thesis). Florida State University, Tallahassee.

Wade, L. M. (2002). A comparison of the effects of vocal exercises/singing versus music- assisted relaxation on peak expiratory flow rates of children with asthma. *Music Therapy Perspectives, 20,* 31–37.

Walworth, D. D. (2005). Procedural-support music therapy in the healthcare setting: A cost-effectiveness analysis. *Journal of Pediatric Nursing, 20,* 276–284.

Whipple, J. (2000). The effect of parent training in music and multimodal stimulation on parent-neonate interactions in the Neonatal Intensive Care Unit. *Journal of Music Therapy, 37,* 250–268.

Whitehead-Pleaux, A., Baryza, M., & Sheridan, R. (2006). The effects of music therapy on pediatric patients' pain and anxiety during donor site dressing changes. *Journal of Music Therapy, 43,* 136–153.

Wolfe, D., & Waldon, E. (2009). *Music therapy and pediatric medicine.* Silver Spring, MD: American Music Therapy Association.

Yinger, O. S. (2012). *Music therapy as procedural support for young children undergoing immunizations: A randomized controlled study* (Unpublished doctoral dissertation). Florida State University, Tallahassee.

Chapter 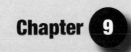 9

Adult Medical/Surgical Music Therapy

Miriam Hillmer, MM, MT-BC

Picture the following situation. The setting is the intensive care unit of a hospital and patient rounds are taking place. The doctor is reporting on a patient who recently suffered a traumatic brain injury. When reporting on the patient's current status, it is mentioned that the patient is agitated and anxious as evidenced by the restless movement and pulling at tubes. The physician looks over at the music therapist in the group and says, "Music therapy?" A referral has just been made, and the patient will be evaluated and treated by the music therapist later that day.

Hospitalizations are on the rise, increasing by 11% between 2000 and 2010 (Hall, Levant, & DeFrances, 2013). Consider these numbers: 35.1 million hospital discharges annually, and 51.4 million procedures performed each year. The average length of stay in the hospital is 4.8 days (Centers for Disease Control and Prevention, 2013). These numbers translate into hundreds of millions of minutes spent in the hospital each year. This is generally an extremely stressful event both for patients and families. Music therapy offers support in (a) coping with these situations, (b) managing symptoms, (c) assisting with recovery, and (d) improving overall perceptions.

While the music therapy profession has been around for over 60 years, it has only become more prominent in the health care setting in the last 20 years. With its ability to address (a) cognitive, (b) physical, (c) emotional, and (d) physiological needs, music therapy has been shown to be effective in addressing a number of goal areas. Recently, insurance reimbursement has become dependent partly on patient satisfaction scores. Music therapy has been shown to improve patient perceptions of their hospital experience (Yinger & Standley, 2011). This information, along with the plethora of research, supports the benefit of the music therapy profession in the health care setting and has aided its increasing prominence in hospitals throughout the country. Table 9.1 highlights common medical music therapy goals and interventions.

Table 9.1. Medical Music Therapy Goals and Interventions			
Music Therapy Goals	**Research Study**	**Evidence-Based Interventions**	**Reseach Study**
Pain	Gutgsell et al., 2012; Li & Dong, 2012	Guided relaxation	Gutgsell et al., 2012
Anxiety/agitation	Davis & Jones, 2012; Singh, Rao, Prem, Sahoo, & Keshav, 2009; Walworth, 2010	Iso-principle	Lee, 2005
Mood	Ghetti, 2011; Zhou, Li, Yan, Dang, & Wang, 2011	Active music making	Ghetti, 2011
Physiological outcomes	Bradt, Dileo, & Grocke, 2010	Singing	Kim, 2010
		Contingent music	Lancioni et al, 2010
		Distraction	Clark et al., 2006; Walworth, 2010
		Song-writing	Nguyen, 2003
		Lyric analysis	Jones, 2005

Reasons for Referral

The hospital environment is fast paced: patients constantly being admitted and discharged, staff providing care, and procedures being done. Patients are dealing with a myriad of issues affecting them physically and emotionally. Families are trying to support their loved ones while dealing with logistical concerns. In the midst of all of this sometimes organized chaos, music therapy can be a comforting and effective presence. Because of the ever-changing nature of the hospital environment, it is often difficult to plan treatment prior to sessions. Music therapists need to address the most immediate need of the patient at the moment. This may or may not be the same need from one session to another and will be dependent on the patient's current physical and mental state, as well as cultural and family dynamics. The therapist determines this goal by (a) asking questions of staff, patients, and family; (b) observation of physiological and behavior clues; and (c) observation of other clues in the environment. It may be helpful to think of this approach to treatment in the mentality of crisis intervention. In crisis intervention therapy, short-term strategies both during and immediately following an event are used to address a person's physical, mental, emotional, and behavioral responses (American Red Cross, 1992). A hospitalization and subsequent treatment is a crisis situation for many patients and families. Therefore, music therapy treatment needs to address the patient's current need, whether it is physical, mental, emotional, or behavioral, and to focus on short-term strategies to help the patient cope with the event.

Pain

It is a fair assumption that individuals in the hospital are experiencing some level of pain. This level will vary depending on the patient and the situation. In the hospital setting, patients typically rate their pain on a scale of 1 to 10: 1 being little pain and 10 being extreme pain. For patients experiencing higher levels of pain, either acute or chronic, it is not uncommon for a music therapy referral to address this. Music therapy can help to ease pain perception as well as address some causes of pain. When determining patient goals for music therapy, one of the first questions asked should be, "Are you experiencing any pain?" and, if so, "Rate this pain on a scale of 1 to 10." If the patient gives a high pain score, this is the immediate need that should be addressed. Expected outcomes of music therapy interventions to address pain include a decrease in reported pain level and/or decrease in level of medication required to manage pain.

Anxiety or Agitation

Symptoms of anxiety or agitation are not uncommon but can manifest for different reasons and present in a myriad of ways. Anxiety may stem from anticipation over a future event, such as an upcoming procedure, test, or diagnosis. Anxious patients generally (a) ask a lot of questions, (b) have difficulty concentrating, (c) are irritable, or (d) experience several of the physical symptoms listed in Table 9.2. Increased anxiety levels are common for patients on ventilator assistance and can lead to an inability to wean off this device or other negative outcomes (Davis & Jones, 2012). Confusion caused by medication or a co-morbid health condition can also lead a patient to present as anxious. In these instances, patients may try to get out of bed, pull out IV lines, or yell at family and staff. Finally, a patient might have a clinical anxiety disorder diagnosis which is not being well controlled.

Music therapy to address anxiety and agitation can provide distraction from (a) anxious feelings, (b) physical manifestations, or (c) confusion. Common outcomes include (a) elevated mood, (b) decrease in irritability, (c) relaxation of the patient, and (d) decrease in undesired behavior from the patient. The following scenario provides a clinical example of music therapy to reduce agitation in a patient at Tallahassee Memorial HealthCare (TMH):

- Patient was constantly anxious and agitated when not medicated.

- Shift documentation on the patient consistently reported yelling and defiant behavior from the patient stemming from confusion.

- During music therapy, the patient was calm.

- The physician ordered music therapy as often as possible, as this was one of the few interventions to have a positive effect on the patient's behavior.

Table 9.2. Physical and Emotional Manifestations of Anxiety	
Physical Manifestations of Anxiety (Andrews et al., 2010)	**Emotional Manifestations of Anxiety (Andrews et al., 2010)**
Nausea	Trouble concentrating
Diarrhea	Feeling tense or jumpy
Shortness of breath	Irritability
Muscle tension	Restlessness
Headaches	
Fatigue	
Insomnia	

Stimulation

Stimulation is a broad term that can encompass a variety of situations and stimulation types. There are many types of stimulation that can be provided: (a) auditory, (b) tactile, (c) visual, and (d) cognitive. *Auditory stimulation* refers to sound (including music), *tactile stimulation* deals with the sense of touch, *visual stimulation* occurs when information is taken in through the eyes, and *cognitive stimulation* is an awareness of one's surroundings. The type of stimulation, the amount required, and how it is presented depends on the medical situation and needs of the patient. On one extreme, patients in a coma or coming out a coma are referred for music therapy as they have received little positive stimulation or structured stimulation. Music strategically layered in and paired with other forms of stimulation can lead to patients opening their eyes, following commands, or moving limbs, sometimes for the first time since being in a coma. Slightly different is a referral for music therapy for tolerance to stimulation. In this instance, the patient is prone to sensory overload, so careful stimulation, again layered in, is provided to build patient tolerance.

Finally, referrals are made to provide cognitive stimulation for patients. Commonly, patients receive little interaction or stimulation other than the television in their room but are perfectly alert and interactive. For instance, at TMH, a referral was made for a long-term patient who had cognitive deficits, had little family support, and was receiving no other therapies due to lack of progress. This individual sat in the hospital room with the television and an occasional staff member entering. Music therapy was able to provide appropriate stimulation and address the patient's awareness of the situation and surroundings.

Mood/Depression

A traumatic event, such as a hospitalization, or a prolonged medical stay can trigger signs of depression or decreased mood. This, in turn, can affect the patient's health outcomes and length of recovery. While any patient is at risk, certain medical conditions are more likely to trigger symptoms of depression. These conditions include (a) heart disease, (b) stroke, (c) diabetes, (d) cancer, and (e) Parkinson's disease (Patten et al., 2005). Signs that a patient might exhibit include (a) flat affect, (b) lack of engagement, (c) decreased appetite, (d) trouble sleeping, (e) excessive sleeping, (f) crying spells, (g) agitation or irritability, and (h) trouble concentrating. Symptoms can be short-term for some individuals, related specifically to hospitalization, or can be a continuation or trigger for a long-term event. Patients exhibiting any signs of depression are good candidates for a music therapy referral, as a music therapist can address all symptoms with carefully tailored interventions. Outcomes with music therapy can include a positive change in affect, increased engagement, focus of attention, and increased relaxation.

Coping Skills

All patients admitted to the hospital are faced with a vast array of issues that they are forced to confront. At the very minimum, a patient is faced with (a) a serious medical problem, (b) new financial concerns, (c) unfamiliar environment, (d) loss of privacy, and (e) disruption of regular patterns. The vast majority of people also deal with additional concerns like family issues or a loss of some sort. Many individuals are able to handle these issues surrounding a hospitalization with little to no problem. Others need support to assist with lessening the burden and to help them process these new issues. Several staff members within the hospital organization are there to assist, including music therapists. Social workers assist with finding community resources and assistance; physicians and nurses attend to the medical needs; physical, occupational, and speech therapists address the physical deficits; and music therapists address the emotional needs. Music therapy sessions can assist the patient in understanding and processing feelings related to:

- a loss of some type—This can be another family member/friend, functionality due to injury, or other perceived personal loss;

- family dynamics—Assistance may be needed in dealing with both supportive or neglectful families;

- a new diagnosis, or coming to terms with a medical condition;

- a long hospitalization;

- financial concerns;

- unrealistic expectations; and

- dealing with staff.

With assistance, patients can express feelings and frustrations, determine questions they have, and develop strategies for moving forward.

Communication

One of the wonderful things about music therapy is that not only is it effective in addressing physiological or psychosocial needs, but it also assists in rehabilitation. Patients who have had a stroke, traumatic brain injury, or other neurological condition may exhibit a deficit in communication. This can manifest in (a) slurred speech, (b) difficulty in word-finding, (c) inability to process incoming language, or (d) trouble coordinating motor functioning (Wong, 2004). Music has the ability to be processed in many areas of the brain (Wong, 2004) and therefore can assist with creating new pathways for information to be processed and transmitted. Therapeutic interventions can lead to improved speech production, strength, word-finding, and motor coordination. Occasionally, music is the first intervention to produce noticeable results following an injury. One such example occurred with a patient at TMH who had recently suffered a debilitating stroke. Upon entering the room, the music therapist quickly determined that the patient was not able to verbally communicate or move various parts of the body. Family members helped identify the patient's preferred music and the therapist started to play a favorite song. The patient almost immediately started to tap a finger. Then the patient started to hum along and, by the conclusion of the session, was making sounds similar to words at the end of the song phrases. The patient had made the first step in the rehabilitation process, which brought an immense sense of hope to both the patient and family.

Motor Deficits

The ability to move about normally can be impaired with a neurological condition or injury. This can be exhibited in a decrease in (a) muscle tone, (b) rigidity, (c) loss of feeling, (d) lack of positioning awareness, (e) decrease in balance, or (f) impaired gait (Wong, 2004). Depending on the severity and location of the damage to the brain, the deficit may affect a portion of the individual's body, a specific side, or a particular extremity. A patient may be able to recover all functionality or only a portion. Regardless, rehabilitation is vitally important, and the sooner it begins following the injury, the better. Music therapy can be effective in administration of or assistance in rehabilitation. The music is motivating and guides the rehabilitation process. Expected outcomes include improved coordination, range of motion, balance, gait, and strength.

Reality Orientation

Hospitalization can cause disorientation in an individual, in certain cases. A person may suddenly become confused or delirious, or have trouble focusing. This can be frightening for the patient and family, can extend the hospital stay, and can lead to poor treatment outcomes. For patients over 65, confusion is the most common complication associated with hospitalization and can affect up to 80% of individuals in the ICU (Harvard Women's Health Watch, 2011). Causes of confusion can include (a) medication, (b) shift in diet, (c) infection, or (d) unfamiliar environment (Harvard Women's Health Watch, 2011). Music therapy is often referred to assist in decreasing patient confusion and help with reality orientation. Frequently, music therapy can offer a much needed reprise for staff members, as patients who are confused often require constant supervision. The music therapist can not only distract the patient for a period of time, but can also put the patient in a state where confusion-related behaviors, such as wandering or agitation, are less present.

Respiratory Issues

Breath is essential to life. When a person has difficulty in this area, it is a serious problem and the cause of much fear and anxiety. Individuals who are unable to breathe on their own are placed on a ventilator, a machine that pushes air into the lungs at periodic intervals. A tube is place in the individual's mouth and down into the lungs. Because this is extremely uncomfortable, patients are often sedated to some extent to minimize discomfort. Long-term side effects of sedation include (a) nausea, (b) respiratory depression, (c) mental status change, (d) delirium, and (e) central nervous system changes. Other side effects of long-term ventilation can include psychological stress and tissue or organ injury. It is a primary goal to wean the patient off of mechanical ventilation as soon as possible. However, the extubation process (removal of the tube) can be a cause of anxiety and fear for patients for various reasons, including unknown expectations or fear of failure. Music therapy interventions for individuals on mechanical ventilation have been shown to decrease anxiety and positively affect physiological outcomes (Bradt et al., 2010). Music can also be effective in addressing respiratory distress for individuals not on ventilators. Feeling short of breath does not always require drastic measures, but can be scary as one feels unable to breathe normally. In these instances, music therapy can help regulate breathing patterns and calm patients.

Relaxation

This is a common goal or reason for referral for patients in the hospital. Assisting an individual in relaxation can have positive effects on (a) perception of pain, (b) anxiety, (c) physiological outcomes, (d) insomnia, (e) tension, (f) nausea, and (g) fatigue.

Physiological Outcomes

Common physiological outcomes measured for individuals in the hospital include (a) blood pressure, (c) heart rate, (d) respiratory rate, and (e) oxygen saturation levels. These indicators can tell a lot about the patient condition, and patients in serious condition are heavily monitored. The goal is for physiological indicators to be within normal limits. Results outside of normal limits can lead to complications for the patient. For instance, high blood pressure can put an individual at higher risk for a stroke, heart problems, or kidney problems (National Heart, Lung, and Blood Institute, 2012). It is important to also understand that physiological measures can be in direct correlation to how the patient is currently feeling. A patient's increased heart rate can be an indication of anxiety, distress, or discomfort. Music therapy can have a positive effect on physiological outcomes. In fact, a review of studies using music therapy with patients on mechanical ventilation consistently showed a positive effect on physiological outcomes, including heart rate, respiratory rate, and blood pressure (Davis & Jones, 2012). This result is consistent across a myriad of research studies examining the use of music with a variety of conditions (Bradt et al., 2010; Standley, 2000). Therefore, music therapy may be referred to help patients improve physiological functioning.

Procedures

It is safe to assume that if individuals are admitted to the hospital, they will undergo a procedure of some type during their stay. Some of these procedures will be minor, and some will be major. Depending on the type, duration, and intensity of the procedure, it can evoke feelings of anxiety, agitation, or be painful. For those patients with a strong negative response to undergoing a procedure, music therapy can be an effective non-pharmacological option. Common hospital procedures that music therapy can assist with are listed in Table 9.3. In all procedures, the common goal for music therapy is to reduce patient anxiety and provide distraction from unpleasant stimuli.

\multicolumn{2}{c}{**Table 9.3. Common Hospital Procedures**}	
Procedure	**Description**
Bone-marrow biopsy	A bone-marrow biopsy is an extremely painful procedure in which a portion of bone marrow is extracted from the patient. Patients are given only a local anesthetic that is often insufficient at masking the pain.
Dialysis	Dialysis is a procedure that a patient must complete 2 to 3 times a week, taking 3 to 4 hours each time. It is required for patients with kidney damage. During the procedure the patient's blood is filtered out of the body and then returned. It often leaves the patient very tired and weak. Patients are required to remain still for the entire procedure. Music therapy can be helpful especially toward the middle to end of the procedure to provide a positive distraction or relaxation for the patient.
IV starts	An IV administers medication or saline solution to the patient over an extended period of time. Administration of this line can be painful and anxiety producing for patients.
Nerve block	A slow drip of numbing medication is administered close to the nerve in the leg to numb the top of the knee following surgery in this area. Administration is typically done in the post-operative care room by the anesthesiologist.
Ventilator	The patient is on a machine that regulates breathing. A tube is placed in the mouth and goes down into the lungs. Some patients experience anxiety when taken off this machine as they fear they will not be able to breathe on their own. If they are too anxious they are at greater risk of having to be placed back on the ventilator. In addition to reducing anxiety before, during, and after the procedure, music therapy can help regulate breathing following extubation.
Wound care	Dressing changes and cleaning of wounds is common throughout the hospital. For more severe wounds this can be a major event causing pain and anxiety.
X-ray	An X-ray machine uses radiation to produce a picture of internal portions of the body (i.e., bones). This test can be administered in patient rooms. It may require repositioning of patients to obtain a good picture and this can be painful in certain circumstances.

Providing Family Support

Patients of all ages may be attended to by their family members. Family involvement can range from families that are mostly absent to those that are overbearing. Sometimes the family is more aware of the patient condition than the patient, sometimes they are charged with decision making, and sometimes they are kept out of the loop. Regardless of the situation, family members are affected by having their loved one being in the hospital and may benefit from support of staff. Music therapy can be a source of this support by addressing the specific need of the family and helping them to cope with the tough situation. Common areas of need for families are found in Table 9.4.

Table 9.4. Common Areas of Need for Families	
Area of Need	**Description**
Unfulfilled expectations	A patient is admitted to the hospital for an elective procedure such as a joint replacement and ends up in the intensive care unit. A procedure that is supposed to be routine ends with an unpredictable result. Support is needed to help adjust to the reality of the situation and feelings of loss.
Traumatic event	A patient is involved in a severe car accident and sustains multiple injuries; the level of recovery is unknown. This is an event that no one can plan for and everyone dreads. Support focuses on helping the family come to terms with the situation and manage stress.
End of life	Death is a natural part of life, but this does not make the death of a loved one easier to handle. It can be even more difficult if family members make the decision to take a loved one off life support. Families benefit from support to cope with their loss and from opportunities for reminiscence of their loved one.
Family dynamics	Each family brings with them a different dynamic. Family dynamics can range from having family members get along well to those who fight with each other. Sometimes support is required to help mediate challenging family dynamics. During one consult at TMH, the music therapist was called to offer support during a terminal extubation. The family involved a wife, the children, and a mistress. The tension in the room was palpable, but the music therapist was able to help focus all parties toward what was needed for the patient at the time.

Evidence-Based Techniques

Music therapists use a variety of techniques and interventions to address the needs of patients in the hospital. These techniques are based on (a) theory and understanding of musical principles, (b) brain mechanisms and behavior, (c) anatomy and physiology, and (d) human preferences and behavior. Research testing the validity of these techniques offers guidance as to the most effective methods of intervention. This is helpful in understanding how to therapeutically approach a patient in a particular situation. However, it is important to keep an open mind in treatment as not everyone responds to even the most well researched techniques in the same manner. Several techniques described below can be effective in addressing a number of different goals, and some goals have a variety of research-based techniques that are effective. It is the job of the music therapist to determine the correct course of treatment based on the individual needs of the patient.

Patient-Preferred Music

Before delving too deep into specific evidence-based techniques, it is important to discuss the use of patient-preferred music in therapeutic interventions. This is the foundation of most music therapy interventions. Research has demonstrated repeatedly that preferred music selected by the patient has the greatest effect (Standley, 2000). For patients who are able to indicate a preference, this can easily be determined. It becomes more difficult when a patient has trouble with communication, is not in reality, or is sedated in some way. In these instances, family or cues in the room (CDs, a Bible, pictures, etc.) can be helpful in deducing music preference. Finally, research has determined that music popular when the patient was in their twenties is most beneficial (Gibbons, 1977). Sometimes the music preference of the patient is not by a well-known artist or a particular type of music. This was observed with a patient in the intensive care unit of TMH. The patient had suffered a severe head injury and had significant cognitive deficits. The first session was conducted using music in the same genre of the patient's preferred band. Before the next session, the music therapist learned a preferred song specifically for the patient. The difference in response from the patient was noticeable. The patient, who was working on verbal communication, sang along with several of the lyrics. The patient was clearly pleased that the song was learned and the therapeutic objective was more easily met.

Music-Assisted Relaxation

For goals such as anxiety or pain, guided relaxation can be an effective intervention. The basic premise of this technique is to guide the patient into a state of relaxation through a combination of (a) verbal suggestions, (b) deep breathing, (c) imagery, and (d) music. Often the therapist will use a "script" of some kind as a guide for the structure of the relaxation. However, this is not necessary for seasoned therapists. Under the umbrella of guided relaxation, there are several approaches that have been found effective: (a) progressive muscle, (b) autogenic, (c) deep breathing, and (d) imagery (a favorite or safe place). Each approach centers on a different aspect, but all guide the patient to concentrate on something specific with the intent of focusing the mind to elicit relaxation. A high cognitive ability is important in this therapeutic technique, as is requires the patient to process information and focus attention.

Music plays an integral part in the guided relaxation. First, it sets the tone for the exercise. Typically, a soothing progression or melody is provided on an instrument of the therapist's choice (though recorded music can also be used). Second, the music assists in supporting different cues for the patient. For instance, a shift from musical tension to release may occur when guiding the patient to exhale the breath. At times, auxiliary instruments are used to further set a soothing tone or augment the mood of the relaxation: ocean drum, steady drum beat, rainstick, bells, etc. A research study conducted with palliative care patients found that just one autogenic relaxation session was effective in lowering pain levels (Gutgsell et al., 2012). Similar positive results, supporting the effectiveness of relaxation in lowering pain and/or anxiety, are found in other studies (Adams, 2005; Good, Anderson, Stanton-Hicks, Gras, & Makii, 2002). At TMH, music-assisted relaxation is used frequently to address pain and anxiety for patients following surgery and undergoing chemotherapy. For more information on music parameters proven to be relaxing, see "Using Music in Perioperative Care" by Gooding, Swezey, and Zwischenberger (2012).

Iso-principle

The music therapy technique of the *iso-principle* is based on the idea of entrainment, the synchronization of two or more independent rhythmic processes. It was first discovered by Christian Huygens in 1665 when he noticed that the pendulum of all clocks in his workshop fell into synchronization, even if he deliberately started them separately (Clayton, Sager, & Will, 2004). This led to the idea of musical entrainment, described by Lee (2005) as the "process of connecting together the feelings conveyed through the music and feeling a sense of commonality with it." The use of music entrainment was first noted in 1948 when a psychiatrist found that matching music to a person's mood and then later shifting the mood of the music altered the individual's state of depression or anxiety (Lee, 2005). People naturally do this in everyday life. It is not uncommon that at the end of a stressful day or when angry, a person will play fast music at a very loud volume. This is a musical illustration of the person's current mood. As the person starts to calm, the music selected will naturally shift to reflect a calmer nature.

As a therapeutic technique, the iso-principle is the use of musical elements, such as tempo and dynamics, to match a patient's pain level or mood, and then a shift of these elements in the desired direction to effect a desired change. This technique has consistently been found to be effective in positively altering a patient's mood and/or pain level (Lee, 2005). In the medical setting, the iso-principle is frequently used. Throughout this process, the therapist constantly assesses behavioral changes in the patient and adjusts accordingly, matching the patient's current state both in verbal and musical interactions. For goals concerning pain, anxiety, mood, and stimulation, the iso-principle is a primary therapeutic technique during the session. When the goal is to reduce pain or anxiety, the dynamics of the music typically start at a higher level and gradually decrease in volume during the session. For individuals in a depressed state or those who require stimulation, the music starts at a lower dynamic level and gradually increases.

Contingent Music

The use of music as a contingency can be an effective intervention for certain situations in the medical setting. The basic premise for this technique is that music serves as a reward following a desired behavior. It should be noted that this is not appropriate in some situations and care needs to be taken when working with adults to make sure it is not presented or perceived as demeaning. For patients who may be confused and/or anxious and consequently act in an undesired way (i.e., pulling on tubes, getting out of bed/chair), contingent music may be effective. Care should be taken that the patient is able to process the condition being presented. At TMH, one patient had a habit of trying to get up and wander, but was not safe walking. This patient thoroughly enjoyed music therapy services. During one session when the patient began to stand up, the therapist indicated the patient needed to sit down for the music to continue. The patient stopped midway, stated "I do not like your terms but accept them," and sat back down.

For patients in a semiconscious or coma state due to injury, contingent music can be effective in eliciting a response from patients. Several studies have found that music used as a reward for responses such as eye movement, lip movement, or hand movement has increased the instances of these responses in patients (Lancioni et al., 2009a, 2009b, 2010). A meta-analysis by Standley (1996) discovered that the use of contingent music in physical rehabilitation had an effect size over five standard deviations greater than control/baseline conditions ($ES = 5.47$) and in medical health the effect size was over two standard deviations greater ($ES = 2.26$).

Active Music Making

In certain cases, patients in the hospital are encouraged or instructed to actively participate in music making. This can be through singing (discussed in another section) or instrument playing. This intervention is effective for a variety of goals that address (a) anxiety, (b) depression, (c) confusion, (d) stress management, (e) movement, and (f) pain. Research has found that playing a musical instrument can affect parts of the human stress response at a genomic level (Bittman et al., 2005). Thus, for patients struggling to cope or who are anxious, active music making assists with stress management, which can affect health outcomes. In addition, active participation requires direct focus from the participant and therefore can distract from unpleasant stimuli or emotions. While active music making has positive effects on stress and mood, it also assists with pain perception. Ghetti (2011) found that for patients who had had liver and kidney transplants, active music making significantly decreased pain levels and negative affect. Instrument playing to work on physical rehabilitation goals is a great option for patients as well. For instance, for a stroke patient whose rehab goals include crossing midline, an instrument is placed past midline as a reference point for the patient. The act itself of hitting the instrument is motivating and a rewarding form of exercise. In addition, the rhythm and other musical properties assist in structuring the movement for greater consistency (Thaut, 2005).

Singing

Engaging patients in the physical act of singing is a great intervention for a wide array of deficits and goals. Singing has a direct positive impact on levels of neurotransmitters in the brain, specifically those associated with pleasure and the immune system (Grape, Sandgren, Hansson,

Ericson, & Theorell, 2003; Kreutz, Bondgard, Rohrmann, Hodapp, & Grebe, 2004). Therefore, participation in singing preferred music elevates patient mood as well as helps the body fight disease. For patients who have suffered a brain injury of some type (stroke, traumatic brain injury), singing can be the gateway to improved communication and cognitive functioning. One symptom often associated with brain injury is an inability to focus. One goal of a music therapy intervention may be to engage the patient in singing to focus his or her attention for the 2 to 3 minute duration of the song. This can be quite an accomplishment for many patients.

Techniques such as having the patient "fill in the blank" or sing the ends of familiar song phrases are other methods of promoting focus of attention. The patient has to attune to what is happening to accurately fill in the correct word. This technique is also effective in achieving goals of word-finding for individuals suffering from aphasia. Singing the correct word may be the first time the patient has successfully communicated since an injury. This can be a wonderful motivation for the patient and can greatly increase self-esteem. Vocal exercises are another intervention for patients with communication deficits. Kim (2010) found that vocal exercises for patients with dysphagia improved respiration, pitch, and speech control. The music is consistent and predictable and therefore helps improve breath control and timing of speech. Finally, more specialized interventions such as Melodic Intonation Therapy (MIT) are effective in improving functional speech for patients with specific forms of aphasia (Schlaug, Marchina, & Norton, 2005). MIT uses rhythm and melodic patterns of speech to transition from singing to speech.

Distraction

Music can be a powerful method of distraction for patients who are anxious, confused, or undergoing procedures. The positive stimuli can shift the patient's attention away from the negative stimuli, thus altering the patient's perceptions in a positive manner. Music therapy interventions to distract pediatric patients during procedures have been used for several years in the hospital setting and have been shown to produce cost-saving results (Walworth, 2005). In recent years, research has started to focus on the benefit of music as distraction for adult patients. In a study with patients undergoing MRI procedures, Walworth (2010) found that live patient-preferred music piped into the MRI tube during the procedure resulted in significantly better perception of the procedure, fewer repeated scans due to movement, and fewer requests for breaks. A separate study looked at the use of live music therapy as distraction for patients undergoing ventilator weaning trials (Hunter et al., 2010). Results indicated that the music intervention was effective in decreasing patient heart and respiratory rates. While live music is most often preferred, in some instances recorded music is the more feasible option due to the nature of the situation. Clark et al. (2006) used recorded music self-selected by patients as a means of distraction during radiation therapy. Patients reported less anxiety and treatment-related distress with the use of music during treatment. Anecdotally, at TMH, music therapy was requested to assist during a bone marrow biopsy. This is an extremely painful procedure in which a needle is inserted down into the bone and marrow is extracted. It is a short procedure with the patient given only local anesthetic. The music therapist used the music as a means of distraction for the patient during the procedure. The therapist met with the patient prior to the procedure and allowed the patient to choose what music would be provided. While pain was not eliminated, music appeared to positively impact the patient's anxiety and perception of the procedure as evidenced by patient comments. At the end of the procedure, the patient hugged the music therapist and thanked her for the music.

Song Writing

One means of involving patients in the therapeutic process is through song writing. This can be done in a variety of ways and can address a myriad of goals. The more structured forms of song writing require the patient to contribute certain words or phrases to already written material. For patients more reluctant about song writing, it can start in a more "Mad Libs" style to engage patients and introduce them slowly in a non-threatening manner. "Piggy-backing" off of a familiar song is another common form of song writing. The familiar melody is used and all or a portion of the words are changed to create the song. Finally, an original melody can be created for patients willing or interested in this option. For all levels of writing, the end product often has a positive impact on patient self-esteem and feelings of accomplishment. Song writing can be done in both a group and individual setting. If a song is written in a group situation, it can be an effective means for promoting social interaction and group cohesion. In both group and individual settings, it is a great outlet for emotional expression. The goals addressed with song writing include improving coping skills, elevation of mood, recognition and expression of feelings, and problem solving. Nguyen (2003) used song writing to create "life celebration" songs with patients on end-of-life care in the hospital setting. Participation in this intervention had a positive impact on patient anxiety. Songs written in this manner are great legacies for patients to leave for family and friends. At TMH, song writing has been used with patients in later stages of recovery from a brain injury. In one situation, song lyrics were changed to a familiar Jimmy Buffet song (the patient's favorite artist). The therapist asked the patient questions relating to the patient's current situation, feelings about the situation, and means of support. The song was a good evaluation of the patient's cognitive skills and insight at the time. In some ways, the patient was aware of the situation and in some ways demonstrated a deficit in insight into the patient's current abilities. Regardless, the patient was extremely proud of the song and viewed the song writing intervention as a great exercise, resulting in a tangible product the patient could share.

Lyric Analysis

One intervention used to facilitate discussion between patient and therapist is lyric analysis. As the name suggests, this technique uses song lyrics as a basis for dialogue—a dialogue about the situation, current feelings, and coping strategies. Song lyrics allow a means to present discussion in a non-threatening manner. When talking about the lyrics, patients are not talking about themselves or their situation, but the situation in the song and the writer's feelings (at least initially). This intervention has long been used and found to be beneficial in psychiatric settings (Clendenon-Wallen, 1991; Jones, 2005; Mark, 1988). In a 2005 study, Jones found that just one group music therapy session employing lyric analysis was effective in increasing feelings of joy and reducing feelings of blame and fear for those who are chemically dependent. It stands to reason that in the medical setting, where a therapist may have only one session with a patient, lyric analysis can serve as a useful approach in addressing goals of mood and coping skills. In addition, lyric analysis can be used to address patient cognitive functioning, particularly the ability to recall and/or decode information sung in a song. For example, a therapist may sing a song verse telling a story and ask the patient to verbalize what is happening in the verse. For a patient with a head injury, this is a challenging task and thus a good exercise. For individuals who struggle with this, the task can be simplified to recalling information from one line of a song. For example, *"On a warm summer's evening, on a train bound for nowhere... Where was the train going?"* When addressing cognitive tasks, the patient must focus attention on the lyrics of the song, retrieve the important information, and accurately verbalize this information. When addressing emotional goals, the lyrics are used as a springboard for a more in-depth discussion with the patient.

Counseling Techniques

Hospitalization is a stressful event and often patients are dealing with a variety of emotions related to their hospitalization, in addition to dealing with the illness itself. Areas for possible emotional support include, but are not limited to (a) a new diagnosis, (b) family dynamics, (c) financial concerns, (d) lack of independence, and (e) lifestyle changes. Music therapists often assist patients in expression and processing of these feeling. This is accomplished through techniques already discussed, such as song writing and lyric analysis. In addition, other counseling techniques are important tools for the music therapist to have. Table 9.5 highlights some effective counseling techniques for incorporation into music therapy sessions.

Table 9.5. Counseling Techniques for Use with Medical Patients		
Technique	**Description**	**Rationale for Use**
Validation and empathy	The therapist makes statements so that the patient feels acknowledged, understood, and heard. People want to feel respected and understood. This does not mean that the therapist needs to agree with the patient but instead recognizes the statements and feelings being verbalized by the patient. A statement such as "It must be scary to not know what is going on" after a patient has expressed fear over an unknown cause of illness is one example of this. The statement lets the patient know that the therapist has heard what is being expressed. Validation and empathy are important because they set the stage for the patient to feel comfortable communicating with the therapist.	In a 1975 article, Peck argued that when one has an understanding of empathy, he or she is better equipped to handle situations in which someone is seeking help. When people feel heard, they are more likely to share their true feelings and thus make progress toward their therapeutic goal.
Reflection	The therapist listens to a patient and summarizes major points or clarifies what a patient is saying/feeling. Usually a feeling word is attached to encourage exploration of emotions (Keeran, n.d.). This technique purposefully rephrases what a patient is communicating to avoid a defensive response. Using the same example of a patient who has expressed fear over an unknown cause of an illness but maybe has not verbalized a specific feeling, a reflective statement would be "It seems that not knowing what is happening has been really scary for you." A patient can either respond that that is an accurate assessment or they can reject the assessment and further clarify his or her feelings. Either way, the patient is being pushed to recognize specific feelings and causes of these emotions. One must be careful of making a reflective statement starting with "I understand" (Keeran, n.d.). Even if the therapist has experience in a similar situation to what the patient is experiencing, the therapist does not have full understanding of what the patient is thinking/feeling.	It allows for exploration of patient feelings in a way that the patient feels heard and understood.
Open-ended questions	It is easy to fall into a trap of asking closed-ended questions and, in some situations, it may be more appropriate to do so (communication or cognitive deficit). However, closed ended questions elicit only short answers from the patient and do not encourage further elaboration. Good open-ended questions start with a statement such as "Tell me more about…," or "What happened…?"	The therapist asks questions in a manner to encourage the patient to elaborate on the topic of discussion. This gives the control to the patient so he or she feels supported.

Recommendations for Clinical Practice

Outside of an understanding of appropriate goals and interventions for music therapy in the hospital setting, there are other important factors to keep in mind when implementing effective medical music therapy sessions and running a successful program. The following points are important considerations for any medical music therapy program:

- *Education*: Despite its 60-plus years as a profession and the recent media attention music therapy has received, the majority of individuals have little to no knowledge about music therapy. Therefore, it is important to educate as many people as possible. For programs both old and new, this education will include administration, physicians, nurses, therapists, social workers, other medical personnel, public relations, family, and patients. A survey given to nursing staff assessing their knowledge and perceptions of music therapy found that increased knowledge and exposure to music therapy had a significant effect on their perceptions of its effectiveness (Hillmer, 2007). With a better understanding of what music therapy is and can do, one is more likely to support the establishment of a program, make referrals, or agree to music therapy services. With high turnover in the medical setting, education is never finished; in-services should be consistently scheduled. Finally, patients often have a misconception of what music therapy is, thinking that the therapist is coming to entertain. When appropriate, the therapist should communicate that music therapy is a referred service and should make clear what the therapeutic goal will be.

- *Visibility*: The common phrase "Out of sight, out of mind" is appropriate in discussing music therapy in a medical setting. Referrals will occur in areas where music therapy is the most present and visible. At TMH, the pain management specialist (a great supporter of music therapy) actually stated, "I love music therapy, but if I don't see you, I forget about you." Therefore, the music therapist needs to take measures to be seen. Attending department rounds is an easy way to remain visible and is one area where one can get the most "bang for the buck," because rounds are attended by a large variety of medical staff. During rounds, it is important to communicate with staff regarding patient progress or to ask questions. This alerts them to the fact that music therapy is part of a specific patient's care and will likely generate referrals for other patients. Another tactic is to participate in appropriate hospital committees; integrative medicine or bereavement councils are areas in which music therapy can lend support while being visible to a variety of hospital area staff.

- *Data collection*: In addition to documentation of patient sessions, it is helpful to collect data to support the benefit of music therapy services. These data should be compiled and submitted to hospital administration and/or other parties to illustrate the impact the program has had on patients and the organization. Patient satisfaction has become a hot topic in the health care world and is becoming a measure for reimbursement from insurance companies. Music therapy has been shown to boost patient satisfaction scores by as much as 3.4 points (Yinger & Standley, 2011). If possible, the music therapist should ensure that music therapy is included in the hospital survey sent to patients. If it is not, an MT can create and distribute a music therapy survey, as allowed. Hospital staff, both administration and medical personnel, are numbers-driven. Therefore, an effective strategy is to track numbers of referrals and sessions to present to the appropriate parties. This will be helpful in supporting the continued need or proposed growth of music therapy.

- *Materials*: Music therapists do not merely use their voice in therapy sessions; they bring materials that will be effective in achieving the therapeutic goal. This usually involves some type of accompanying instrument. Therapists have their preferred instrument, but the guitar is recommended as it is easily portable, fits readily into tight spaces, and minimizes the sense of a barrier between patient and therapist. It is also helpful to carry a few smaller instruments to offer the patient: maraca, tambourine, paddle drum, etc. Finally, on a regular basis, an item that holds a variety of chord sheets/sheet music of differing genres is needed, such as a binder or tablet device (iPad). The benefit of using an electronic device like a tablet is that it is light and portable and can hold other applications useful in the hospital setting, such as a communication board, music apps for music creation, translator tools, tuner, etc. With these basic materials, a therapist can be effective in the hospital setting and can bring in other items as needed.

- *Memorized music*: While music therapists always want to be equipped with chord/sheet music at their disposal, it is not always feasible to have music out during a session. Sometimes the set-up of the room does not provide a place to put music. Occasionally, the therapist does not have time to take out the music before needing to start the session. Additionally, it can be distracting and therapeutically destructive to flip through music. In these instances, it is important that the therapist have an arsenal of memorized music to draw from. As a variety of genres are played in the hospital setting, it is important that the therapist has music memorized in all of these genres. This takes time but is worth the effort.

- *Room set-up*: Every hospital room is set up differently, even those on the same unit. Some rooms are roomy with places to sit and place music; others are so small there is no space available for sitting or setting up music. In each room, therapists need to quickly assess the room set-up and position themselves in the best place therapeutically. Priorities for set-up should be the ability to maintain eye contact with the patient to be able to elicit a positive response from the patient. The music therapist should avoid putting music on the floor; a table or lap is better (or even the patient's bed, if permission is granted). Items may be moved around to make the set-up successful but must be returned to their place before leaving the room.

- *Physiological indicators*: Patients in all intensive care units and occasionally on the regular floor may be hooked up to monitors measuring their heart rate, respiratory rate, oxygen saturation level, and blood pressure. The music therapist must pay attention to these monitors, document them, and respond to significant changes, as they indicate how the patient is responding (particularly patients who are verbally or behaviorally less responsive). Music therapy has consistently been shown to positively impact these indicators (Davis & Jones, 2012; Singh et al., 2009). It is easy to forget about these important numbers and the music therapist should be careful to note them.

Case Example 1: The phone rings in the music therapy office. A nurse is calling to refer a patient who is emotionally upset and distressed. "Please come see her as soon as possible," the nurse pleads. The music therapist heads over to see the patient and is confronted with the symptoms the nurse described. Over the course of the next 45 minutes, the therapist listens to the patient verbalize her problems, offers validation and empathy, counsels, and uses music to process with the patient and uplift. By the end of the session, the patient is in a calm state. At the next session, the patient thanks the music therapist, stating how helpful the previous visit had been during a difficult time.

Case Example 2: During a rehab center interdisciplinary team meeting, music therapy is referred to see a patient who is not performing up to a desired level in therapy. "It appears the patient is depressed and giving up" is the comment made by staff members. During the music therapy assessment, it is learned that the patient is a musician, a guitar player. The patient is given a guitar to play and practice, both during and outside of music therapy sessions. The patient and music therapist decide to "work up" some songs to perform for other rehab patients and they organize a performance. Staff starts to report a change in the patient's mood and motivation in therapies. Treatment goals are starting to be reached and attitudes have shifted. The patient has been given a purpose with the performance goal. The concert for the center is a success and provides a wonderful change of pace for both patients and staff. One music therapy referral had a positive impact, not only on the patient but on the whole center.

Case Example 3: An inpatient cancer patient is taken for radiation treatment planning. This involves uncomfortable transportation, making of an immobilizing device for treatment, and a CT scan. The patient has been anxious and nauseous all morning. To the patient's surprise, a music therapist greets the patient and plays preferred music during the planning process and subsequent CT scan. The music therapist continues while waiting on transport back to the patient room. The music therapist notes the patient's physically relaxed state as the music plays—a sharp contrast to how the patient presented when arriving for treatment planning. The patient's family reports that the music was a wonderful surprise and assisted in making the procedure tolerable for the patient.

Conclusion

These examples illustrate the impact music therapy has in the medical setting. It distracts, motivates, and comforts patients, families, and staff. The information presented has outlined the evidence-based techniques found to be effective in addressing a myriad of potential goals for patients in the hospital. Music therapy is not a "one size fits all" prescription. The wonderful thing about the profession is that it is tailored to the needs and preferences of the patient. Medical music therapists must keep updated on the research and use their knowledge to create the most effective therapeutic interventions. However, they need to be willing to adapt to the situation and the immediate needs of the patient. This will allow the best therapeutic outcome to occur. Music therapy is needed in medical settings, and more hospitals are starting to realize this. As music therapy continues to grow in this area, there will be more goals that emerge, more research that is conducted, and more interventions that are devised. The potential for continued music therapy in medicine is exponential.

References

Adams, K. S. (2005). *The effect of music therapy and deep breathing on pain in patients recovering from gynecologic surgery in the PACU* (Unpublished master's thesis). Florida State University, Tallahassee.

American Red Cross. (1992). *Disaster services regulations and procedures: 3077-IA.* Washington, DC: American Red Cross.

Andrews, G., Hobbs, M. J., Borkovec, T. D., Beesdo, K., Craske, M. G., Heimber, R. G., et al. (2010). Generalized worry disorder: A review of DSM-IV generalized anxiety disorder and options for DSM-V. *Depression and Anxiety, 27*(2), 134-147.

Bittman, B., Berk, L., Shannon, M., Sharah, M., Westengard, J., Guegler, K. J., & Ruff, D. W. (2005). Recreational music-making modulates the human stress response: A preliminary individualized gene expression strategy. *Medical Science Monitor, 11*, 31–40.

Bradt, J., Dileo, C., & Grocke, D. (2010). Music interventions for mechanically ventilated patients. *Cochrane Database of Systematic Review, 2010 Dec 8*(12), CD006902. doi:10.1002/14651858. CD006902.pub2

Centers for Disease Control and Prevention. (2013, May 30). *FastStats: Hospital utilization.* Retrieved from http://www.cdc.gov/nchs/fastats/hospital.htm

Clark, M., Issacks-Downton, G., Wells, N., Redlin-Frazier, S., Hepworth, J. T., & Chakravarthy, S. (2006). Use of preferred music to deduce emotional distress and symptom activity during radiation therapy. *Journal of Music Therapy, 43*, 247–265.

Clayton, M., Sager, R., & Will, U. (2004). In time with the music: The concept of entrainment and its significance for ethnomusicology. *ESEM CounterPoint, 1*, 1–45.

Clendenon-Wallen, J (1991). The use of music to influence the self-confidence and self-esteem of adolescents who are sexually abused. *Music Therapy Perspectives, 9*, 73–79.

Davis, T., & Jones, P. (2012). Music therapy: Decreasing anxiety in the ventilated patients: A review of the literature. *Dimensions of Critical Care Nursing, 31*, 159–166.

Ghetti, C. (2011). Active music engagement with emotional-approach coping to improve well- being in liver and kidney transplant recipients. *Journal of Music Therapy, 48*, 463–485.

Gibbons, A. C. (1977). Popular music preference of elderly people. *Journal of Music Therapy, 14*, 180–189.

Good, M., Anderson, G. C., Stanton-Hicks, M., Gras, J. A., & Makii, M. (2002). Relaxation and music reduce pain after gynecologic surgery. *Pain Management Nursing, 3*, 61–70.

Gooding, L. F., Swezey, S., & Zwischenberger, J. B. (2012). Using music interventions in perioperative care. *Southern Medical Journal, 105*, 486–490.

Grape, C., Sandgren, M., Hansson, L. O., Ericson, E., & Theorell, T. (2003). Does singing promote well-being? An empirical study of professional and amateur singers during a singing lesson. *Integrative Physiological Behavioral Science, 38*, 65–74.

Gutgsell, K. T, Schlucher, M., Margevicius, S., DeGolia, P. A., McLaughlin, B, Harris, M., et al. (2012). Music therapy reduces pain in palliative care patients: A randomized controlled trial. *Journal of Pain and Symptom Management, 45*, 822–831.

Hall, M. J., Levant, S., & DeFrances, C. J. (2013). *Trends in inpatient hospital deaths: National Hospital Discharge Survey, 2000–2010.* NCHS data brief, no 118. Hyattsville, MD: National Center for Health Statistics.

Harvard Women's Health Watch. (2011, May). When patients suddenly become confused. Retrieved April 28, 2013, from www.health.harvard.edu/newsletters/Harvard_Womens_Health_Watch/20110May

Hillmer, M. (2007). *Survey of nurses' attitudes and perceptions toward music therapy in the hospital setting* (Unpublished master's thesis). University of Kansas, Lawrence.

Hunter, B., Oliva, R., Sahler, O. Z., Gaisser, D., Salipante, D. M., & Arezina, C. H. (2010). Music therapy as an adjunctive treatment in the management of stress for patients being weaned from mechanical ventilation. *Journal of Music Therapy, 47*, 198–219.

Jones, J. (2005). A comparison of songwriting and lyric analysis techniques to evoke emotional change in a single session with people who are chemically dependent. *Journal of Music Therapy, 42*, 94–110.

Keeran, D. (n.d.). *Effective counseling skills.* Retrieved from http://www.ctihalifax.com/images/CounselingSkillsArticle.pdf

Kim, S. J. (2010). Music therapy protocol development to enhance swallowing training for stroke patients with dysphagia. *Journal of Music Therapy, 47*, 102–119.

Kreutz, G., Bondgard, S., Rohrmann, S., Hodapp, V., & Grebe, D. (2004). Effects of choir singing or listening on secretory immunoglobulin A, cortisol, and emotional state. *Journal of Behavioral Medicine, 27*, 632–635.

Lancioni, G. E., O'Reilly, M. F., Singh, N. N., Buonocunto, F., Sacco, V., Collonna, F., et al. (2009a). Evaluation of technology-assisted learning setups for undertaking assessment and providing intervention to persons with a diagnosis of vegetative state. *Developmental Neurorehabilitation, 12*, 411–420.

Lancioni, G. E., O'Reilly, M. F., Singh, N. N., Buonocunto, F., Sacco, V., Colonna, F., et al. (2009b). Technology-based intervention options for post-coma persons with minimally conscious state and pervasive motor disabilities. *Developmental Neurorehabilitation, 12*, 24–31.

Lancioni, G. E., Saponaro, F., Singh, N. N., O'Reilly, M. F., Sigafoos, J., & Oliva, D. (2010). A microswitch to enable a woman with acquired brain injury and profound multiple disabilities to access environmental stimulation with lip movements. *Perceptual and Motor Skills, 110*, 488–492.

Lee, H. J. (2005). The effect of live music via the iso-principle on pain management in palliative care as measured by self-report using a graphic rating scale (GRS) and pulse rate. *Electronic Theses, Treatises and Dissertations,* Paper 3199.

Li, Y., & Dong, Y. (2012). Preoperative music intervention for patients undergoing cesarean delivery. *International Journal of Gynecology and Obstetrics, 119*, 81–83.

Mark, A. (1988). Metaphoric lyrics as a bridge to the adolescent world. *Adolescence, 23,* 313–323.

National Heart, Lung, and Blood Institute. (2012, August 2). What is high blood pressure? Retrieved from http://www.nhlbi.nih.gov/health/health-topics/topics/hbp/

Nguyen, J. T. (2003). *The effect of music therapy on end-of-life patients' quality of life, emotional state, and family satisfaction as measured by self-report (*Unpublished master's thesis). Florida State University, Tallahassee.

Patten, S. B., Beck, C. A., Kassam, A., Williams, J., Barbul, C., & Metz, L. M. (2005). Long-term medical conditions and major depression: Strength of association for specific conditions in the general population. *The Canadian Journal of Psychiatry, 50,* 195–202.

Peck, T. (1975). Counseling skills applied to reference services. *RQ, 14,* 233–235.

Schlaug, G., Marchina, S., & Norton, A. (2005). Evidence for plasticity in white-matter tracts of patients with chronic Broca's aphasia undergoing intense intonation-based speech therapy. *Annals New York Academy of Sciences, 1169,* 385–394.

Singh, V. P., Rao, V., Prem, V., Sahoo, R. C., & Keshav, P. K. (2009). Comparison of the effectiveness of music and progressive muscle relaxation for anxiety in COPD: A randomized controlled pilot study. *Chronic Respiratory Disease, 6,* 209–216.

Standley, J .M. (1996) A meta-analysis on the effects of music as reinforcement for education/therapy objectives. *Journal of Research in Music Education, 44,* 105–133.

Standley, J. M. (2000). Music research in medical treatment. In American Music Therapy Association (Ed.), *Effectiveness of music therapy procedures: Documentation of research and clinical practice* (3rd ed., pp. 1–64). Silver Spring, MD: American Music Therapy Association.

Thaut, M. H. (2005). The future of music in therapy and medicine. *Annals New York Academy of Sciences, 1060,* 303–308.

Walworth, D. (2010). Effect of live music therapy for patients undergoing magnetic resonance imaging. *Journal of Music Therapy, 47,* 335–350.

Walworth, D. D. (2005). Procedural-support music therapy in the healthcare setting: A cost-effectiveness analysis. *Journal of Pediatric Nursing, 20,* 276–284.

Wong, E. (2004). *Clinical guide to music therapy in adult physical rehabilitation settings.* Silver Spring, MD: American Music Therapy Association.

Yinger, O. S., & Standley, J. M. (2011). The effect of medical music therapy on patient satisfaction: As measured by the Press Ganey Inpatient Survey. *Music Therapy Perspectives, 29,* 149–156.

Zhou, K., Li, X., Yan, H., Dang, S., & Wang, D. (2011). Effects of music therapy on depression and duration of hospital stay on breast cancer patients after radical mastectomy. *Chinese Medical Journal, 124,* 2321–2327.

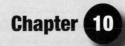

Chapter 10

Music Therapy and Older Adults in the Medical Setting
Olivia Swedberg Yinger, PhD, MT-BC, and Andrea Cevasco-Trotter, PhD, MT-BC

Over 40 million adults age 65 and older currently live in the United States. Between 2000 and 2010, growth in the U.S. population age 65 and older occurred at a faster rate (15.1%) than growth of the total U.S. population (9.7%) (Werner, 2011). Although adults age 65 and over represented only 13% of the U.S. population in 2010, they represented 38.7% of patients discharged from hospitals (National Center for Health Statistics, 2013; Werner, 2011). In 2011, 16.9% of adults age 65 and over had one or more hospital stays (National Center for Health Statistics, 2013).

The term *geriatric* is an adjective that relates to the process of aging and to older adults. Geriatric medicine is that branch of medicine that deals with the problems and diseases of old age and aging people ("Geriatric," 2013). For the purpose of this chapter, the term *older adult* will be used in place of the noun *geriatric* to refer to those over age 65 (Hooyman & Kiyak, 2008). Older adults may experience changes in vision, touch, hearing, and cognition, as well as physical and psychosocial functioning, which are typical of the process of aging. Other common concerns for older adults include insomnia, physical pain, delirium, dementia, and challenges due to multiple medications. The likelihood of contracting certain chronic conditions also increases with age. This chapter will first describe typical changes related to aging and common concerns for older adults, followed by brief descriptions of several common age-related conditions that music therapists working in medical settings may encounter. It should be noted that although these changes become more prevalent as people age, not everyone ages at the same rate. There is great variation in the level, extent, and timing of the occurrence of age-related changes among individuals.

Sensory Changes Associated With Aging

Sensation is the process of using the sense organs to bring in information (Hooyman & Kiyak, 2008) through vision, hearing, touch, taste, and smell. Although aging tends to affect all five senses, each person experiences these changes differently and an individual's senses may be affected to different degrees. Minimal age-related changes occur in taste and smell (Fisk, Rogers, Charness, Czaja, & Sharit, 2009), whereas visual, haptic (the term for changes in touch), and hearing changes tend to be more extensive. Perceptual changes also occur as people age, changing the way that the brain processes sensory information (Hooyman & Kiyak, 2008). Table 10.1 describes areas of sensory impairment that occur with age, along with recommended modifications.

	Table 10.1. Areas of Sensory Impairment		
Area	**Impairment**	**Activity Limitation**	**Modification**
Visual Changes	Reduced pupil opening (Hooyman & Kiyak, 2008)	Poor vision in low light and difficulty adjusting to ambient light changes. Difficulty reading small print (Saxon, Etten, & Perkins, 2010)	Provide adequate lighting Large print with high contrast (Hooyman & Kiyak, 2008)
Haptic (touch) Changes	Decreased sensory receptors in the vestibular system. Decreased touch receptors on soles of feet (Saxon, Etten, & Perkins, 2010)	Decreased stability of movement and greater fall risk. Older adults compensate by moving more slowly and/or walking with a wider gait (Fisk et al., 2009; Saxon et al., 2010)	Remove objects from traffic flow and encourage use of assistive devices. Move objects such as wires, floor mats, tables, chairs, and furniture out of the traffic flow. Define the edges and corners of obstacles (such as stairs, walls, and doors) with contrasting colors or textures (Fisk et al., 2009)
Hearing Changes	The pinna, external ear canal, membranes of the middle ear, and ossicles become stiffer and lose flexibility. Segments of the cochlea deteriorate (Saxon et al., 2010)	Hearing losses may impair social interaction (Fisk, Rogers, et al., 2009). Presbycusis makes it more difficult to perceive high frequencies at first, later affecting lower frequencies (Hooyman & Kiyak, 2008)	Find a quiet room, free from environmental noise. Structure spoken messages in a clear, systematic way. Speak slowly and clearly, without exaggerating speech or shouting. Use a lower pitched, but not monotonous, voice. Avoid talking for long stretches of time (Fisk et al., 2009)

Cognitive Changes Associated With Aging

Cognition is the process by which the brain takes sensory input and transforms, reduces, elaborates, stores, recovers, and uses it (Fisk et al., 2009). Areas of cognition that may be affected by the process of aging include memory, language comprehension, visual attention, and multi-tasking. Table 10.2 describes cognitive changes that occur with age, along with recommended modifications.

	Table 10.2. Cognitive Changes that Occur with Age	
Cognitive Area	**Activity Limitation**	**Modification**
Memory	Short-term, working, and prospective memory decline with age	Provide written reminders for events. Use event-based cues rather than time-based cues when asking them to remember to do something in the future.
Language Comprehension	Older adults store smaller "chunks" of information when reading or processing speech, making it more difficult to draw inferences	Slow the pacing of conversation or instruction and give older adults more time to respond or follow directions. Make transfer of information explicit.
Attention	Dynamic visual attention becomes more difficult, since older adults may need more time to orient their attention. Often perform tasks that require multi-tasking more slowly and with less accuracy	Break down tasks that require doing multiple things at one time into more simple tasks that require a single focus of attention.

Physical Changes Associated With Aging

Changes in motor control also occur with aging and contribute to older adults' increased risk of falling. As people age, the ability to control movements becomes more difficult, causing older adults to move more slowly and with less precision, performing movements one and a half to two times more slowly than younger adults (Fisk et al., 2009). In addition to increasing the risk of falling, cognitive and motor changes associated with aging can lead to changes in activities of daily living (ADLs) and instrumental activities of daily living (IADLS). Across time, older adults might experience changes in ADLs, which are the basic skills for independent living, including mobility, transferring, dressing, bathing, hygiene, toileting, continence, and feeding (Besdine, 2013). Eventually older adults evince changes in IADLs, which involve complex tasks such as traveling, managing finances, housekeeping, and other day-to-day tasks.

Frailty

Frailty is often a primary or secondary diagnosis and is commonly used to describe an occurrence in the elderly (Ahmed, Mandel, & Fain, 2007); disease, loss of activity, poor nutrition, stress, and/or physiologic changes of aging can result in frailty (Ahmed et al., 2007). Normal age-related changes, combined with all other factors, contribute to frailty (Heuberger, 2011). Common clinical symptoms include weight and muscle loss, physical exhaustion and weakness, and slow gait and lower levels of activity and functionality (Heuberger, 2011). Patients experience a progressive increase of problems, self-propagated by the individual; the disability is the outcome of the functional decline. Older adults who are frail have a greater risk for falls, fractures, and medical complications, all which increase the probability of institutionalization and result in accruing health care expenses (Heuberger, 2011). Eventually the patient will experience failure to thrive and, eventually, the end of life after a period hospitalization and institutionalization (Ahmed et al., 2007; Heuberger, 2011).

Failure to Thrive

Failure to thrive is a diagnosis involving decline and deterioration that occurs at the end of life (Institute of Medicine, 1991; Lonergan & Krevans, 1991; Robertson & Montagnini, 2004). Patients evince loss of vitality, decline in will to live, and are unable to thrive in current setting. While patients complain of "just not feeling well," family members state their loved ones are "going downhill" for seemingly no reason (Rocchiccioli & Sanford, 2009).

Four broad areas commonly evinced by individuals who are failing to thrive include impaired physical functioning, malnutrition, depression, and cognitive impairments (Robertson & Montagnini, 2004). It is often defined as a condition of weight loss, decreased appetite and poor nutrition, and inactivity. Furthermore, depression, dehydration, low cholesterol levels, and immune system decline also occur (Lonergan & Krevans, 1991). Death is the final byproduct (Robertson & Montagnini, 2004).

Psychosocial Changes Associated With Aging

Life changes that occur with age, such as retirement, the death of a loved one, or loss of functioning, may cause psychosocial changes. Depression and isolation are two experiences that older adults may face, commonly leading to changes in psychosocial functioning.

Depression

Major depressive disorder consists of a depressed mood or loss of interest, desire, and/or difficulty in enjoying life. Other symptoms include changes in weight and appetite, changes in sleep, psychomotor agitation or retardation, fatigue or loss of energy, feelings of guilt or worthlessness, loss of concentration or indecisiveness, and thoughts of suicide or even suicide attempts (American Psychiatric Association, 2013). Persistent depressive disorder, or *dysthymia*, is a mild, although long-term, type of depression (lasting at least two years) that interferes with functioning and enjoyment of life. Individuals with persistent depressive disorder are often considered pessimistic, humorless, lethargic, introverted, critical of self and others, and complaining (Coryell, 2009).

Late-life depression is the term used to describe individuals who first experience depression after the age of 60 (Fiske, Wetherell, & Gatz, 2009) or 65 (Rodda, Walker, & Carter, 2011). There are multiple reasons for depression in later life, including physical health/disabilities, bereavement, cognitive impairments, and sleep disturbance, as well as isolation, loneliness, and lack of social supports (Fiske et al., 2009; Rodda et al., 2011).

Depression is one area of great concern regarding older adult medical patients. Many different contributing factors, as well as individual past, present, and future experiences, determine the outcome. One such factor involves patients' experience of pain. Researchers have determined that many older adults who have pain commonly have depression; interestingly, social network and functional status tended to predict depression more than the severity of pain in non-disabled older adults who reside in community dwellings (Lliffe et al., 2009). Those who experience pain might not be as engaged in the community, and it directly impacts their ability to be functionally independent. Furthermore, older adult medical patients who have depression have poor prognosis (Cole & Bellavance, 1997). This is due to a low recovery rate and high mortality rate. Severe depression, serious physical illness, and symptoms of depression prior to admission all contributed to poor outcomes (Cole & Bellavance, 1997). Thus, this results in a cyclical problem, which is often difficult to stop.

Isolation

Another concern of the aging population is social isolation; there is not only a concern about the isolation that occurs and even seems to magnify with the normal process of aging, but also with the isolation that occurs during the hospitalization period. This includes individuals who might be hospitalized across time in a long-term care unit or those residing in contact isolation due to mandatory infection control policies. Loneliness seems to be one major issue that affects and escalates aging-related decline in physiological resistance (Hawkley & Cacioppo, 2007). It affects health behaviors, stress appraisal and coping, psychological stress responses, and recuperative processes (Hawkley & Cacioppo, 2007). Of course, patients with family networks and good parameters of quality of life (QOL) were less likely to be isolated (Giuli et al., 2012).

The impact of social isolation is quite severe; researchers found that social isolation predicted re-hospitalization (Giuli et al., 2012). Furthermore, social isolation also predicts morbidity and mortality from cancer, cardiovascular disease, and other causes in older adults (Hawkley & Cacioppo, 2007). It is important to realize that women perceive their social supports worse than men, to a significant degree (Giuli et al., 2012). This might be an important consideration when prioritizing referrals.

There has been an exponential growth in the number of multi-drug resistant organisms; thus, mandatory infection control programs exist and provide rules and regulations to protect patients. Most patients who are placed under contact isolation experience greater depression, anxiety, anger, fear, and loneliness than non-isolated patients; these behaviors tended to increase across time (Abad, Fearday, & Safdar, 2010). Furthermore, health care workers usually spent less time with these patients, and recorded incomplete or no vital sign recordings and no nursing narratives or physician progress notes in their charts. These patients were also twice as likely as non-isolated patients to have adverse preventable events. Supportive care failures were eight times more likely for patients in contact isolation; this included falls, ulcers, and fluid and electrolyte abnormalities. The uncertainty and loss of control result in psychologically adverse effects.

Other Common Considerations for Older Adults

Insomnia, physical pain, delirium, dementia, and complications due to multiple medications are other factors that may be of concern to older adults. It is important for music therapists working with older adults to be aware of these considerations to adapt their treatment appropriately.

Insomnia

People who have insomnia have problems initiating sleep, maintaining sleep, or engaging in sleep that seems inadequate or not refreshing. Often individuals are fatigued during the day and have problems functioning. While insomnia can be a disorder of its own with no obvious cause, others might have insomnia due to irregular sleep–wake schedules, poor sleep habits, physical disorders, use or withdrawal of drugs, alcohol consumption in the evening, or emotional problems, anxiety, and stress.

Over half of the people over the age of 80 say they have problems with sleep (Abeles, 1998). Those who have medical illness are at greater risk for sleep problems due to disruptions in sleep and impairments in alertness (Lopez, 2008). Treatment regimens for individuals vary and include cognitive-behavioral techniques, sleep restriction, and stimulus control approaches (Doghramji, 2008; Lopez, 2008).

Physical Pain

Pain indicates that there is something wrong with the body. The onset of pain can be slow or sudden, can range from mild and occasional to severe or constant, and can be classified as acute or chronic. Acute pain occurs due to disease, inflammation, or damage to tissue. It typically lasts less than six months and ceases when the cause of pain has been treated or healed (National Institutes of Health, 2013). Examples of acute pain include burn pain, acute headache, post-operative pain, interventional pain due to diagnostic and therapeutic procedures, post-traumatic pain, spinal cord injury, etc. (Kumar, 2007). Opioid analgesics are often used to provide relief of acute pain.

If acute pain has not been treated or resolved, it can lead to chronic pain. Chronic pain often persists even when the injury has healed, although some people who experience chronic pain do not have any past injury or indication of damage to the body. Within the nervous system, pain signals continue to fire (National Institutes of Health, 2013). Examples of chronic malignant pain include cancer, HIV/AIDS, advanced chronic obstructive heart failure, advanced congestive heart failure, Parkinsonism, etc. Musculoskeletal pain (spinal pain, various types of arthritis, bone pain, etc.), neuropathic pain, and visceral pain are examples of chronic non-malignant pain (Kumar, 2007).

Long-term physical effects of pain include tense muscles, limited mobility, lack of energy, and even changes in appetite; emotional effects include depression, anger, anxiety, and fear of re-injury (Abeles, 1998; National Institutes of Health, 2013). Expectations of pain and discomfort often increases anxiety; furthermore, the anticipation and belief that this pain will not be easy to handle, as well as unexpected and unplanned pain, also result in increased stress (Nichols, 2003). Boredom, loneliness, and bereavement also influence the perception of pain. Behavior related to pain may be reinforced by family members who give more attention to loved ones when they complain about pain.

Delirium (Acute Confusional State)

Delirium refers to a reversible and transient fluctuating disturbance that occur with a rapid onset, causing a disturbance of consciousness that affects an individual's ability to focus, sustain, or shift attention. Changes in cognition can also occur, such as memory deficit, disorientation, language disturbance, or development of a perceptual disturbance that is not better accounted for; results indicate that the changes are from a medical condition (Abeles, 1998; American Psychiatric Association, 2013; Fong, Tulebaev, & Inouye, 2009). *Sundowning* is the term used to describe delirium-related confusion and agitation that occur later in the day (Abeles, 1998). A variety of factors affect delirium, including older age, metabolic disturbances, medications/polypharmacy, infections, anesthesia, hip fractures, unfamiliar surroundings accompanied by a change in daily routine, lack of sensory stimulation, overstimulation, sensory impairments, changes in the sleep-wake cycle, a history of dementia or brain injury, surgery, pain, acute neurological diseases, and other types of physical or psychological stressors (Abeles, 1998; Fong et al., 2009). Delirium is often the result and cause of hospitalization (Fong et al., 2009).

Dementia

Whereas delirium involves a sudden onset in confusion and is reversible, dementia tends to have a more gradual onset and is irreversible. Symptoms of dementia include multiple disturbances in neurological, psychological, and social functioning. Multiple cognitive deficits, including memory, aphasia, apraxia, agnosia, and difficulty with executive functioning, are characteristic of dementia, as is significant impairment in social or occupational functioning that is markedly different from one's previous level of functioning (Saxon, Etten, & Perkins, 2010). Alzheimer's disease is the most common type of primary dementia, accounting for 50–80% of all cases of dementia (Alzheimer's Association, 2013). Although the incidence of Alzheimer's disease and related dementias increases with age, mostly affecting adults over age 65, it is important to note that serious mental decline is not a normal part of aging. One in eight people (13%) over the age of 65 are estimated to have Alzheimer's disease, compared to less than half (45%) of those over age 85 (Alzheimer's Association, 2012).

Medications

With the advancement of modern medicine, diseases and conditions can be detected, prevented, and treated. Despite the positive advancements of medications, older adults often experience medication-related problems due to physiological changes, such as body weight, digestive changes, circulation system, etc. All of these changes impact the way medications are absorbed and used (Cameron, 2004; U.S. Food and Drug Administration, 2012). Over-the-counter, prescription, and herbal remedies/alternative medicines all contribute to problems (Cameron, 2004). Individuals who take multiple medications at one time, called polypharmacy, are at risk for drug interactions; other potential problems occur with drug-condition interactions (when certain drugs interact with a pre-existing medical condition), drug-food interactions, and drug-alcohol interactions (Cameron, 2004).

Common Causes of Hospitalization for Older Adults

In addition to typical, non-pathological changes that occur with aging, older adults are at greater risk for certain acute and chronic conditions that may require hospitalization. Several of the leading causes of hospitalization for older adults (Foltz-Gray, 2012; National Center for Health Statistics, 2013) are described here. The following causes of hospitalization are listed in order of their frequency among older adults.

1. *Heart disease.* Heart disease includes ischemic heart disease, heart attacks, arrhythmias, and heart failure. Coronary atherosclerosis is a blockage of blood flow to the heart from the build-up of fatty plaque, which could cause a heart attack, heart damage, or chest pain. Cardiac arrhythmias are irregularities such as atrial fibrillation, which can cause palpitations and sudden drops in blood pressure. In turn, palpitations and changes in blood pressure could lead to unconsciousness, strokes, or cardiac arrest. Congestive heart failure (CHF) is a condition caused by heart disease, which weakens heart muscle tissue.

2. *Infections.* As people age, their immune system weakens, making older adults more susceptible to infections. In addition, the effects of such infections can be more serious for older adults. Common infections that result in hospitalization for adults over age 65 include pneumonia, septicemia, and urinary tract infections.

3. *Injuries.* Normal changes of aging, such as difficulty maintaining one's balance and decreased bone strength increase the risk of injury from falling. Fractures, particularly hip fractures, due to falling are one of the most common types of injuries that occur among adults over age 65.

4. *Cerebrovascular accident (CVA or stroke).* The technical term for when a blood vessel leading to the brain forms a clot or begins to bleed is *cerebrovascular accident* (CVA), since these involve the brain's vascular system. CVAs are frequently referred to as strokes. The effects of strokes vary based on the location and extent of the damage that is caused by loss of oxygen to the brain. Effects of strokes may include aphasia (impaired expressive and/or receptive language abilities), paralysis or loss of functioning in one or more limbs (often only on one side of the body), and impaired cognitive functioning.

5. *Cancer.* Cancer results from an abnormal production of cells, which form a mass or tumor. Cancer may affect various parts of the body. The most common cancers that result in hospitalization for older adults are those of the breast, prostate, and lung. Cancer is one of the leading causes of hospitalization for those between the ages of 65 and 84, but adults over age 85 are hospitalized more frequently for reasons other than cancer.

6. *Osteoarthritis.* Many people refer to osteoarthritis, an age-related hardening of one's cartilage, as OA or simply arthritis, although it must be differentiated from rheumatoid arthritis, an autoimmune condition. Osteoarthritis may seriously affect one's ability to perform tasks of daily living when certain movements become too painful. Modern technology allows for certain joints that have become arthritic to be replaced. Hip replacements and knee replacements are two common orthopedic procedures that increase mobility for many older adults and may require hospitalization.

7. *Chronic obstructive pulmonary disease (COPD).* This respiratory condition is an umbrella term that refers to the co-occurrence of emphysema with chronic bronchitis. Smoking is the primary cause of COPD. Shortness of breath and labored breathing are common unpleasant symptoms of COPD.

8. *Iatrogenic complications, complications of care, and adverse effects.* This category may include adverse drug events, misadventures, and complications of medical care or surgical procedures. When older adults have difficulty with medications that cause hospitalization, it is frequently the results of corticosteroids, blood thinners, sedatives, and/or sleep aids (Foltz-Gray, 2012). *Iatrogenic complications* is the terminology that refers to any problems that occur due to a diagnostic procedure, any form of therapy, or even a harmful event that is not normally a result of the patient's current diagnosis; older adults are at a greater risk of experiencing iatrogenic complications (Pacala, 2009). Patients who have iatrogenic disease experience loss in psychomotor skills and adverse changes to their social needs (Permpongkosol, 2011). Furthermore, the hospital environment and pacing may have negative impact on a patient's status; this includes an individual's mental, physical, and social activities of daily life.

9. *Kidney disease.* The kidneys are organs that filter blood plasma, help maintain an acid/base balance, and regulate the concentration of urine. Chronic renal failure, the technical name for kidney disease, occurs when the kidneys shrink and their functioning deteriorates over time to the point that they are no longer able to produce urine. Chronic renal failure may require treatment with dialysis, which uses an external filtration system to perform the task that the kidneys are no longer able to do. Kidney transplantation is also an option for some with chronic renal failure. Infection, metabolic disorders (including diabetes), and dehydration are all factors that may contribute to the occurrence of chronic renal failure. Common symptoms include excessive urination—particularly at night, insomnia, weakness, loss of appetite, nausea, and increased blood nitrogen levels.

10. *Non-insulin-dependent diabetes mellitus (type 2 diabetes).* Type 2 diabetes has also been referred to as adult-onset diabetes. It is a deficiency of insulin that is often treated with oral hypoglycemic drugs. Because risk factors for developing type 2 diabetes include being overweight and inactive, changes in lifestyle are frequently recommended to help manage type 2 diabetes. Adults over age 45 are also at an increased risk of developing type 2 diabetes. The effects of type 2 diabetes can be widespread. Common diabetes-related reasons for hospitalization among older adults include strokes, heart attacks, ulcers, and dehydration from elevated blood sugar levels.

It is important for music therapists working in medical settings to be familiar with the changes that occur with aging, whether the result of the typical aging process or a chronic health condition. In addition, music therapists should be aware of the needs of those caring for older adults, since caregivers face many challenges, particularly when their loved one is hospitalized. The following sections provide an overview of the medical music therapy literature as it pertains to older adults, including information on expected outcomes of music therapy treatment, research-based techniques, and recommendations for clinical practice.

Case Example 1: A nurse stops you in the hallway of the internal medicine unit. "I need to check Ms. Jones's vital signs and give her some medication in about 10 minutes," she says. "Ms. Jones has dementia and is very confused. Sometimes she tries to hit me when I get close to her. Do you think you could help keep her calm?" Ms. Jones's daughter is standing by the bedside adjusting a blanket when you enter the hospital room. Ms. Jones calls out in confusion as her daughter approaches her. "Stop it!" Ms. Jones shouts. Her daughter backs away and looks at you, with frustration and sadness on her face. You briefly introduce yourself and tell why you are there. "My mother loves gospel music," says the daughter, smiling slightly. Making eye contact with Ms. Jones and smiling, you begin playing the guitar and singing, "Glory, glory, hallelujah, since I lay my burdens down." Ms. Jones stops shouting and, after looking at you for a moment, a smile breaks out on her face. During the first verse of the song, she claps her hands lightly to the beat and during the chorus, she starts to sing with you. When the nurse enters, you smile at her and tell Ms. Jones, "She is here to help you feel better. Let's sing together. 'I feel better, so much better, since I lay my burdens down.'" The nurse smiles as she approaches Ms. Jones and even begins humming along as she checks Ms. Jones's vital signs. When it is time for her to give Ms. Jones her medication, you tell Ms. Jones, "This will help you feel so much better," and she takes her medication without complaint.

Case Example 2: A nurse referred Mr. Smith, 71 years of age, for music therapy for pain management, but she also thought he and his wife would benefit because an argument five minutes ago. The previous day the music therapist had a lively session with the couple as they celebrated their last night in the hospital; however, he fell during the night and was now required to stay a few extra days rather than being discharged that morning. When the music therapist entered the room, she sensed tension between the husband and wife. The music therapist asked Mr. Smith how he was doing and if he wanted to start the session with a song that might express how he was feeling today. He asked her to play "If You Knew Susie" from the 1920s. After a few minutes, he sang along and glanced sweetly at his wife, Susan. He reached out for her hand and she grasped his fingers tightly as tears filled her eyes. As the song ended, he told her that he always sang that song to his "Susie" with his off-key voice. She chuckled and said that he sang the song to her on her first date and from that moment on she was smitten. Mrs. Smith asked the therapist to sing "Side by Side." After the song was finished the therapist asked if there was a reason for the song. Mrs. Smith said that she wanted her husband to understand that she planned to be side-by-side with him through the good and bad times; she didn't mind staying with him at the hospital a few extra days, and she wanted to take care of things at home while he recovers, even after discharge. Once she finished, Mr. Smith said that he was worried about his Susie taking on too much while he was at the hospital. She was quite a gal, but she was working too hard to keep everything going around the house, paying bills, etc. He also felt bad that he was not taking care of her and their home. Once they expressed those feelings, the music therapist guided them in discussing how to resolve their concerns about the recovery process and what might be feasible for each of them during this time period. They happily decided that the session should end with "For Me and My Gal."

Reasons for Referrals and Expected Outcomes

The reasons why older adults are referred for music therapy are often similar to those of other adults in medical settings (Chapter 9) and in emergency care (Chapter 11). Reasons for referral may include management of pain or anxiety, decreasing agitation, promoting coping skills, procedural support, family support, and end-of-life care. Outcomes of music therapy treatment for older adults include improvements in physical and psychosocial functioning. Improvements in physical functioning may include decreases in heart rate, respiratory rate, blood pressure, and reported pain, as well as improved ambulation. Improvements in psychosocial functioning may include anxiety reduction; improved mood, self-esteem, and quality of life; increases in positive social behaviors; and improvements in cognitive functioning, including alertness, memory, and reality orientation. Although the reasons for music therapy referrals may be similar for older and younger adults, the considerations mentioned previously tend to affect older adults to a greater degree and may make it necessary to adapt music therapy treatment to meet the unique needs of older adults. Table 10.3 shows the outcomes from several studies and meta-analyses in which music therapy treatment was used with patients affected by conditions that commonly result in hospitalization for older adults.

Table 10.3. Older Adult Research		
Population	**Expected Outcomes**	**Research Study**
Cancer	Anxiety reduction Improved mood Improved quality of life Decreased heart rate Decreased respiratory rate Decreased blood pressure Pain reduction	Bradt, Dileo, Grocke, & Magill, 2011
COPD	Improved diaphragmatic breathing Improved mental and social health	Engen, 2005
Dementia	Increase positive social behaviors [a] Improved cognition [b, e] Increased alert responses in late-stage dementia [c] Decreased confusion [e] Decreased stress hormones [d, e, f, g] Improved language skills [e] Decreased irritability [e] Improved ability to control bladder and bowel [f] Decreased agony [f] Decreased paranoid/delusional ideation [f] Decreased systolic blood pressure [g] Increased recall of familiar and new material [h]	[a] Ziv, Granot, Hai, Dassa, & Haimov, 2007 [b] Bruer, Spitznagel, & Cloninger, 2007 [c] Clair, 1996 [d] Kumar et al., 1999 [e] Suzuki et al., 2004 [f] Suzuki et al., 2007 [g] Takahashi & Matsushita, 2006 [h] Prickett & Moore, 1991
Depression	Decreased depression [a, b] Decreased distressed [b] Improved self-esteem [b] Elevated mood [b]	[a] Ashida, 2000 [b] Hanser & Thompson, 1994
Heart disease	Decreased blood pressure Decreased heart rate Decreased respiration rate Pain reduction	Bradt & Dileo, 2009
Osteoarthritis	Decreases in discomfort Improvement in finger strength and dexterity Increased socialization	Zelazny, 2001
Stroke	Improved ambulation [a] Improved swallowing within treatment for dysphagia [b] Decreased depression [c]	[a] Magee, Dileo, Wheeler, & McGilloway, 2010 [b] Kim, 2010 [c] Kim et al., 2011

Evidence-Based Techniques

Many of the music therapy techniques described elsewhere in this book are also recommended for older adults (see chapters by Gooding, Hillmer, and Negrete for descriptions of the techniques). Music-assisted relaxation, the iso-principle, contingent music, active music making, singing, distraction, song writing, lyric analysis, music listening, and counseling techniques all have applications for older adults in medical settings. One approach that has been found to be very helpful with older adults who have dementia is *Validation*. Validation consists of 14 techniques specific to helping older adults in various stages of dementia, one of which includes using music that is familiar to the individual. A full description of the Validation approach can be found in Dr. Naomi Feil's (2002) book, *The Validation*

Breakthrough. A summary of techniques found in the music therapy literature to be effective with older adults is included in Table 10.4.

Table 10.4. Effective Techniques for Older Adults		
Technique	**Outcomes**	**Research Study**
Listening to recorded music	Increases in positive behaviors while under restraints [a] Decreases in repetitive, disruptive vocalizations [b] Decreased episodes of confusion and delirium [c] Increased length of exercise time and decreasing rate of perceived exertion [d]	[a] Janelli & Kanski, 1997 [a] Janelli, Kanski, & Wu, 2002 [b] Casby & Holm, 1994 [c] McCaffrey & Locsin, 2004 Ziv et al., 2007 [d] Thornby, Haas, & Axen, 1995
Music and stress reduction techniques	Decreased depression and distress; elevated mood and self-esteem	Hanser & Thompson, 1994
Therapeutic instrumental music playing	Decreased rate of perceived exertion and perceived fatigue level	Lim, Miller, & Fabian, 2011
Active group music therapy interventions (playing instruments, singing, reminiscing, moving to music, etc.)	Decreased depressive symptoms and increasing interactions. [a] Short-term improvements in cognitive functioning [b] Improvements in neuroendocrine parameters [c] Decreased stress responses; improved language; decreased irritability [d]	[a] Ashida, 2000 [b] Bruer, Spitznagel, & Cloninger, 2007 [c] Kumar et al., 1999 [d] Suzuki et al., 2004
Live music listening	Increased alert responses	Clair, 1996
Active music therapy with family members/caregivers	Decreased psychopathology, dementia problem behavior, agitation, and cognitive problems As negative behaviors decreased, caregivers state anxiety decreased	Brotons & Marti (2003)

Recommendations for Clinical Practice

Music therapy has many potential benefits for older adults in medical settings, but it is important for music therapists to be aware of the individual needs of their older clients. When working with older adult clients who are not able to communicate verbally as the result of dementia or a stroke, determining their music preference can be a challenge. This section will include recommendations on selecting music and music therapy interventions for older adults, as well as suggestions on using nonverbal communication and asking questions appropriate to the individual's level of understanding.

Music Preference

Older adults. Singing and listening activities are preferred by older adults compared to other activities (Gilbert & Beal, 1982; Hylton, 1983). A review of the research literature across the past 30 years reveals subtle changes regarding music preferences of the aging population. Initial research indicated that older adults preferred popular music from their young adult years, the time period when an individual is 18–25 years (Bartlett & Snelus, 1980; Gibbons, 1977; Jonas, 1991). Moore, Staum, and Brotons (1992) found older adults expressed the greatest preference for patriotic music, followed by hymns, popular music from their young adult years, and folk music. In Jonas's (1991) study, older adults most preferred country music, followed by traditional jazz and art music, whereas current popular music was least preferred.

A recent survey indicates that music therapists are using songs that do not adhere to the young adult years hypothesis (Cevasco, VanWeelden, & Bula, in press). Furthermore, a compilation of research indicates older adults have heard, named, preferred to sing, and liked music from before their young adult years "a lot" compared to music from their young adult years (Cevasco & VanWeelden, 2012; VanWeelden & Cevasco, 2009, 2010). The authors suggested music therapists might consider other factors when choosing repertoire for older adults.

Educational level, the size of the community where one grew up, and one's musical training outside of the school setting were factors that influenced musical preference (Jonas, 1991). Participants who grew up in smaller communities and had lower levels of education tended to have higher preferences for country music and current popular music, and higher overall preference scores. Participants who had undergone musical training outside of school tended to have higher preferences for art music.

Jonas (1991) recommended that music therapists working with older adults find ways to give their clients responsibilities, offer choices, and ask for their personal opinions, since many older adults have decreased control. Asking older adults about their musical preferences is also important since various studies on musical preferences of elderly clients have found varying results. Jonas suggested that this could be done either through the use of a formal questionnaire or through informal conversation.

The optimal comfortable singing range for older adults was determined to be between F3 and C5 for women and an octave lower for men (Moore et al., 1992). Vocal range decreased with age, from 20 semitones on average at age 60, to 15 semitones at age 90. Greenwald and Salzburg (1979) found that 75% of older adults had a much narrower range, extending from A# below middle C to G above middle C; they considered this an optimal range to reduce stress and strain on the vocal chords.

Older adults prefer slow tempi over medium or fast tempi, although preferences for tempo may have been related to the types of music used in the study by Moore et al. (1992). With regard to accompanying instruments, older adults reported preferring live singing with autoharp or omnichord accompaniment the most, followed by recorded singing with the melody and chordal accompaniment played on the piano, and recorded singing with basic guitar accompaniment. Participants made negative comments about recorded singing with only the melody played on the piano, as well as recorded singing with a full electronic accompaniment. Results of their study indicated that live singing with an accompaniment that is musically responsive and not too simple is most likely to be preferred by older adults (Moore et al., 1992).

Older adults with dementia and other cognitive challenges. There is not a lot of clinical guidance regarding memory and recall of songs for older adults with dementia, especially when music therapists might encounter individuals who cannot provide preferences due to cognitive challenges. This was evident in a study by Bartlett, Halpern, and Dowling (1995), in which they found healthy elderly participants showed better recognition for traditional tunes than for novel tunes, whereas older adults with Alzheimer's disease showed equally as many "false alarms" in terms of recognition for traditional and novel tunes.

In this situation, music therapists might consult several resources published in *Music Therapy Perspectives*, including song lists for five genres (popular, musicals, patriotic, hymn, and folk music), as suggested by music therapists working with older adults, in the VanWeelden and Cevasco (2007) article. Another source includes songs alphabetically listed by decade from the 1900s to 1960s for four song book series (Cevasco & VanWeelden, 2010). Lastly, a popular song list for working with three subpopulations of older adults (Alzheimer's/dementia, geriatric clients, and well elderly) was compiled by Cevasco, VanWeelden, and Bula (in press), based on suggestions from music therapists.

Regarding instrumental accompaniment, Cevasco and Grant (2006) investigated the effects of instrumental accompaniments on individuals with moderate to severe cognitive decline. They found that singing with a djembe accompaniment or a cappella singing resulted in the greatest number of individuals singing or singing and moving (tapping feet, clapping hands, tapping fingers, etc.) during sessions. Regarding complexity and type of accompaniment, Groene (2001) determined there were more compliments and applause after the live singing versus the recorded sessions for individuals with dementia, and there were significant differences in participants' rates of leaving before and after simple guitar accompaniment sessions; in other words, individuals demonstrated greater participation for reading the lyrics, attention after, compliments after, and applause for sessions involving complex guitar conditions.

When working with individuals with dementia, VanWeelden and Cevasco (2010) recommended singing multiple repetitions of the song to aid individuals in recalling the lyrics. Cevasco and Grant (2006) suggested transposing songs down when songs are in the upper range, especially when songs extend beyond the range suggested by researchers (Greenwald & Salzburg, 1979; Moore et al., 1992).

While several studies have noted that older adults expressed preferences for singing and listening to music (Gilbert & Beale, 1982; Hylton, 1983), a study by Brotons and Pickett-Cooper (1994) indicated that older adults with dementia actually showed greater participation in music activities that involved playing instruments and moving/dancing. They found significantly less participation in composing/improvising than in playing instruments, dancing, or playing games, although participants reported enjoying activities fairly equally. Groene, Zapchenk, Marble, and Kantar (1998) also found that individuals with moderate to severe cognitive decline participated more to exercise-to-music than in singing. Another study confirmed individuals in middle to late stages of dementia participated more in rhythm interventions (83%), followed by movement (51%), and then singing (49%) (Cevasco & Grant, 2006).

In settings in which music therapists use live music during singing, movement, and rhythm-based interventions, participation was highest during a cappella singing (63%), followed by singing with djembe accompaniment (61%), keyboard accompaniment (60%), guitar and djembe accompaniment as well guitar accompaniment (57%), and autoharp accompaniment (54%) (Cevasco & Grant, 2006). It is possible that music therapists might want to monitor the amount of stimulation, especially since a cappella singing, regardless of the intervention, seemed to result in greater participation from individuals with dementia.

Cevasco and Grant (2003) suggested music therapists provide multi-sensory stimulation, in the form of constant auditory and visual cues, to provide meaningful exercise for individuals with dementia. Furthermore, they found that exercising to instrumental music resulted in greater participation than using vocal music. Exercising with instruments to vocal music resulted in the least participation. They believe the vocal music provided competing stimuli to the verbal cues, resulting in less participation. They also stated that the lower participation during exercise with instruments might have been due to the competing response of grasping, manipulating, and playing instruments while also following the music therapist. This includes having individuals reach up and down while playing a maraca or turning from side to side while playing a paddle drum. In other settings, it is possible that playing instruments might motivate individuals to move and engage in exercise.

When designing rhythm interventions, Cevasco and Grant (2006) found that rhythmic accuracy was highest when the therapist used a djembe to present rhythm patterns, followed by a paddle drum, maraca, and then claves. Individuals imitated eight eighth-note patterns the most accurately, followed by four quarter-note patterns and the two eighth notes followed by a quarter note, repeated. Gibbons (1983) suggested simple and repetitive rhythm patterns to provide opportunities for success; however, complex rhythms can be introduced following simple patterns, especially when cues and opportunities to practice are provided (Cevasco & Grant, 2006). Individuals participate longer when playing a drum on their lap versus a drum held in front of them; this is due to the vibrotactile feedback (Clair & Bernstein, 1990).

Brotons and Pickett-Cooper (1994) recommended that music therapists working with older adults employ a variety of activities to engage participants with dementia to stimulate multiple senses and provide novelty in order to maintain interest. In addition, they emphasized the importance of being able to adapt activities for adults with dementia on the spot and the necessity of observing participants' behavior instead of relying solely on their verbal reports of what they prefer, which songs they know, or what they can do. The authors also cautioned music therapists not to let their expectations what clients with dementia can do limit opportunities for their clients to participate in music therapy activities.

Nonverbal Communication

Music therapists are often actively engaged in singing and playing instruments throughout music therapy sessions; thus, careful attention to nonverbal behavior is necessary while therapists are musically engaged. This is especially salient when working with older adults; as people age, their ability to encode and decode changes, possibly due to neurological changes in the frontal and temporal areas (Calder et al., 2003; Ruffman, Henry, Livingstone, & Phillips, 2008; Sprengelmeyer et al., 2003). Recently, a meta-analysis indicated that older adults have problems recognizing emotions (happiness, surprise, anger, sadness, fear, disgust) when examining faces, voices, bodies/contexts, and matching faces to voices (Ruffman et al., 2008). They often take verbal information and restructure the content to match the nonverbal information provided through facial expressions (Thompson, Aidinejad, & Ponte, 2001).

Nonverbal research in health care indicates that professionals' nonverbal behavior not only impacts patient satisfaction, but it also affects long-term cognitive, physical, and emotional well-being (Ambady, Koo, Rosenthal, & Winograd, 2002; Griffith, Wilson, Langer, & Haist, 2003). Cevasco (2010) found that therapists' affect and proximity directly impacted the affect and participation of older adults with dementia. Belgrave (2009) found that expressive touch, defined as touch to communicate support, comfort, and care, was more effective for eliciting and maintain alert behavior states than instrumental touch (touch used to assist an individual with a task) or no contact for the initial session of individuals with late-stage dementia of the Alzheimer's type. Belgrave theorized that patients initially experienced increased alertness at the onset of touch, but across time it might result in relaxation of the individuals and decreased alert rates. Table 10.5 summarizes recommended accommodations that may be helpful when using nonverbal communication with older adults. As noted previously, the changes that occur with age will vary from person to person, and accommodations should be based on the individual's needs.

Table 10.5. Accommodations
Accommodating Changes in Nonverbal Communication

• Utilize changes in affect, but make sure affective state is congruent with content of message.
• Examine body position when working with older adults.
   - Remove barriers between you and the individuals in the room.
   - Engage in closer proximity, including leaning forward, to provide greater increased attentiveness to positively impact communication and enjoyment.
Affect and proximity together had greatest impact on affect and participation of adults with dementia, followed by affect only. Engaging in proximity without affect resulted in less participation and fewer smiles than the no proximity and no affect conditions (Cevasco, 2010).

Table 10.6 summarizes general considerations when designing music therapy interventions for older adults.

Table 10.6. Considerations
General Considerations When Designing Music Therapy Interventions for Older Adults
Musical selections: • Use songs that are familiar and preferred by your patients. • Ask them which genres and/or specific songs they prefer. • If a patient cannot tell you his or her preferred music, ask a family member. • If a family member is unavailable or does not know the patient's preferred music, consider the person's age and select music that would have been popular when he or she was a young adult (between 18 and 25). • See *Music Therapy Perspectives* article by VanWeelden and Cevasco (2007) to find top 10 recommended songs used by music therapists for popular, musicals, patriotic, hymn, and folk music. See Cevasco and VanWeelden (2010) for a list of popular songs and materials music therapists might need when utilizing singing interventions in music therapy sessions; songs are alphabetically listed by decade from the 1900s to 1960s from four song book series. • Popular music (from the early to mid-20th century), patriotic music, country music, and hymns have been found to be highly preferred by older adults in various regions of the United States; however, age and regional variations in preference make it necessary to consider each person's preferences individually. The size of the community where individuals grew up, their level of education, and whether or not they received music instruction outside of school are also factors that influence music preference.
Range: • To encourage patients to sing along, present songs with a range between F3 and C5 for women, and one octave lower for men.
Tempo: • Consider your patient's current status and therapeutic objectives when deciding whether to use fast (stimulative) or slow (sedative) music. • When using the iso-principle, a music therapist matches the tempo of the music to the person's current emotional and physiological state and gradually changes the tempo and character of the music to bring about therapeutic change.
Accompaniment: Use live singing accompanied by: (most to least effective): • Piano with melody and chordal accompaniment • Guitar • Autoharp or omnichord   **For those with dementia (most to least effective):** • A cappella singing • Djembe accompaniment • Keyboard • Guitar or guitar with djembe • Autoharp

Mode of participation:
• Offer multiple ways for patients to participate meaningfully, even if they lack verbal language skills or do not wish to sing.
• Some older adults may be self-conscious about singing in front of others and may be unsure of what to do when asked to compose/improvise.
• Recommended types of musical activities include:
    - Playing musical instruments
    - Moving/dancing to music
    - Playing musical games
    - Singing
    - Listening to music
• Model the desired response, especially for playing instruments or movement/exercise for rehabilitation goals.
• Constantly monitor patient's responses to determine if verbal and/or visual cuing is necessary and when it is overstimulating.
• Utilize active interventions for individuals in late stage dementia,
  including multi-sensory experiences involving touch, singing, and instrument playing.

Talking and reminiscing about music: *Provide opportunities for reminiscence related to music by:* • Asking the patient open-ended questions • Commenting on lyrical content of the song • Commenting on the singer/songwriter • Commenting on historical events that occurred when the song was popular • Using original pictures of sheet music or pictures of items from the time period to cue reminiscing

When talking to individuals with dementia, it is important to ask questions that are appropriate, given their cognitive and communicative abilities. Asking questions that are too challenging can be frustrating and fruitless, whereas asking questions that are too simple will not provide appropriate cognitive stimulation and may be embarrassing for the individual. There are two general categories of questioning: recall and recognition. **Recall** involves retrieving or generating information, such as when answering a fill-in-the-blank or short answer question on a test. **Recognition**, on the other hand, involves selecting the answer from several choices, such as in a multiple choice or true/false question. In general, it is easier to recognize an answer from a limited number of choices than it is to recall an answer without options to choose from. As people age, recall tends to be more difficult than recognition (Salthouse, 2010).

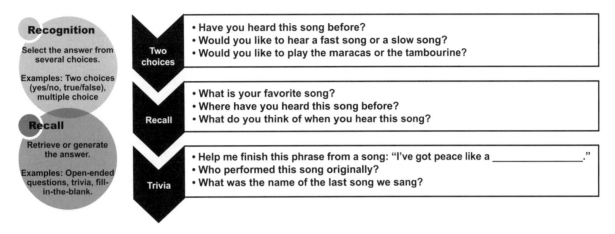

*Figure 10.1.*Recognition and Recall

Caregivers of Older Adult Patients

Loss of functioning that occurs with aging and age-related conditions may make it necessary for older adults to use the services of a full- or part-time caregiver or series of caregivers, particularly when an older adult's ability to perform activities of daily living is impaired. Caregivers are frequently family members. Within the medical setting, spouses, siblings, children, grandchildren, and other family members might be visiting. Family dynamics are quite complex; however, with the complications and stress of hospitalization or a complex diagnosis, caregivers experience a range of emotions. Table 10.7 includes recommendations for working with caregivers of older adult patients.

Table 10.7. Recommendations
Recommendations for Working with Patients and Their Caregivers

Reasons for inclusive music therapy services:
Music therapy services are primarily for the patient, although there are times in which there may be a direct referral for services to assist with family or the initial assessment reveals that direct involvement of the caregiver will assist the overall care of the patient. Specific instances include:
• When caregivers evince extremely high levels of anxiety or stress. Oftentimes, the patients also experience the caregiver's anxiety and stress due to emotional contagion.
• When caregivers experience stress during the transition of a loved one to a new hospital, unit, floor, etc. Stress during transitions usually results in additional staff time and resources being devoted to the family member(s), and the new hospital/unit/floor wants to portray a positive environment. Thus, music therapy can assist the patient and family during the transitional period and portray the new environment in a positive manner.
• When caregivers' personal needs and fears keep patients from learning information about the diagnosis when their loved ones want to be fully informed. Sometimes caregivers project their personal needs and fear onto the patient. At times, withholding information from the patient results in patient fear and poor outcomes.
• When caregivers are experiencing grief, guilt, or distress over the conditions of their loved one. Music therapy can provide opportunities for the caregiver to express emotions that are not easy to discuss.
• When patients and caregivers need to express the unexpressed to each other.
• When caregivers need a positive opportunity to be involved in the patient's care/life. Music therapy can provide opportunities for the family member to feel like a positive part of the patient's life/treatment.

Interventions:
• Utilize a variety of interventions to meet the varying needs of the patient and caregiver.
• Program lyric rewrite and other complex interventions to discuss unexpressed emotions of caregivers and individuals who do not evince cognitive problems.
• Provide opportunities for active engagement (such as playing instruments or moving to music) to gain the greatest participation from individuals with dementia.
• Encourage the caregiver to provide positive tactile (touch) and auditory stimulation (through singing) during music therapy and at other times during the day for individuals who might not be responsive.

Suggestions:
• Always look at and address the patient.
• When necessary, use the caregiver as needed. (e.g., to help you understand a patient's request).
• Based on the referral and initial assessment, determine the patient's individual needs and then determine the caregiver and patient dynamics. Prioritize the goals for the session.
• Sometimes family members are bored and will interject comments into the session and even dominate the conversation. Acknowledge them, but make sure the session is focused on the patient (unless there is a need to give attention to the caregiver).

Conclusion

Older adults face many challenges when undergoing medical treatment, and music therapy is one way to help improve their health care experiences. As author Andrew O'Hagan (2008) once wrote,

> *Empathy with old people is not just a do-gooder's philosophy—it is a form of self-interest. With any luck, we will all have our turn at shuffling down the high street. A culture that does not know how to look after its elderly is a brutal one, a vicious one, and ultimately, a self-defeating one.*

Using music therapy to support the health and wellness of older adults receiving medical treatment not only helps others in the present, it also helps ensure a better future.

References

Abad, C., Fearday, A., & Safdar, N. (2010). Adverse effects of isolation in hospitalized patients: A systematic review. *Journal of Hospital Infection, 76*, 97–102.

Abeles, N. (1998). *What practitioners should know about working with older adults*. American Psychological Association. Retrieved from http://www.apa.org/pi/aging/resources/guides/practitioners.pdf

Ahmed, N., Mandel, R., & Fain, M. J. (2007). Frailty: An emerging geriatric syndrome. *The American Journal of Medicine, 120*, 748–753.

Alzheimer's Association. (2012). 2012 Alzheimer's disease facts and figures. *Alzheimer's & Dementia, 8*, 1–72.

Alzheimer's Association. (2013). What is Alzheimer's? Retrieved from http://www.alz.org/alzheimers_disease_what_is_alzheimers.asp

Ambady, N., Koo, J., Rosenthal, R., & Winograd, C. H. (2002). Physical therapists' nonverbal communication predicts geriatric patients' health outcomes. *Psychology and Aging, 17*, 443–445.

American Psychiatric Association. (2013). *Diagnostic and statistical manual of mental disorders* (5th ed.). Arlington, VA: Author. Retrieved from http://dsm.psychiatryonline.org

Ashida, S. (2000). The effect of reminiscence music therapy sessions on changes in depressive symptoms in elderly persons with dementia. *Journal of Music Therapy, 37*, 170–182.

Bartlett, J. C., & Snelus, P. (1980). Lifespan memory for popular songs. *American Journal of Psychology, 95*, 551–560.

Bartlett, J. C., Halpern, A. R., & Dowling, W. J. (1995). Recognition of familiar and unfamiliar melodies in normal aging and Alzheimer's disease. *Memory and Cognition, 23*, 531–546.

Belgrave, M. (2009). The effect of expressive and instrumental touch on the behavior states of older adults with late-stage dementia of the Alzheimer's type and on music therapists perceived rapport. *Journal of Music Therapy, 46*, 132–146.

Besdine, R. W. (2013). Evaluation of the elderly patient. *The Merck Manual*. Retrieved August 1, 2013, from http://www.merckmanuals.com/professional/geriatrics/approach_to_the_geriatric_patient/evaluation_of_the_elderly_patient.html?qt=ADLs&alt=sh#top

Bradt, J., & Dileo, C. (2009). Music for stress and anxiety reduction in coronary heart disease patients. *Cochrane Database of Systematic Reviews, 2*, Art. No. CD006577. doi:10.1002/14651858.CD006577.pub2

Bradt, J., Dileo, C., Grocke, D., & Magill, L. (2011). Music interventions for improving psychological and physical outcomes in cancer patients. *Cochrane Database of Systematic Reviews, 8*, Art. No. CD006911. doi:10.1002/14651858.CD006911.pub2

Bradt, J., Magee, W., Dileo, C., Wheeler, B. L., & McGilloway, E. (2010). Music for acquired brain injury. *Cochrane Database of Systematic Reviews, 7*, Art. No. CD006787. doi:10.1002/14651858.CD006787.pub2

Brotons, M., & Marti, P. (2003). Music therapy with Alzheimer's patients and their family caregivers: A pilot project. *Journal of Music Therapy, 40*, 138–150.

Brotons, M., & Pickett-Cooper, P. (1994). Preferences of Alzheimer's disease patients for music activities: Singing, instruments, dance/movement, games, and composition/improvisation. *Journal of Music Therapy, 31*, 220–233.

Bruer, R. A., Spitznagel, E., & Cloninger, C. R. (2007). The temporal limits of cognitive change from music therapy in elderly persons with dementia or dementia-like cognitive impairment: A randomized controlled trial. *Journal of Music Therapy, 44*, 308–328.

Calder, A. J., Keane, J., Manly, T., Sprengelmeyer, R., Scott, S., Nimmo-Smith, I., & Young, A. W. (2003). Facial expression recognition across the adult life span. *Neuropsychologia, 41*, 195–202.

Cameron, K. (2004). *Medications: A double-edged sword.* National Center on Caregiving at Family Caregiver Alliance. Retrieved September 12, 2013, from http://www.caregiver.org/caregiver/jsp/content_node.jsp?nodeid=1104

Casby, J. A., & Holm, M. B. (1994). The effect of music on repetitive disruptive vocalizations of persons with dementia. *The American Journal of Occupational Therapy, 48*, 883–889.

Cevasco, A. M. (2010). Effects of the therapist's nonverbal behavior on participation and affect of individuals with Alzheimer's disease during group music therapy sessions. *Journal of Music Therapy, 47*(3), 282–299.

Cevasco, A. M., & Grant, R. E. (2003). Comparisons of different methods for eliciting exercise-to-music for clients with Alzheimer's disease. *Journal of Music Therapy, 40*, 41–56.

Cevasco, A. M., & Grant, R. E (2006). Value of musical instruments used by the therapist to *Music Therapy, 43*, 226–246.

Cevasco, A. M., & VanWeelden, K. (2010). An analysis of songbook series for older adult populations. *Music Therapy Perspectives, 28*, 37–78.

Cevasco, A. M., & VanWeelden, K. (2012). *Older adults' preferences for popular songs from the 1900s–1960s to use in singing activities: An ongoing analysis.* American Music Therapy Association National Conference Research Poster Session, St. Charles, IL.

Cevasco, A. M., VanWeelden, K., & Bula, J. A. (in press). Music therapists' perception of top ten popular songs by decade (1900s–1960s). *Music Therapy Perspectives.*

Clair, A. A. (1996). The effect of singing on alert responses in persons with late stage dementia. *Journal of Music Therapy, 33*, 234–247.

Clair, A. A., & Bernstein, B. (1990). A comparison of singing, vibrotactile, and non-vibrotactile instrumental playing responses in severely regressed persons with dementia of the Alzheimer's type. *Journal of Music Therapy, 27*, 119–125.

Cole, M. G., & Bellavance, F. (1997). Depression in elderly medical inpatients: A meta-analysis of outcomes. *Canadian Medical Association Journal, 157*, 1055–1060.

Coryell, W. (2009). Depressive disorders. Mood disorders. Available from http://www. merckmanuals.com/professional/psychiatric_disorders/mood_disorders/depressive_disorders. html?qt=dysthymia&alt=sh

Doghramji, K. (2008). Insomnia. Sleep disorders. Available from http://www.merckmanuals.com/ home/brain_spinal_cord_and_nerve_disorders/sleep_disorders/insomnia.html

Engen, R. L. (2005). The singer's breath: Implications for treatment of persons with emphysema. *Journal of Music Therapy, 42*, 20–48.

Feil, N. (2002). *The validation breakthrough: Simple techniques for communicating with people with "Alzheimer's-type dementia"* (2nd ed.). Baltimore, MD: Health Professions Press.

Fisk, A. D., Rogers, W. A., Charness, N., Czaja, S. J., & Sharit, J. (2009). *Designing for older adults: Principles and creative human factors approaches* (2nd ed.). Boca Raton, FL: CRC Press.

Fiske, A., Wetherell, J. L., & Gatz, M. (2009). Depression in older adults. *Annual Review of Clinical Psychology, 5*, 363–389.

Foltz-Gray, D. (2012). Most common causes of hospital admissions for older adults. *AARP Bulletin.* Retrieved July 10, 2013, from http://www.aarp.org/health/doctors-hospitals/info-03-2012/ hospital-admissions-older-adults.html

Fong, T. G., Tulebaev, S. R., & Inouye, S. K. (2009). Delirium in elderly adults: Diagnosis, prevention and treatment. *Nature Reviews Neurology, 5*, 210–220.

Geriatric. (2013). In *Merriam-Webster.com*. Retrieved from http://www.merriam-webster.com/ dictionary/geriatric

Gibbons, A. C. (1977). Popular music preferences of elderly people. *Journal of Music Therapy, 14*, 180–189.

Gibbons, A. C. (1983). Item analysis of the primary measures of music audiation in elderly care home residents. *The Journal of Music Therapy, 20*, 201–210.

Gilbert, J. P., & Beal, M. R. (1982). Preferences of elderly individuals for selected music education experiences. *Journal of Research in Music Education, 30*, 247–253.

Giuli, C., Spazzafumo, L, Sirolla, C., Abbatecola, A. M., Lattanzio, F., & Postacchini, D. (2012). Social isolation risk factors in older hospitalized individuals. *Archives of Gerontology and Geriatrics, 55*, 580–585.

Greenwald, M. A., & Salzburg, R. S. (1979). Vocal range assessment of geriatric clients. *Journal of Music Therapy, 16*, 172–179.

Griffith, C. H., Wilson, J. F., Langer, S., & Haist, S. A. (2003). House staff nonverbal communication skills and standardized patient satisfaction. *Journal of General Internal Medicine, 18*, 170–174.

Groene, R. (2001). The effect of presentation and accompaniment styles on attentional and responsive behaviors of participants with dementia diagnoses. *Journal of Music Therapy, 38*(1), 36–50.

Groene, R., II, Zapchenk, S., Marble, G., & Kantar, S. (1998). The effect of therapist and activity characteristics on the purposeful responses of probable Alzheimer's disease participants. *Journal of Music Therapy, 35*, 119–136.

Hanser, S. B., & Thompson, L. W. (1994). Effects of a music therapy strategy on depressed older adults. *The Journal of Gerontology, 49*, P265–269.

Hawkley, L. C., & Cacioppo, J. T. (2007). Aging and loneliness: downhill quickly? *Current Directions in Psychological Sciences, 16*, 187–191.

Heuberger, R. A. (2011). Review: The frailty syndrome: A comprehensive review. *Journal of Nutrition in Gerontology and Geriatrics, 30*, 315–328.

Hooyman, N. R., & Kiyak, H. A. (2008). *Social gerontology: A multidisciplinary perspective* (8th ed.). Boston, MA: Pearson.

Hylton, J. (1983). Music programs for the institutionalized elderly in a Midwestern metropolitan area. *Journal of Music Therapy, 20*, 211–223.

Institute of Medicine. (1991). *Extending life enhancing life: A national research agenda on aging* (E. T. Lonergan, ed.). Committee on a National Research Agenda on Aging. Washington, DC: National Academy Press.

Janelli, L.M., & Kanski, G. W. (1997). Music intervention with physically restrained patients. *Rehabilitation Nursing, 22*, 14–19.

Janelli, L. M., Kanski, G. W., & Wu, Y. W. B. (2002). Individualized music: A different approach to the restraint issue. *Rehabilitation Nursing, 27*, 221–226.

Jonas, J. L. (1991). Preferences of elderly music listeners in nursing homes for art music, traditional jazz, popular music of today, and country music. *Journal of Music Therapy, 28*, 149–160.

Kim, S. J. (2010). Music therapy protocol development to enhance swallowing training for stroke patients with dysphagia. *Journal of Music Therapy, 47*, 102–119.

Kim, D. S., Park, Y. G., Choi, J. H., Im, S. H., Jung, K. J., Cha, Y. A., Jung, C. O., & Yoon, Y. H. (2011). Effects of music therapy on mood in stroke patients. *Yonsei Medical Journal, 52*, 977–981.

Kumar, A. M., Tims, F., Cruess, D. C., Mintzer, M. J., Ironson, G., Loewenstein, D., et al. (1999). Music therapy increases serum melatonin levels in patients with Alzheimer's disease. *Alternative Therapeutic Health Medicine, 5*, 49–57.

Kumar, N. (2007). *Report of Delphi Study to determine the need for guidelines and to identify the number and topics of guidelines that should be developed by WHO.* WHO Normative Guidelines on Pain Management. Geneva. Retrieved September 12, 2013, from http://www.who.int/medicines/areas/quality_safety/delphi_study_pain_guidelines.pdf

Lim, H. A., Miller, K., & Fabian, C. (2011). The effects of therapeutic instrumental music performance on endurance level, self-perceived fatigue level, and self-perceived exertion of inpatients in physical rehabilitation. *Journal of Music Therapy, 48*, 124–148.

Lliffe, S., Kharicha, K., Carmaciu, C., Harari, D., Swift, C., Gillman, G., & Stuck, A. E. (2009). The relationship between pain intensity and severity and depression in older people: Exploratory study 2009. The Cochrane Controlled Trials Register (CCTR/CENTRAL). In *Cochrane Library*, Issue 1, 2012.

Lonergan, E. T., & Krevans, J. R. (1991). A national agenda for research in aging. *New England Journal of Medicine, 324*, 1825–1828. doi:10.1056/NEJM199106203242527

Lopez, M. A. (2008). *Older adults and insomnia resource guide.* American Psychological Association. Retrieved from http://www.apa.org/pi/aging/resources/guides/insomnia.aspx

McCaffrey, R., & Locsin, R. (2004). The effect of music listening on acute confusion and delirium in elders undergoing elective hip and knee surgery. *Journal of Clinical Nursing 13*(S2), 91–96.

Moore, R. S., Staum, M. J., & Brotons, M. (1992). Music preferences of the elderly: Repertoire, vocal ranges, tempos, and accompaniments for singing. *Journal of Music Therapy, 29*, 236–252.

National Center for Health Statistics. (2013). *Health, United States, 2012: With special feature on emergency care.* Retrieved from http://www.cdc.gov/nchs/hus.htm

National Institutes of Health. (2013). *Pain: Hope through research.* Retrieved September 12, 2013, from http://www.ninds.nih.gov/disorders/chronic_pain/detail_chronic_pain.htm#215763084

Nichols, K. A. (2003). *Psychological care for ill and injured people: A clinical guide.* Philadelphia: Open University Press.

O'Hagan, A. (2008, February 12). Ignoring old age won't keep you young. *The Telegraph.* Retrieved from http://www.telegraph.co.uk/comment/columnists/andrewo_hagan/3554902/Ignoring-old-age-wont-keep-you-young.html

Pacala J. T. (2009). Prevention of iatrogenic complications in the elderly. *Geriatrics.* Retrieved September 3, 2013, from http://www.merckmanuals.com/professional/sec23/ch342/ch342e.html

Permpongkosol, S. (2011). Iatrogenic disease in the elderly: Risk Factors, consequences, and prevention. *Clinical Interventions in Aging, 6*, 77–82.

Prickett, C. A., & Moore, R. S. (1991). The use of music to aid memory of Alzheimer's patients. *Journal of Music Therapy, 28*, 101–110.

Robertson, R. G., & Montagnini, M. (2004). Geriatric failure to thrive. *American Family Physician, 70*, 343–350.

Rocchiccioli, J. T., & Sanford, T. S. (2009). Revisiting geriatric failure to thrive. *Journal of Gerontological Nursing, 35*, 18–24.

Rodda, J., Walker, Z., & Carter, J. (2011). Depression in older adults. *British Medical Journal, 343*, 683–687.

Ruffman, T., Henry, J. D., Livingstone, V., & Phillips, L.. (2008). A meta-analytic review of emotion recognition and aging: Implications for neuropsychological models of aging. *Neuroscience and Biobehavioral Reviews, 32*, 863–881.

Salthouse, T. A. (2010). *Major issues in cognitive aging.* Oxford: Oxford University Press.

Saxon, S. V., Etten, M. J., & Perkins, E. A. (2010). *Physical change and aging: A guide for the helping professions* (5th ed.). New York: Springer.

Sprengelmeyer, R., Young, A. W., Mahn, K., Schroeder, U., Waitalla, D., Buttner, T., Kuhn, W., & Przuntek, H. (2003). Facial expression recognition in people with medicated and unmedicated Parkinson's disease. *Neuropsychologia, 41*, 1047–1057.

Suzuki, M., Kanamori, M., Nagasawa, S, Tokiko, I., & Takayuki, S. (2007). Music therapy-induced changes in behavioral evaluations, and saliva chromogranin A and immunoglobulin A concentrations in elderly patients with senile dementia. *Geriatrics Gerontology International, 7*, 61–71.

Suzuki, M., Kanamori, M., Watanabe, M., Nagasawa, S., Kojima, E., & Ooshiro, H. (2004). Behavioral and endocrinological evaluation of music therapy for elderly patients with dementia. *Nursing and Health Sciences, 6*, 11–18.

Takahashi, T., & Matsushita, H. (2006). Long-term effects of music therapy on elderly with moderate/severe dementia. *Journal of Music Therapy, 43*, 317–333.

Thompson, L. A., Aidinejad, M. R., & Ponte, J. (2001). Aging and the effects of facial and prosodic cues on emotional intensity ratings and memory reconstructions. *Journal of Nonverbal Behaviors, 25*, 101–125.

Thornby, M. A., Haas, F., & Axen, K. (1995). Effect of distractive auditory stimuli on exercise tolerance in patients with COPD. *CHEST, 107*, 1213–1217.

U.S. Food and Drug Administration. Council on Family Health. (2012). *Medicines and you: A guide for older adults.* Retrieved from http://www.fda.gov/drugs/resourcesforyou/ucm163959.htm

VanWeelden, K., & Cevasco, A. M. (2007). Repertoire recommendations by music therapists for geriatric clients during singing activities. *Music Therapy Perspectives, 25*, 4–12.

VanWeelden, K., & Cevasco, A. M. (2009). Geriatric clients' preferences for specific popular songs to use during singing activities. *Journal of Music Therapy, 46*(2), 147–159.

VanWeelden, K., & Cevasco, A. M. (2010). Recognition of geriatric popular song repertoire: A comparison of senior citizens and music therapy students. *Journal of Music Therapy, 47*, 84–99.

Werner, C. (2011). *The older population: 2010 census briefs.* Retrieved from http://www.census.gov/prod/cen2010/briefs/c2010br-09.pdf

Zelazny, C. M. (2001). Therapeutic instrumental music playing in hand rehabilitations for older adults with osteoarthritis: Four case studies. *Journal of Music Therapy, 38*, 97–113.

Ziv, N., Granot, A., Hai, S., Dassa, A., & Haimov, I. (2007). The effect of background stimulative music on behavior in Alzheimer's patients. *Journal of Music Therapy, 44*, 329–343.

Chapter 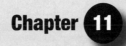 11

Music Therapy in the Emergency Department
Brianna Negrete, MM, MT-BC

As I walked into the emergency department, someone was yelling at a staff member, asking why a doctor wasn't seeing their son. After listening to the conversation, I knew that music therapy could help this child. When I was able to step into the conversation, I asked the nurse and family member if I could provide music therapy for the child. They both agreed, and I entered the examining room. The child just stared at me. He had shut down and would not speak or follow any directions from the staff. They needed him to move his fingers on his broken arm to ensure there wasn't any nerve damage and that the bone was reset properly. The staff asked if I could get him to move his fingers so they wouldn't have to forcibly do it. Learning that his favorite song was "Old McDonald" and knowing that using instruments might overwhelm him, I sang the song and included his favorite stuffed animal he held. He didn't join in, but he followed me with his eyes. After a few minutes of singing, he began to shake his head yes or no when I would ask questions—a definite improvement. When the staff reentered the room, they asked me to test whether he could move his fingers. I began to include body parts in the song: "Old McDonald had some toes . . . with a wiggle wiggle here . . ." He happily wiggled his toes. Feeling I had built a strong rapport with him, I put a shaker in front of his hand of the injured arm. He immediately grabbed it with the fingers that we needed to check and smiled as he started shaking it. Success!

From 1999 to 2009, the number of people visiting the emergency department (ER) increased 32% (Hing & Bhuiya, 2012). Although people of all ages are admitted to the emergency department, the most frequently admitted age range is 25–44 years old (Centers for Disease Control and Prevention [CDC], 2009). Individuals of low socioeconomic status are twice as likely to require ER visits as individuals of higher socioeconomic status (Kangovi et al., 2013). Reasons for coming to the ER vary drastically, but the top three reasons are (a) stomach pains or cramps, (b) fever, or (c) chest pain. The increase in ER visits has led to new challenges, and the CDC identifies the waiting room as one of the areas most affected in the ER (CDC, 2009). Based on 2009 data, the average length of time spent in the emergency department was 4 hours and 7 minutes. There are many concerns related to long wait times in the emergency department, one of which is that patients grow tired of waiting and leave. This results in the patient retuning when the situation has worsened and leads to a more critical emergency than originally presented (American College of Emergency Physicians, 2012).

Music Therapy in the ER

Music therapists in inpatient settings work with patients who have already been admitted and have a better understanding about their situation, or who have contacted family or friends to assist them during this stressful time. The emergency department is a completely different situation, in which people have not planned weeks or days in advance to take time off from work to receive medical care.

Reasons for an ER visit range from the expected—having severe stomach pains, breaking a bone, or having chest pains with symptoms of a heart attack, to the unexpected—for example, a child who has eaten the dog's flea medication. Individuals who cannot obtain timely access to primary care are also likely to visit the ER, resulting in more severe illnesses with complications (Tang, Stein, Hsia, Maselli, & Gonzalez, 2010).

Music therapy in the emergency department is an emerging area and, as such, a limited amount of research is available on the subject. However, there are a number of studies on the use of music in the ER by non-music therapy professionals. (See Young, Griffin, Phillips, & Stanley, [2010], and Short, Ahren, Holdgate, Morris, & Sidhu [2010] for examples.) Some of the earliest music therapy research in the ER involved children receiving (a) intravenous starts/restarts, (b) venipunctures, (c) injections, or (d) heel sticks in an after-hours unit in an ER (Malone, 1996). A more recent study by Barton (2008) involved children in the emergency department undergoing both invasive and non-invasive procedures. In this study, children who had music therapy exhibited fewer negative behaviors during the procedures than did children who did not have music therapy. Additionally, Negrete (2011) studied the effects of music therapy on adults who had been admitted to the emergency department and determined that patients who received music therapy services showed a significant decrease in their pain scores and a significant increase in comfort. Both studies found that 100% of the participants stated they wanted to have music therapy again if they ever returned to the emergency department. Finally, a 2013 study (Hartling et al., 2013) investigated the effect of music selected by a music therapist and played via ambient speakers on children undergoing intravenous placement. Results suggested that the music intervention led to decreased distress scores and decreased pain scores. Parents' satisfaction scores in the music group were different than non-music parents, and the health care providers working with patients in the music group reported it was easier to perform the procedure and they were more satisfied with their work (Hartling et al., 2013). These results suggest that music therapy in the emergency department is an untapped resource that would benefit from additional research.

Reasons for Referrals

Music therapy referrals in the ER can be initiated by a variety of sources, depending on the structure of the music therapy referral system. Figure 11.1 highlights possible referral sources based on referrals received at Tallahassee Memorial Hospital between August 2010 and July 2013. Not only do referral sources vary, but so do reasons for referral. Some common reasons include (a) pain, (b) anxiety, (c) agitation, (d) coping, (e) procedural support, (f) family support, and (g) end-of-life care.

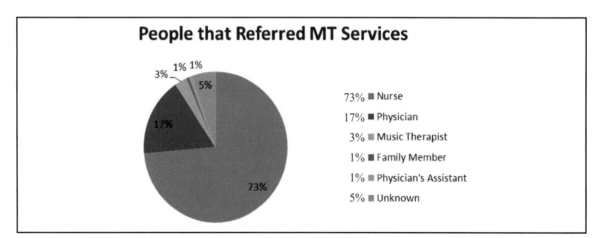

Figure 11.1. Referral sources.

Pain

A typical misconception is that a patient's pain is under control once he or she is admitted to the emergency department. Johnston et al. (1998) surveyed patients who had been admitted to the emergency department and found that a large percentage felt that they left in more pain than when they arrived. When working with patients who have a large amount of pain, many times, especially if the patient is unable to speak, the music therapist must also communicate with caregivers to determine how the patient is handling the pain. It is important to note that one study found that patients rate their pain on a higher level than their caregivers perceive their pain to be (Guru & Dubinsky, 2000). This may be an important factor to consider when addressing pain during music therapy services. In addition, 49% of patients feel no pain relief once in the emergency department.

Pain is one of the most common reasons for music therapy referral in the emergency department. Figure 11.2 highlights data collected from Tallahassee Memorial Hospital from August 2010 to July 2013. As seen in the graph, pain was the second most common referral for music therapy services. Preliminary research suggests that music therapy has the potential to be effective in reducing pain in the emergency department. In fact, Negrete (2011) determined that live music therapy techniques were effective in significantly reducing a patient's perception of pain.

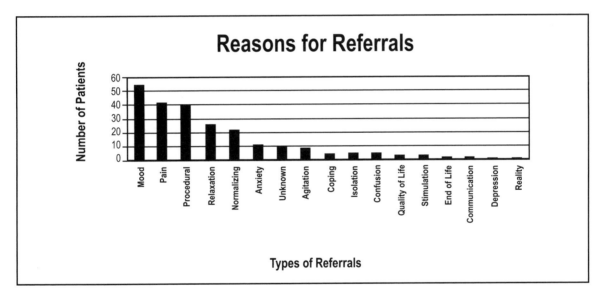

Figure 11.2. Reasons for music therapy referrals in the ER.

Anxiety

According to Yoon and Sonneveld (2010), the top reasons for anxiety in the emergency department waiting room are uncertainty and fear. Music may be able to reduce anxiety in this high-risk area. Holm and Fitzmaurice (2008) found that playing recorded music in the emergency department waiting room significantly reduced anxiety of waiting patients compared to aromatherapy. Although music therapy may not eliminate this anxiety, it can assist in decreasing patients' anxiety and distracting them before they are seen by the doctor. In addition, music therapy can also be used with the families to help reduce their anxiety.

Agitation

Agitation is found in many forms in the emergency department. Often agitation is manifested toward staff members in the emergency waiting room or in a treatment room after admission. An agitated person in the emergency department can have a domino effect. Once one person begins to express his or her concerns and frustrations loudly, suddenly everyone wants to voice issues with the staff and the ER. Music therapy can be very effective in this setting as well. The music therapist can use counseling techniques to listen to and validate what the patient or family member is saying and even assist in helping the patient with that problem.

El-Mallakh et al. (2012) found that crowding in the emergency department waiting area increases the need to use medications or restraints for agitated patients in the waiting room. Staff in the emergency department use different techniques to work with out-of-control, agitated patients, including verbal and/or physical restraints. Sometimes staff can calm down patients by talking to them. If the staff needs to use physical restraint (which is rare, but it does happen), as many as five people or the use of chemical restraints (medication) may be necessary (Gallego, Perez, Aquilino, Angulo, & Estarlich, 2009). A music therapist may be able to distract an agitated patient, avoiding the use of physical or chemical restraints. For this reason, it is beneficial to have music therapy in the emergency department.

Sometimes patients become very agitated because they are confused. Although some are confused before they come to the ER, once they are admitted their agitation increases because they do not understand where they are and why they are there. Many times staff members try to explain what is going on, but because they have numerous patients to help, they cannot focus on one patient for a long period of time. Music therapy has been shown to be effective in reducing agitation in individuals (like those with dementia) who can be confused (Brotons & Marti, 2003).

Coping
Studies by Robb (2000) and Robb et al. (2008) suggest that music therapy interventions can be used to facilitate coping and to encourage coping-related behaviors during difficult medical situations. In the emergency department, patients may face difficult situations, as when given a diagnosis such as cancer or another serious disease. Music therapy can be used during these types of circumstances to address patients' concerns related to their diagnosis. For example, the music therapist may help the patient create an action plan or use lyric discussion to talk through concerns in this beginning stage of the treatment process.

Procedural Support
Providing music therapy during procedural support is another common referral received in the emergency department. With procedural support, staff members can experience firsthand the effectiveness of music therapy, and many times not only do the patients benefit, but so do families and staff (Walworth, 2005). Procedures in the emergency department can vary from non-invasive procedures, such as taking a patient's temperature or having a patient receive an EKG, to invasive procedures like intubations and lumbar punctures. The top three procedures that were performed in the ER in 2009 were (a) IV starts for fluids, (b) placing splints or wraps, and (c) using the nebulizer (CDC, 2009). MacLean, Obispo, and Young (2007) found that even simple procedures can be distressful and accompanied by pain, yet there is a gap between knowledge of effective pain management procedures and actual implementation of these procedures. Music therapy may be an effective pain management tool that does not place additional burden on the medical staff. With this in mind, bringing music therapy to a procedure can only help the patient and provide a more positive outcome.

Procedural support with children. The majority of procedural support experiences are with children, due to the fact that children typically have more anxiety about procedures. As stated previously, one of the earliest music therapy studies in the ER involved IV starts and other procedures (Malone, 1996). Overall, the main goal of procedural support is successful completion of the procedure. If the child needs to remain still for the procedure, the goal for the music therapist is to keep the child still using music-based interventions to distract the child from the procedure. If the child cannot stay still on his or her own, then extra staff is used to keep the child still. This usually involves nurses and nursing assistants holding the child down so that the procedure can be completed. Even if restraining needs to occur, music therapy can play a major role in helping to keep the child (and family, if they are in the room) calm and the situation from escalating so the procedure can be completed.

While nursing staff and physicians prepare for a procedure, the family of the patient can respond in various ways. Boie, Moore, Brummett, and Nelson (1999) surveyed family members of children undergoing invasive procedures in the emergency department. Results suggested that most parents want to be in the room during invasive procedures, although the more invasive the procedure is, the less likely a parent is to express a desire to be in the room. In fact, Beckman et al. (2002) found that the more the invasive the procedure is (e.g., intubations), the less likely the physician is to ask the family to remain in the room. It is important to recognize that the families' wants and needs may change due to the severity of procedure; as a result, it is vital to communicate with the family throughout this process.

Procedural support for adults. Procedural support is also used with adults. As stated earlier, older adults, in particular, may arrive at the emergency department confused about both their medical condition and their surroundings. As a result, procedural support for confused adults may be a possible referral reason. Because the patient is already confused, an unfamiliar person performing an invasive procedure can be extremely frightening or upsetting. Music therapy is an effective way to assist with the procedure and work with the patient so the procedure can be successfully completed.

Family Support

In crisis situations like car accidents, strokes, or heart attacks, patients are often rushed to the trauma area of the emergency department via ambulance. In the trauma area, patients receive immediate care, including surgery and other emergency procedures. When a patient is brought in, a social worker, a police officer, or another staff member notifies the patient's family. When the family members arrive, music therapy can be an effective way to provide family support during that very stressful time. In an ER setting, this may include (a) using counseling techniques to validate the family members and what they are going through, (b) providing music for relaxation, and (c) facilitating communication between the family and staff.

End-of-Life Care

Unfortunately, patients and their families can be faced with end-of-life situations in the emergency department. Because these situations are often crisis-based, the family may not be prepared to handle the situation and the decisions that accompany it. In his work with imminently dying patients, Krout (2003) highlights the ability of music therapists to meet the needs of family members, providing comfort when needed. Consider the following example: A family called EMTs to transport their mother to the emergency department, but they could not handle being in the room during the patient's last moments of life. The music therapist was paged to provide music for the patient. The chaplain was also paged to be with the patient, and the two providers alternated back and forth until the patient died. Sometimes families are not ready to face death, and in this situation, the music therapist was able to support both the family and patient.

Case Example 1: Distraction—When working in the emergency department one afternoon, a doctor asked me, "Are you the music therapist that can help during procedures?" When I answered, "Yes," his response was, "Prove it." The patient was an 8-year-old boy who was having a lumbar puncture, a procedure used most commonly to diagnose meningitis. The child was asked to lie on his side with his legs brought up to his chest. This position is used so the doctor can extract the fluid from the patient's lower spine. I was positioned at the head of the bed next to the child's head. Because his hands were free, he could engage in playing with small instruments with me. I distracted the child with activities that included (a) copying rhythms, (b) naming the instrument, (c) "Simon Says" and (d) filling in the blank in familiar and popular songs. The child was completely engaged with me from the beginning of the session, which made the procedure much easier for the doctor. During the session, the doctor commented that he had never had a child hold so still for this procedure. He then proceeded to invite other staff members to come in and observe the lumbar puncture procedure and describe medically what he was doing to the staff who had never seen the procedure done before. All of this was done as I was distracting this 8-year-old boy using music therapy.

Evidence-Based Techniques

Iso-principle

The iso-principle has been shown to be effective in reducing pain with patients in the hospital (Lee, 2005). The iso-principle utilizes a technique called *entrainment* or the process of matching the energy or pain level of the patient and using music to bring the patient to the pain level or energy level where you want him or her to be. For example, if a patient were screaming in pain, then the therapist would play music very loudly to match the intensity of the patient's pain. Once the pain level has been matched, the music is brought down slowly to bring down the patient's pain through the music. This has been shown to be effective with children after surgery in decreasing pain. Bradt (2001) found that live music combined with the iso-principle with children after surgery resulted in a significant decrease in pain and increase in mood.

Contingent Music

Confused adults are admitted frequently in the emergency department. According to Samaras, Chevalley, Samaras, and Gold (2010), older adults make up about 25% of all visits in emergency departments. The contingent use of music has been shown to be effective in reinforcing therapy objectives (Standley, 1996). Much of the research on contingent music in the medical setting has focused on premature infants (Standley, 2003); however, the concept can be transferred to other medical populations, including the emergency department.

Distraction

A study by Young, Griffin, Phillips, and Stanley (2010) was conducted on the use of music for distraction in the emergency department, although the music was not performed by a board-certified music therapist. The researchers found that using iPods with preferred music helped distract patients who were undergoing painful procedures. In addition, Sinha, Christopher, Fenn, and Reeves (2006) studied the use of various forms of distraction (video games, bubbles, etc.) during laceration repairs with children in the emergency department. Significant reductions in anxiety were found for children older than the age of 10. Additionally, 65% of these children chose listening to music on an iPod as their distracter of choice during the laceration repair. These studies did not include board-certified music therapists; however, music has been shown to be effective in distracting children in the emergency department and preferred by children older than 10 years. Although much of the research has been done with children and distraction in the ER, adults may also benefit from distraction.

Case Example 2: Contingent Music—I was asked by a nurse to help with an older woman who had dementia and was brought to the emergency department by an ambulance from an assisted living center. She had no family or staff with her that she knew, and she did not understand where she was and why someone wanted to give her an IV. The nurse had been trying to start an IV for quite some time; the patient resisted the staff and would not let them near her. I was asked to work with the patient so the staff could put the IV in and give the patient some medicine. When I walked in the room, I immediately introduced myself to the patient and explained who I was. The patient told me her preferred music, and after the first song the patient was singing and reminiscing about the song we just sang. The staff then entered the room and I began to use contingent music to assist staff in getting an IV started for the patient. This meant that I would stop singing when the patient did not do what the staff asked. I first explained exactly what the staff was going to do during the procedure so there would not be any surprises. The staff asked the patient to hold out her arm. When the patient followed the directions and held out her arm for the staff, I continued singing until the patient stopped holding out her arm. When the patient pulled away her arm, I stopped singing until the patient followed the directions given to her by the staff. When the patient held out her arm and followed directions, I continued singing. This process took only one song; by the time it was over, the IV had been started and the patient was happily singing with me. Without the technique of contingent music, this procedure would not have been completed in the emergency department.

Relaxation

Music therapy and relaxation can be done in a variety of ways with different populations. Relaxation may be used with patients to assist them with reducing their stress emotionally or physiologically. Research has also been conducted on reducing stress and increasing relaxation for hospital staff members. Cooke, Holzhauser, Jones, Davis, and Finucane (2007) found that pairing massage with recorded music for nursing staff in the emergency department increased their relaxation and helped in decreasing stress. Hopefully, decreasing staff stress can help decrease stress for patients who interact with the staff.

Case Example 3: Iso-principle—One afternoon I played continuous music in the waiting room per the staff's request because it was a very busy day. There was a middle-aged woman who was wheeled in by a nurse tech. She described being in a significant amount of pain and continued to moan and yell very loudly, sharing with everyone how much pain she was in. After the patient's information was taken, she exclaimed, "Put me next to the girl with the guitar!" The staff happily wheeled the patient toward me and I asked about her preferred music. I then used the iso-principle to take the woman from screaming to no longer screaming to falling asleep. I did this by first playing very loudly to match her volume; then I slowly brought the volume of the guitar and my singing down until I was picking on the guitar and singing softly. Having music therapy in the waiting room provided the patient with a one-on-one music therapy session, which calmed her down and helped her fall asleep. This not only benefited the patient, but also regained some calmness for the other patients and staff in the waiting room.

Case Example 4: Relaxation—Arriving at a hospital via an ambulance can be a very stressful experience, especially for a child, and music therapy and relaxation can help calm not only a patient, but also the attending staff. As I entered the emergency department one day, I could hear screaming in the hallway, and I had a feeling that music therapy would be very effective in whatever situation was taking place. When I walked up to the first unit where the patients come straight from the ambulance, the charge nurse asked me to please help. There was an 8-year-old boy lying on a stretcher as tense as could be, just screaming. I was told that the child had been brought in due to seizures, and that the child had been diagnosed with autism and was nonverbal. The emergency medical technicians (EMTs) who brought the child into the room looked rather frazzled themselves, and as I followed them I turned off the lights in the room to calm the child. Four EMTs were in the room, in addition to the child and me. They needed to stay until they delivered their report. I closed the door to shut out any outside noise, and then I began to hum (a relaxation technique that I have found to be effective). The EMTs immediately became quieter (and started looking calmer themselves), and the child's screaming became more of a cry and a pause rather than a constant scream. I brought out an ocean drum and played the ocean drum's soothing sounds as I continued to hum. The pauses between each of the cries became longer and longer until soon the child was lying still with his eyes closed. When the nurses came into take the patient's blood pressure, I hummed a little louder and quietly cued the staff to remain as quiet as possible, pointing out that the child was no longer screaming. All that could be heard were the calming sounds of the ocean drum and my humming. When family entered the room, the child was no longer screaming and was relaxed and sound asleep.

Recommendations for Clinical Practice

Any emergency department would benefit tremendously by having a music therapist on staff.

Materials

The emergency department is a fast-paced environment in which any type of situation may occur at any time. Figure 11.3 indicates that patients seen between August 2010 and July 2013 at Tallahassee Memorial Hospital ranged in age from 0 to 82. Thus, it is important to be prepared with materials appropriate for both children and adults. A variety of instruments is important and should include small drums and hand percussion. In addition to instruments, familiar children's books, scarves, and puppets are also important to include. Because the music therapist must carry these materials around the emergency department, they need to be as streamlined and lightweight as possible. A music therapist primarily leads one-on-one sessions in the emergency department, so multiples of any one instrument are typically not needed.

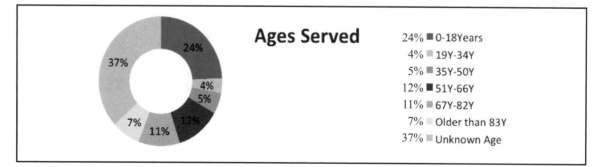

Figure 11.3. Ages served in the ER.

Guitar is the ideal accompaniment instrument for use in the emergency department because of its portability. It allows the therapist freedom to move around the room while playing, which is helpful when trying to stay out of the staff's way. It also provides the flexibility to sit and play, which is needed during a procedure in which the therapist needs to be seated near the patient's face. A therapist must have music memorized; in the emergency department there may be room enough only for the music therapist and the guitar. Having music memorized is necessary to make sessions work and meet the goals of the patient. In addition, it is also important to have a variety of music organized in an iPad or notebook for easy access during a session, to help build rapport with the patient and achieve the goal of using the patient's preferred music.

Scheduling for Music Therapy Service

Understandably, due to the number of music therapists on staff and their various locations throughout the day, adding emergency department patients to a music therapist's caseload could prove to be difficult. Ideally, a music therapist should be scheduled exclusively to the emergency department to handle any referrals. One scheduling solution is to have the music therapist in the emergency department during a specific block of time on a certain day each week. This helps remind the staff that music therapy is there consistently and can provide services for patients during that time. Education about music therapy is a crucial part of working in the emergency department due to the high staff volume. If music therapists devote time to the emergency department, they need to be given appropriate referrals.

In addition, the more a music therapist is present, educating about music therapy and discussing appropriate music therapy referrals, the more likely it is that the staff will page or call the music therapy department during urgent situations. A simple way to encourage this is to provide a one-page summary that explains (a) what music therapy is, (b) what appropriate referrals are, (c) the hours of the music therapist, and (d) contact information. When the music therapist is not constantly in the emergency department, staff may forget that the service is available. An information sheet posted at the nursing station is a friendly reminder for the staff about all that music therapy has to offer and how to contact music therapy.

Referrals

Receiving appropriate referrals in the emergency department varies, based on the type of emergency department and what works best for the staff. At Tallahassee Memorial, the music therapist sought out referrals. After reviewing patients' charts, appropriate referrals were discussed with medical staff. Music therapy was explained briefly and appropriate reasons for referral were highlighted. Suggestions for appropriate patients were also given. Giving specific examples to staff also helps in receiving referrals. For example, explaining that music therapy can assist during procedures such as IV starts, or that music therapy can be provided for patients who are in pain and will not be receiving pain medication soon can help increase the amount and appropriateness of referrals.

Conclusion

Music therapy in the emergency department has many rewards, for both the patient and the therapist. Due to its fast-paced environment, it is not always possible to make the same connections with ER patients as with patients in other departments in the hospital that are seen by the therapist on a day-to-day basis. However, the music therapist still can impact a patient's hospital experience, even though the time spent with the patient is brief.

I learned that this was true at a restaurant one night with a group of friends. I recognized a couple at a corner table as the parents of the boy with the broken arm (see vignette at the beginning of this chapter), but was unable to acknowledge them due to HIPAA regulations. Later in the evening, the couple sent a round of drinks to our table to thank me for what I had done for their son in the emergency department. When they later spoke to me, they said that after I had left their son, he opened up and that they were able to complete more procedures that could not have been accomplished prior to the music therapy session.

The presence of music therapy in the emergency department is powerful. Music therapy in the emergency department can do more to create a positive experience for the staff and patients than any other intervention provided. The emergency department is a growing and developing area for the medical music therapy community. Hopefully, more hospitals and medical music therapists will expand into the emergency department, making a difference for both the patients in the ER and their families.

References

American College of Emergency Physicians. (2012). *Emergency department wait times, crowding and access fact sheet.* Retrieved from http://www.acep.org/uploadedFiles/ACEP/News_Room/ NewsMediaResources/Media_Fact_Sheets/FINAL%20Wait%20Times%20Crowding%20 and%20Access.pdf

Barton, S. (2008). *The effect of music on pediatric anxiety and pain during medical procedures in the main hospital or the emergency department* (Unpublished master's thesis). Florida State University, Tallahassee.

Beckman, A. W., Sloan, B. K., Moore, G., Cordell, W. H., Brizendine, E. J. . . . Geninatti, M. R. (2002). Should parents be present during emergency department procedures on children, and who should make that decision? A survey of emergency physician and nurse attitudes. *Academic Emergency Medicine, 9*(2), 154–158.

Boie, E. J., Moore, G. P., Brummett, C., & Nelson, D. R. (1999). Do parents want to be present during invasive procedures performed on their children in the emergency department? A survey of 400 parents. *Annals of Emergency Medicine, 34*(1), 70–74.

Bradt, J. (2001). *The effects of music entrainment on postoperative pain perception in pediatric patients* (Unpublished doctoral dissertation). Temple University, Philadelphia, PA.

Brotons, M., & Marti, M. (2003). Music therapy with Alzheimer's patients and their family caregivers: A pilot project. *Journal of Music Therapy, 40*, 138–150.

Centers for Disease Control and Prevention. (2009). *National hospital ambulatory medical care survey: 2009 emergency department summary tables.* Retrieved from http://www.cdc.gov/ nchs/data/ahcd/nhamcs_emergency/2009_ed_web_tables.pdf

Cooke, M., Holzhauser, K., Jones, M., Davis, C., & Finucane, J. (2007). The effect of aromatherapy massage with music on the stress and anxiety levels of emergency nurses: Comparison between summer and winter. *Journal of Clinical Nursing, 16*(9), 1695–1703.

El-Mallakh., R. S., Whiteley, A., Wozniak, T., Ashby, M., Brown, S., Colbert-Trowel, D., . . . Terrell, C. L. (2012). Waiting room crowding and agitation in a dedicated psychiatric emergency service. *Annals of Clinical Psychiatry, 24*(2), 140–142.

Gallego, V. F., Perez, E. M., Aquilino, J. S., Angulo, C. C., & Estarlich, M. C. G. (2009). Management of the agitated patient in the emergency department. *Emergencias, 21,* 121–132.

Guru, V., & Dubinsky, I. (2000). The patient versus caregiver perception of acute pain in the emergency department. *The Journal of Emergency Medicine, 18*(1), 7–12.

Hartling, L., Newton, A. S., Liang, Y., Jou, H., Hewson, K., Klassen, T. P., & Curtis, S. (2013). Music to reduce pain and distress in the pediatric emergency department: A randomized clinical trial. *JAMA Pediatrics, 167*, 826–835. doi:10.1001/jamapediatrics.2013.200

Hing, E., & Bhuiya, F. (2012, August). *Wait time for treatment in hospital emergency departments: 2009* (NCHS Data Brief No. 102). Hyattsville, MD: National Center for Health Statistics.

Holm, L., & Fitzmaurice, L. (2008). Emergency department waiting room stress: Can music or aromatherapy improve anxiety scores? *Pediatric Emergency Care, 24*(12), 836–838.

Johnston, C. C., Gagnon, A. J., Fullerton, L., Common, C., Ladores, M., & Forlini, S. (1998). One-week survey of pain intensity on admission to a discharge from the emergency department: A pilot study. *Journal of Emergency Medicine, 16*(3), 377–382.

Kangovi, S., Narg, F. K., Carter, T., Long, J. A., Shannon, R., & Grande, D. (2013). Understanding why patients of low socioeconomic status prefer hospitals over ambulatory care. *Health Affairs, 32*, 1196–1203. doi:10.1377/hlthaff.2010.0825

Krout, R. E. (2003). Music therapy with imminently dying hospice patients and their families: Facilitating release near the time of death. *American Journal of Hospice & Palliative Care, 20*, 129–134.

Lee, H. J. (2005). *The effect of live music via the iso-principle on pain management in palliative care as measured by self-report using a graphic rating scale (GRS) and pulse rate* (Unpublished master's thesis). Florida State University, Tallahassee.

MacLean, S., Obispo, J., & Young, K. D. (2007). The gap between pediatric emergency department procedural management treatments available and actual practice. *Pediatric Emergency Care, 23*(2), 87–93.

Malone, A. B. (1996). The effects of live music on the distress of pediatric patients receiving intravenous starts, venipunctures, injections, and heel sticks. *Journal of Music Therapy, 33*, 19–33.

Negrete, B. (2011). *The effect of music therapy in the emergency department for pain and anxiety management* (Unpublished master's thesis). Florida State University, Tallahassee.

Robb, S. L. (2000). The effect of therapeutic music interventions on the behavior of hospitalized children in isolation: Developing a contextual support model of music therapy. *Journal of Music Therapy, 37,* 118–146.

Robb, S. L., Clair, A. A., Wantanabe, M., Monahan, P. O., Azzouz, F., Stouffer, J. W., . . . Hannan, A. (2008). Randomized controlled trial of the active music engagement (AME) intervention on children with cancer. *Psycho-Oncology, 17,* 699–708.

Samaras, N., Chevalley, T., Samaras, D., & Gold, G. (2010). Older patients in the emergency department: A review. *Annals of Emergency Medicine, 56*(3), 261–269.

Short, A. E., Ahren, N., Holdgate, A., Morris, J., & Sidhu, B. (2010). Using music to reduce noise stress for patients in the emergency department: A pilot study. *Music and Medicine, 5*, 201–207. doi:10.1177/1943862110371808

Sinha, M., Christopher, N. C., Fenn, R., & Reeves, L. (2006). Evaluation of nonpharmacologic methods of pain and anxiety management for laceration repair in the pediatric emergency department. *Pediatrics, 117*(1), 1162–1168.

Standley, J. M. (1996). A meta-analysis on the effects of music as reinforcement for education/therapy objectives. *Journal of Research in Music Education, 440*, 105–133.

Standley, J. M. (2003). The effect of music-reinforced nonnutritive sucking on feeding rate of premature infants. *Journal of Pediatric Nursing, 18*(3), 169–173.

Tang, N., Stein, J., Hsia, R. Y., Maselli, J. H., & Gonzalez, R. (2010). Trends and characteristics of US emergency department visits, 1997–2007. *JAMA, 304*, 664-670. doi:10.1001/jama.2010.1112

Walworth, D. D. (2005). Procedural-support music therapy in the healthcare setting: A cost-effectiveness analysis. *Journal of Pediatric Nursing, 20*, 276–284.

Yoon, J., & Sonneveld, M. (2010, January 25–27). Anxiety of patients in the waiting room of the emergency department. Retrieved from http://tei-conf.org/10/uploads/Program/p279.pdf

Young, T., Griffin, E., Phillips, E., & Stanley, E. (2010). Music as distraction in a pediatric emergency department. *Journal of Emergency Nursing, 36*(5), 472–473.

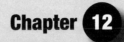

Chapter 12

Music Therapy for End-of-Life Care in the Hospital
Natalie Wlodarczyk, PhD, MT-BC

Hospital work attracts many music therapists because of the range of ages and diagnoses they could potentially encounter. A medical music therapist has the opportunity to work with patients from the cradle to the grave, all in a single day's work, and end-of-life (EOL) care represents the latter part of the continuum. *EOL* is an umbrella term that can take many forms. A music therapist will typically encounter three basic types of EOL patients in the hospital: (a) hospice patients, (b) non-hospice palliative care patients, and (c) non-palliative EOL patients. The terms *hospice* and *palliative care* are often used interchangeably; however, there are distinct differences in the medical care provided for patients in each category. Also, several different situations can result in an individual becoming a non-palliative EOL patient in the hospital, which will be explored further in this chapter. Music therapy interventions used will likely be consistent amongst EOL patients in general (i.e., song writing could be used for a hospice patient and a non-palliative patient). The aim of the first section in this chapter is to explain key differences between the three EOL patient types, such as reasons for hospitalizations, common medical procedures, and legal and ethical considerations. The latter section discusses reasons for music therapy referral, research-based music therapy interventions, and expected clinical outcomes.

Hospice

Hospices care for 1.65 million patients and their families each year (National Hospice and Palliative Care Organization [NHPCO], 2013a). Hospice patients are enrolled in a hospice program that is most often unaffiliated with a hospital. Hospice is a type of palliative care that is widely recognized as the standard of care for those with a life-limiting illness. Hospice employees are considered by the medical community to be experts in pain and symptom management. While all hospice patients are palliative care patients, not all palliative care patients are enrolled in hospice. The term *hospice* refers to a philosophy of care, not a physical place, as hospice patients are most often cared for in their private homes. Patients may also receive hospice care in (a) nursing homes; (b) assisted living facilities; (c) inpatient hospice facilities; (d) correctional, forensic, and psychiatric facilities; and (e) hospitals. Essentially, the hospice staff will visit patients wherever they currently reside (Belgrave, Darrow, Walworth, & Wlodarczyk, 2011).

Though not an exhaustive list, common hospice diagnoses include cancer, Alzheimer's disease, Parkinson's disease, Amyotrophic Lateral Sclerosis (ALS), and heart/lung disease. In order to be enrolled in a hospice program, a patient's doctor and the hospice's medical director must certify that the patient has 6 months or less to live if curative treatment is discontinued and the disease is left to run its normal course. Patients are then recertified every 3 months if the disease progression continues, but can be discharged from hospice care if their prognosis improves. Length of hospice service is not limited to 6 months as long as the patient's disease progression meets recertification standards.

Eligibility requirements should not be confused with length of service; however, in recent years, Medicare has become increasingly strict regarding documentation of patients' decline for recertification. Currently, it is less common to have patients in hospice care for 2 or more years, a frequent occurrence in the past. The Medicare Hospice Benefit, initiated in 1983 under Medicare Part A, is available to patients enrolled in a Medicare-approved hospice program. Currently, over 90% of hospices nationwide are certified by Medicare and must meet their Conditions of Participation for non-curative medical and support services for patients and their families. Medicare pays the hospice program a per diem rate to cover all (and only) the expenses related to the patient's terminal illness. Additionally, Medicare-certified hospices are required to provide all services to any hospice patient regardless of ability to pay, even if the patient is not a Medicare recipient (Centers for Medicare & Medicaid Services, 2013; NHPCO, 2013b).

The overall goal of hospice care is to maintain the highest possible quality of life for each patient for as long as possible (Hilliard, 2005a) with a holistic plan of care—encompassing (a) physical, (b) psychosocial, and (c) spiritual goals of comfort. Thus, hospices utilize an interdisciplinary team (IDT) approach in which several different disciplines work together, each using its own skill set, on the same plan of care for an individual patient. The Hospice Medicare Benefit provides for the following IDT members to work toward these goals: (a) physicians, (b) nurses, (c) home health aides, (d) social workers (typically called family support counselors), (e) chaplains, (f) volunteers, and (g) bereavement counselors. The Hospice Medicare Benefit also provides for the following services: medical equipment and supplies, medication for symptom management and pain relief, and short-term inpatient and respite care (Centers for Medicare & Medicaid Services, 2013; NHPCO, 2013b). Hospice music therapists are considered to be members of the IDT by their hospice coworkers, though they are not covered by the Medicare Hospice Benefit (Wlodarczyk, 2008).

Reasons for Hospitalization of Hospice Patients

Since hospice care is designed to be non-curative, in-home care, it may seem counterintuitive to see a hospice patient in the hospital. However, there are circumstances under which hospitalization of a hospice patient may occur. The first scenario involves miscommunication among the patient's family members. Once admitted to hospice care, patients and family members are instructed to call the hospice if a problem arises, instead of calling 911 for emergency medical services (EMS). Even when the patient's assigned nurse is off-duty, an on-call nurse can always be reached 24 hours a day. Despite this information, family members sometimes panic and call EMS if there is a sudden change in the patient's breathing or pain level, or if an alarming new symptom presents itself (Jones et al., 2012). In other cases, out-of-town family or visitors may call EMS because they are unfamiliar with the protocol. In these situations, the hospice is usually called and a hospice nurse will often meet the patient at the hospital. The patient usually returns home quickly once the symptom has been brought under control.

A more common scenario involves the hospice patient who is admitted to the hospital for symptom management that cannot be controlled at home. In some cases, hospice patients may experience uncontrolled pain, nausea and vomiting, or terminal agitation that requires continuous monitoring or intravenous (IV) medications. Many hospices today have their own inpatient facility or hospice house where this care can take place, but if such a facility is not available or has no open rooms, the hospice patient will be admitted to the hospital for symptom management. If the symptoms can be brought under control, the patient will usually return home and continue routine home care. In some cases, symptoms will remain intense and the patient will die in the hospital (NHPCO, 2013a).

Palliative Care

Palliative care broadens the philosophy of hospice to include a wider range of patients, such as those in earlier stages of their disease process. Palliative care patients may opt for less aggressive treatment, but they generally experience longer survival (Temel et al., 2010). Although both hospice and palliative care teams strive for improved quality of life through pain relief and symptom management, palliative care does not exclude any therapies or treatments (NHPCO, 2013a). Instead, palliative care is designed to work with the primary treatment to ease suffering while treatment is still being received

Chapter 12 • Music Therapy for End-of-Life Care in the Hospital 193

that seeks to cure the illness. This includes reducing common treatment side effects such as pain and nausea (National Institute of Nursing Research, 2009). Palliative care is characteristically provided in the hospital after a doctor's referral to the palliative care team, which is similar to the hospice IDT in that several disciplines work together on the same goals for the patient. Most types of insurance, including Medicare and Medicaid, will cover palliative care in the hospital. If the patient is no longer responding to curative treatments or all other options have been exhausted, palliative care patients are usually discharged from the hospital and sent home with hospice care (National Institute of Nursing Research, 2009; NHPCO, 2001, 2013a).

Comfort measures only. Some palliative care patients in the hospital may reach a point at which treatment is no longer a viable option, but rather than going home with hospice care, they remain in the hospital as a comfort-measures-only or comfort-care-only patient. Some hospitals view these to be outdated terms and prefer the broader term of *palliative care*. There also seems to be a lack of consensus on the usage and definitions of these terms among hospital staff, but despite the inconsistencies, *comfort measures only* would indicate that curative treatment has been discontinued in favor of pain and symptom management in the hospital (L. Camire, personal communication, June 27, 2013; J. McNaughten, personal communication, June 27, 2013; Zanartu & Matti-Orozco, 2013). However, research suggests that patients who receive orders for palliative care instead of comfort measures only have better outcomes regarding pain and symptom management at the end of life (Walker, Nachreiner, Patel, Mayo, & Kearney, 2011; Walker, Peltier, Mayo, & Kearney, 2010).

Non-Palliative End-of-Life

The reality is that any patient admitted to the hospital could potentially become an EOL patient. While hospice and palliative care patients are diagnosed with a terminal or life-limiting illness, non-palliative EOL patients are usually fighting for survival until the last moment of life. These patients usually die suddenly, often without affording time for traditional palliative care interventions (Mosenthal & Murphy, 2003). A variety of critically ill or injured patients fall into this category. Examples include heart attack and stroke patients in the intensive care unit (ICU), patients who experience complications from surgery or childbirth, trauma patients resulting from accidents or natural disasters, and victims of violence. Studies show that 10 to 20% of trauma patients admitted to hospital will die from their injuries (Mosenthal et al., 2008). Many of these patients are previously healthy individuals whose deaths are neither expected nor peaceful. While palliative care embraces a holistic approach toward managing the last phase of life, hospital staff must make rapid decisions intended to prolong the lives of critically ill or injured patients, no matter the risk (Jacobs, Burns, & Jacobs, 2010; Mosenthal & Murphy, 2003; Mosenthal et al., 2008).

Heroic measures and life support. In these cases of critically ill or injured patients, doctors and nurses often intervene with heroic measures. Simply put, heroic measures are risky last-resort procedures that could potentially harm the patient, yet without these procedures, the patient has no chance of survival. *Cardiopulmonary resuscitation* (CPR), emergency surgery or amputation, intubation, and defibrillation are common examples. When life-saving treatments are unsuccessful, patients often die with painful symptoms or are placed on some type of life support (Walling et al., 2010), which can be counterintuitive to the palliative care philosophy of safeguarding quality of life.

Life support is a broad term that includes several interventions meant to sustain life. One type of life support, intubation, involves inserting an endotracheal tube in the patient's windpipe in order to maintain an open airway or to provide mechanical ventilation when a patient can no longer breathe on his or her own. A second type of life support, heart and lung bypass machines, can temporarily take over the functions of the heart and lungs. Additionally, tube feeding can provide hydration and nutrition to patients indefinitely (American Thoracic Society, 2013a, 2013b; Wong, 2004).

Ethical dilemmas often arise when patients survive as a result of heroic measures, only to exist with poor quality of life (D'Amico, Krasna, Krasna, & Sade, 2009; Gerstel, Engleberg, Koepsell, & Curtis, 2008; Hite & Weiss, 2003; Jones et al., 2012; Mosenthal et al., 2008; Walling et al., 2010). Studies show that a high percentage of patients spend their final days in the ICU on life support because doctors did not understand their resuscitation preferences (Walling et al., 2010). CPR, first introduced in the 1960s, can result in broken ribs and further trauma to the body, especially in patients over the age of 60 (Hite & Weiss, 2003; Mosenthal & Murphy, 2003). Mechanical ventilation can result in collapsed or damaged lungs and also carries a high risk of infection since the endotracheal tube in the windpipe makes it much easier for bacteria to enter the lungs (American Thoracic Society, 2013a). Many critically ill patients who are put on a ventilator will never be able to breathe on their own. In these cases, the ventilator is only prolonging inevitable death, and the patient is now considered an EOL patient (American Thoracic Society, 2013b; Gerstel et al., 2008).

Withdrawal of life support. Studies have shown that the majority of critically ill patients dying in the ICU have some form of life support withdrawn before death, yet there is no consistent pattern regarding when and how these decisions are made for the patient (American Thoracic Society, 2013b; D'Amico et al., 2009; Gerstel et al., 2008; Mosenthal & Murphy, 2003). Withdrawal of life support is not the same as causing the patient's death, nor is it considered physician-assisted suicide or euthanasia. Simply put, it is removing artificial means of sustaining life and allowing natural death to occur (American Thoracic Society, 2013b). Structured communication between patients, families, and physicians is paramount in reaching an early consensus regarding EOL decisions, which leads to better outcomes for both the patient and family (Limehouse, Feeser, Bookman, & Derse, 2012; Mosenthal et al., 2008).

The decision to withdrawal life support is naturally very traumatic for family members, especially if the patient is non-responsive and the family is unsure as to the patient's final wishes (Gerstel et al., 2008; Quinn et al., 2012). Again, as many trauma and critical care patients are young and were previously healthy, discussion of EOL preferences with family members have rarely occurred prior to hospitalization (Mosenthal & Murphy, 2003). Older adult patients are more likely to have advance directives in place to indicate their wishes to their family, but age does not necessarily ease the burden of the decision (Jones et al., 2012; Mosenthal & Murphy, 2003). Increasingly, doctors suggest a compromise of removing one life support measure at a time over a period of several days, rather than all at once, to minimize the trauma for the patient's family. This practice, commonly referred to as sequential withdrawal, may also improve the family's satisfaction with their hospital experience (Gerstel et al., 2008; National Institutes of Health, 2008). Palliative care is usually administered both during and after the withdrawal of life support. Table 12.1 summarizes the types of end-of-life care provided in the hospital setting.

Advance Directives

The knowledge of whether an individual would want heroic measures or specific types of life support can save family members the excruciating task of having to make those decisions for them (Limehouse et al., 2012). *Advance directives* are legal written documents that provide instructions to doctors regarding the specific medical care that patients would wish to receive in the event that they are unable to communicate or make those decisions for themselves. The best time to complete advance directives is when a patient is healthy so that their true wishes can be carefully considered.

Legal requirements for advance directives vary from state to state, but most states require that the documents be signed in the presence of one or more witnesses. It is also important to understand that some states may not recognize advance directives from other states, which may cause problems (i.e., a patient is critically injured while vacationing in a state in which they do not reside). There are two types of advance directives: a living will and a durable power of attorney, also known as a medical power of attorney. Since a living will may not cover every medical situation that could arise, it is sensible for a patient to have both legal documents in place (American Cancer Society, 2013a; Mayo Clinic, 2013; National Cancer Institute, 2013).

Living wills. Living wills are legal written documents that clearly outline what types of medical treatment that individuals do or do not want in the event that they cannot communicate. The most common medical treatments that are addressed in living wills are the use of CPR, ventilators, respirators, dialysis, tube feeding, and organ and tissue donation. Sometimes a *Do Not Resuscitate* (DNR) order is included in a living will; however, a living will is not required in order to have a DNR. Instead, a DNR can simply be a stand-alone document in the patient's medical chart. A DNR instructs the medical staff to not perform CPR if the patient's breathing or heartbeat stops (American Cancer Society, 2013a; Hite & Weiss, 2003; Mayo Clinic, 2013; National Cancer Institute, 2013).

More about DNR. A DNR is not required for hospice or palliative care to be initiated; however, most hospice patients are strongly encouraged to have a DNR on file within several weeks of admission. Although rules vary from hospice to hospice, some hospice nurses are not permitted to perform CPR even if a DNR is not on file. In these situations, the patient's family would have to call EMS if they wanted the patient to be resuscitated (NHPCO, 2013a). Non-hospice palliative care patients may have a DNR on file, but it is much less likely that a trauma or ICU patient would come into the hospital with a DNR already in place, unless he or she is an older adult (Jones et al., 2012; J. McNaughten, personal communication, June 27, 2013).

Additionally, there is growing interest from the medical community for the language to be changed from *Do Not Resuscitate* to *Allow Natural Death*. Those who advocate for the language change propose that *Allow Natural Death* (AND) focuses on what the medical staff is going to do, rather than what they are *not* going to do. Opponents of the change posit that *AND* is too ambiguous and may create confusion regarding what medical interventions will and will not be given. Despite the dissent, some hospitals are already using DNR and AND interchangeably. Some initial studies report that both patients and family members are more open to the language of the AND versus the DNR, suggesting that semantics do influence a patient's willingness to sign the order (Chen & Youngner, 2008; Hite & Weiss, 2003; Reed, 2009; Venneman, Narnor-Harris, Perish, & Hamilton, 2006).

The Five Wishes document. Though other types of advance directives vary from state to state, 42 states currently recognize a type of living will called *The Five Wishes* document. This document covers a wider range of situations in addition to EOL, including short-term unconsciousness or cognitive impairment due to Alzheimer's disease or other types of dementia. The Five Wishes document outlines a patient's wishes in five areas: (1) who should make health care decisions for the patient if he or she cannot, (2) the type of medical treatment a patient wants, (3) comfort preferences, (4) how the patient wants to be treated, (5) and what the patient would like their family to know. This document has gained popularity due to its straightforward language and the ease with which it can be filled out (Aging with Dignity, 2012).

Durable power of attorney. A *durable power of attorney*, also known as a medical power of attorney or a health care proxy, is a legal document used to name an individual who will make health care decisions for the patient in the event that he or she is unable to do so. A power of attorney is not only practical for EOL decisions; the document goes into effect in any situation that may arise in which a doctor determines that the patient is unable to make medical decisions (American Cancer Society, 2013a; Hite & Weiss, 2003; Mayo Clinic, 2013; National Cancer Institute, 2013).

Table 12.1 provides a summary of the different types of advance directives.

Table 12. 1. Types of Advance Directives	
Advance Directive	**Description**
Living Will	
Do Not Resuscitate Order	Instructs not to perform CPR if the patient's breathing or heart-beat stops
The Five Wishes Document	Outlines patient's wishes in five areas
Durable Power of Attorney	
Medical Power of Attorney	Legal document naming an individual who will make health care decisions
Health Care Proxy	

Most Americans participate in the death-denying culture that society has created over time (Worden, 2009). It is problematic that EOL patients and their family members rarely discuss decisions regarding the last phase of life until it becomes necessary. Hospice patients, non-hospice palliative care patients, and non-palliative EOL patients may have different reasons for hospitalization, but many of their needs and symptoms will be similar. It is beneficial for music therapists who encounter these patients to have a basic understanding of advance directives and life support options so that they can anticipate probable phases of treatment during the course of hospitalization. Understanding the weight of the decisions patients must make in their final days can be advantageous when planning individual music therapy treatment. The next section of this chapter will explore research-based interventions music therapists could apply for EOL care in the hospital. Additionally, recommendations for clinical practice will be addressed for physical, psychosocial, and spiritual goals.

Music Therapy for End-of-Life Care in the Hospital

Over the last three decades, music therapy has become a valued discipline in EOL care (Bradt & Dileo, 2010; Mandel, 1993; Munro & Mount, 1978; O'Callaghan, 2009). Hospice has become one of the fastest growing job markets for music therapists (Belgrave et al., 2011; Berger, 2006; Hilliard, 2005a, 2005b). Additionally, hospital palliative care teams make frequent referrals for medical music therapy (O'Callaghan, 2009; O'Kelly, 2007). The positive outcomes of music therapy have been documented in the literature for the physical, psychosocial, and spiritual needs of patients with a life-limiting illness (Belgrave et al., 2011; Bradt & Dileo, 2010; Hilliard, 2005a, 2005b; O'Callaghan, 2009). Music therapy has shown to be effective in (a) reducing perception of pain and improving physical comfort, (b) improving mood, (c) reducing fatigue, (d) facilitating relaxation, (e) increasing self-expression, and (f) promoting spiritual well-being for EOL patients (Belgrave et al., 2011; Hilliard, 2005a, 2005b; O'Kelly, 2007). Music therapists use their distinctive ability to blend live patient-preferred music interventions and counseling skills to enhance each patient's plan of care and contribute to an overall improved quality of life in the last phase of life (Abbott, 1995; Belgrave et al., 2011; Choi, 2010; Hilliard, 2003, 2005a, 2005b; O'Kelly, 2007).

Reasons for Music Therapy Referral

EOL patients in the hospital experience a wide range of multidimensional symptoms that are best understood when categorized into three goal areas: (a) physical, (b) psychosocial, and (c) spiritual (Belgrave et al., 2011; Hilliard, 2005a; O'Callaghan, 2009). Medical music therapists may receive referrals for several different objectives from one or more goal areas. All music therapy goals and objectives for EOL patients in the hospital should be consistent with the hospice and palliative care philosophy of primarily providing comfort. The following sections will explore each goal area and outline appropriate objectives for a music therapy referral. All goal areas fall under the larger umbrella category of improved quality of life, a key concept of EOL care (Abbott, 1995; Belgrave et al., 2011; Choi, 2010; Hilliard, 2003, 2005a, 2005b; O'Callaghan, 2009; O'Kelly, 2007).

Physical goals. Although EOL care embraces a holistic (i.e., physical, psychosocial, and spiritual) approach, dying is predominantly a physical process. "I'm not afraid of dying; I'm afraid of being in pain" is a common sentiment heard from EOL patients (DiMaio, 2010, p. 106). When patients are invited to discuss their personal goals and fears in terms of comfort at the end of life, they will often share physical goals first as a result of this pervasive fear (Anderson, Kools, & Lyndon, 2013; Nissim et al., 2012). EOL patients may experience (a) pain, (b) discomfort, (c) nausea, (d) vomiting, (e) anxiety, and (f) agitation. While anxiety and agitation have emotional components, they also produce physical symptoms such as (a) shortness of breath, (b) heart palpitations, (c) restlessness, and (d) insomnia. Unfortunately, many patients enter into a cycle of pain and anxiety; they experience pain, which makes them feel anxious, and they become increasingly more anxious as they anticipate more intense pain.

Music therapy referrals are common for physical objectives such as (a) decreased perception of pain, (b) decreased discomfort, and (c) increased relaxation (DiMaio, 2010; Groen, 2007; Hilliard, 2001, 2005a, 2005b; O'Callaghan, 1996b). EOL patients in the hospital will often be removed from life support, such as mechanical ventilation, and music therapists can be referred for procedural support during extubation (Orellano, 2009).

Physical signs of imminent death. As EOL patients get closer to the moment of death, there will be physical changes in the body that will indicate that death is imminent. Hospice organizations actually refer to actively dying patients as imminent patients to indicate that death is imminent (Krout, 2003). Patients near death may sleep progressively more, until periods of wakefulness are infrequent. They often become non-responsive in their final days or hours; this is especially characteristic of cancer patients. Changes in breathing patterns may also occur. Some patients exhibit patterns of shallow, irregular breaths, with periods of no breath that can last up to 30 seconds long. This pattern of breathing can be especially disturbing for the family, as they must continuously wonder if the last breath has taken place. Breathing may also become noisy as mucous and secretions build up in the lungs and throat; this is the explanation behind the colloquial term "death rattle." This type of breathing can be disconcerting for the patient's family, but is usually not painful for the patient (American Cancer Society, 2013b; Haskins, Reilly, & Wlodarczyk, 2007; Krout, 2003). Music therapists can be referred to increase relaxation in EOL patients, which can have a positive effect on irregular breathing common with the dying process.

As the body begins the process of shutting down, it needs less nutrition and hydration, so it is common for appetite and fluid intake to decrease at the end of life. Urine output and bowel movements also become less frequent as a result of the decreased liquid and food intake. Within days of death, the patient's urine will also become exceedingly concentrated and dark in color; this can be a visible indicator of approaching death if the patient is using a Foley catheter and urine collection bag. The patient's body temperature may fluctuate, and his or her physical appearance can change dramatically from day to day as skin becomes taut due to dehydration (American Cancer Society, 2013b; Haskins et al., 2007; Krout, 2003). Again, music therapists are referred for relaxation for the patient and also emotional support for the family as these physical changes take place.

Psychosocial goals. EOL patients need an abundance of emotional support as they contemplate the end of their lives. As described previously in this chapter, some EOL patients in the hospital will already be hospice patients who may have been struggling with a terminal illness for quite some time, while other patients may be facing the end of their lives abruptly • as a result of trauma or a sudden illness. The emotional state and acceptance level of each EOL patient will largely depend on the circumstances surrounding their illness and hospitalization. Patients with long-term illness will often go through emotional stages as they face their mortality, such as in Kübler-Ross's stages of (a) denial, (b) anger, (c) bargaining, (d) depression, and (e) acceptance (Belgrave et al., 2011). EOL patients who face death unexpectedly due to trauma or sudden illness will obviously not have much time to process their feelings and emotions, nor will their family members. Psychosocial reasons for music therapy referral in hospitalized EOL patients include emotional support, opportunities for self-expression and relationship completion, anxiety reduction, opportunities to process loss of autonomy and control, and caregiver bonding (Hilliard, 2005a; Krout, 2005; Nguyen, 2003; O'Callaghan, 1996a, 1997, 2008, 2009; Whitall, 1991; Wlodarczyk, 2009).

Psychosocial signs of imminent death. It is normal for EOL patients to become increasingly withdrawn, confused, or restless as they near death (Callanan & Kelly, 1992). Patients may also begin to exhibit behaviors and communication styles that seem atypical. Some patients claim that they see or hear deceased family members. This is usually not frightening for the patient and can actually be a comforting experience as they transition away from the living. It is also common for patients to talk of travel or transportation, such as the need to catch a train, bus, or boat. It is important not to contradict the patient; instead, ask patients to tell you more about what they are experiencing and reassure them that everything will be taken care of (Callanan & Kelly, 1992; Wlodarczyk, 2007).

Spiritual goals. There is a natural connection between spirituality and the end of life (Foxglove & Tyas, 2000; Wlodarczyk, 2007). Regardless of spritiual background, EOL patients commonly explore questions about the meaning of life, what will happen to them when they die, and whether there is an afterlife. Patients will also contemplate whether they were a "good person" and whether their lives had meaning. In some cases, patients or family members will express anger at a higher power for allowing them to get sick or become injured. Hospital chaplains and the patient's own spiritual leader are best equipped to address these types of concerns; however, music therapists commonly receive referrals for goals such as (a) increased spiritual support through music, (b) opportunities for worship, and (c) opportunities for spiritual self-expression (Belgrave et al., 2011; Foxglove & Tyas, 2000; Wlodarczyk, 2007). Table 12.2 provides a summary of the physical, psychosocial, and spiritual signs of imminent death.

Table 12. 2. Signs of Imminent Death		
Physical	**Psychosocial**	**Spiritual**
Increased sleep; may become non-responsive	Withdrawal, confusion, or restlessness	Question the meaning of life, the afterlife
Changes in breathing pattern/body temperature	Atypical communication	
Decreased need for nutrition/hydration	May see/hear deceased relative	
Decreased urine output; dark in color	Symbolic talk of travel	
Skin becomes taut		

Evidence-Based Interventions and Recommendations for Clinical Practice

Music therapy interventions for physical goals. Music therapists do not claim to cure physical ailments; however, music can help in many ways to alleviate physical symptoms such as (a) pain, (b) discomfort, (c) anxiety, (d) restlessness, (e) agitation, and (f) nausea. Since music therapy interventions will typically be consistent regardless of the patient's specific EOL diagnosis, the following section categorizes interventions by symptoms rather than diagnoses. Yet, it is important to remember that each patient must be treated as an individual—what benefits one may not benefit all. By and large, there is substantial research that indicates music therapy is a valuable treatment modality for the physical goals of EOL patients (Groen, 2007; Hilliard, 2001, 2005b; Krout, 2001; O'Callaghan, 1996b, 2009).

Pain and anxiety. Pain is a subjective experience, influenced by a variety of demographic and historical factors (DiMaio, 2010; Groen, 2007; O'Callaghan, 1996b; Standley, 2000). Pain can range from mild to severe and can be acute (lasting a relatively short time) or chronic (present for long periods of time). Pain assessment is commonly done using a numeric rating scale (i.e., patients are verbally asked to rate their pain level on a scale of 1–10). Music therapists routinely incorporate formal pain assessment into their sessions (Groen, 2007), typically at the beginning and again at the end to measure any change that has taken place. Because perception of pain is subjective, music therapists should note that a pain rating of 10 for one patient could be equivalent to a pain rating of 3 for another.

There are several verbal and nonverbal indicators of pain to watch for, including (a) crying/ yelling, (b) grimacing/wincing, (c) furrowed brow, (d) clenched fists, (e) touching/holding a body part, (f) restlessness, and (g) irritability. Pain may also manifest as agitation or combativeness, particularly in lower-functioning patients. There is also an emotional component to pain that may cause patients to feel anger, depression, irritability, or mood swings, or have suicidal thoughts. In accordance with the holistic approach to palliative medicine, research suggests that pain will be resistant to standard treatment if emotional issues are not addressed (Groen, 2007).

Music therapy can enhance the patient's pain management plan to aid in maintaining a balance between comfort and alertness (Bailey, 1986; Gfeller, 2008; Krout, 2001). Many EOL patients initially resist high doses of pain medication because they are afraid of becoming addicted, although this could be considered a non-issue at the end of life. Additionally, patients worry that pain medication will make them too drowsy to make decisions or to have quality interactions with family members. To address these concerns, the palliative care team, including the music therapist, seeks an optimal regimen of pain medication that meets each patient's individual needs.

Although it is widely accepted that listening to preferred music can increase pain tolerance (Beck, 1991; Mitchell & MacDonald, 2006; Mitchell, MacDonald, Knussen, & Serpell, 2007; Trauger-Querry & Haghighi, 1999), it is not an equally successful technique in all contexts. Specifically, music is most effective for mild to moderate pain, becoming less effective as pain becomes severe (Standley, 2000). According to Gfeller (2008), music can contribute to pain and anxiety management in four ways: (a) as a stimulus for focus of attention or distraction, (b) to facilitate relaxation, (c) as a masking agent, and (d) as a positive environmental stimulus (p. 319). Live patient-preferred music can redirect attention from pain and function as a distraction during the time between the delivery of medication and relief. Using the iso-principle to facilitate relaxation can also assist with pain management through the principles of music therapy entrainment (DiMaio, 2010). Promoting both a physical and emotional relaxation response through music can, in effect, reduce patients' perception of pain, elevate mood, and improve their sense of control (Groen, 2007; Krout, 2001; Kwekkeboom,

2003; Lee, 2005; Longfield, 1995; Magill, 2001; Magill-Levreault, 1993; Michel & Chesky, 1995; O'Callaghan, 1996b). There has also been some investigation into the practice of patients engaging in singing to enhance coping with chronic pain (Kenny & Faunce, 2004); however, this may not be a practical intervention for hospitalized EOL patients with acute pain.

A survey by Groen (2007) identified music therapy interventions and techniques most commonly used to address pain in the hospice setting. Respondents cited music listening for relaxation as the primary intervention used by music therapists for pain management. Additional techniques cited were (a) music as distraction, (b) music paired with deep breathing, (c) music-assisted progressive muscle relaxation (PMR), and (d) music-assisted cognitive reframing. Meditation, autogenics, and guided imagery were also mentioned as viable techniques. Furthermore, Groen (2007) found that music listening was most often used for chronic pain, while music as distraction was most often used for acute pain. It is more likely that critically ill and injured patients in the hospital will be experiencing acute pain; therefore, medical music therapists should be skilled in the use of live, patient-preferred music to distract, relax, and focus attention away from pain.

It is difficult to discuss music therapy interventions for pain and anxiety separately, since the two symptoms are closely related and often intertwined. Again, the aforementioned cycle of pain and anxiety is common for EOL patients. Gfeller's (2008) above functions of music for pain and anxiety management suggest that the iso-principle can be used to systematically decrease symptoms of anxiety, agitation, and restlessness by promoting a relaxation response (Curtis, 1986; Hilliard, 2001; Horne-Thompson & Grocke, 2008; Kim, 2006; Krout, 2001). Additionally, live music can serve as a positive focus of attention away from anxiety-producing stimuli. Music therapists should recognize the importance of uncovering and addressing the source of patients' anxiety rather than simply treating its physical manifestations. It is also critical to recognize the need for music therapists to be effective in a single EOL session, as the possibility exists that there may not be additional sessions (Calovini, 1993; Horne-Thompson & Grocke, 2008; Krout, 2001).

Terminal extubation. Medical music therapists routinely provide procedural support, primarily by using live patient-preferred music as distraction during painful or anxiety-inducing procedures (Hunter et al., 2010; Walworth, 2005). One common procedure is extubation, which is the removal of the endotracheal tube from the patient's windpipe that was used to provide mechanical ventilation. This type of removal of life support is referred to as *terminal* extubation when it is understood that the patient will die within minutes to hours as a result (Campbell, Bizek, & Thill, 1999; Orellano, 2009; Willms & Brewer, 2005). Procedural support for terminal extubation is a common reason for music therapy referral in EOL care (Hunter et al., 2010; Orellano, 2009; R. Moats, personal communication, July 10, 2013; J. Peyton, personal communication, June 19, 2013).

Existing research has demonstrated that the use of music and music therapy can reduce stress and anxiety in hospitalized patients receiving mechanical ventilation (Chlan, Engeland, Anthony, & Guttormson, 2006; Chlan & Heiderscheit, 2009; Chlan, Tracy, Nelson, & Walker, 2001; Korhan, Khorshid, & Uyar, 2011; Lee, Chung, Chan, & Chan, 2005), as well as assist with the weaning process (Hunter et al., 2010). To date, only one study has explored the use of music therapy for terminal extubation (Orellano, 2009). This post-hoc analysis investigated the effect of music therapy during terminal extubation on length of life following the removal of mechanical ventilation. No significant differences in length of life post-extubation were found between the music therapy group and the control group, though the sample size was small, making generalized claims difficult. Despite the clear need for research on this topic, terminal extubation is a viable clinical application of music therapy (R. Moats, personal communication, July 10, 2013; J. Peyton, personal communication, June 19, 2013).

Since terminal extubation results in the patient's death, this procedure can cause strong emotional reactions from both the family and the patient. Music therapy is an ideal modality to address these emotional needs, due to the inherent connection between music and emotion.

Terminal extubation can cause physiological symptoms for the patient as well. Increased stress and anxiety are possible, whether the patient is alert or unresponsive; however, patients are usually completely unresponsive by this point (Campbell et al., 1999; Willms & Brewer, 2005). The iso-principle can be used to promote relaxation and comfort for the patient during the physical act of extubation. The music therapist should be prepared for the patient to possibly expel some oral secretions as the tube is removed.

Following extubation, the music therapist should use preferred songs that were meaningful to the patient and family to facilitate the communication of final messages and goodbyes (Haskins et al., 2007; Krout, 2003). Therefore, the removal of life support also functions as a grief ritual, which can aid the family members in their grief process (Wlodarczyk, 2011, 2013). During the final minutes before death, live music can create a metaphorical safety net or sacred space within which these final goodbyes may take place. One medical music therapist who utilizes this technique quoted a family member as saying, "I can't imagine going through that with just silence and crying" (R. Moats, personal communication, July 10, 2013).

If the patient dies during the session, the music therapist should not immediately exit. By continuing to play music after death has occurred, the music therapist directly engages the emotional needs of the family, allowing the safe environment already created for final goodbyes to now function as a safe space for the family during their initial displays of active grief (i.e., crying, embracing the patient, etc.). Taking nonverbal cues from the family, the music therapist should use the iso-principle to slowly fade the music out and exit the hospital room after the initial displays of grief have begun to subside (Haskins et al., 2007).

Music therapy interventions for psychosocial goals. While traditional hospice patients may have months to process the emotions associated with their terminal diagnosis, critically ill or injured patients in the hospital may have only days or hours to do the same. A number of palliative care patients will have been battling their illnesses for some time and may have reached the point at which they are ready to cease their corporeal struggle and instead focus on spending their remaining time with family. Other patients may be young and previously healthy, dealing with the anger associated with a random accident and injuries that they will not survive. There are countless circumstances for hospitalized EOL patients that can result in a wide spectrum of emotional responses. It is likely that the music therapist may see these patients only once or just a handful of times; therefore, rapid assessment and treatment skills are essential to provide maximum benefit in the time available. Research has demonstrated that music therapy at the end of life can provide opportunities to engage in life review, process anticipatory grief, express feelings, find closure in relationships, enhance caregiver bonding, and leave a legacy for loved ones (Clements-Cortes, 2004, 2011; Hilliard, 2005a; Krout, 2005; Magill, 2009; Nguyen, 2003; O'Callaghan, 1996a, 1997, 2008, 2009; Whitall, 1991; Wlodarczyk, 2009).

Life review. The capacity for music to evoke memories and trigger emotions is vast and powerful. Music therapists working in hospice and palliative care routinely engage patients in musical life review, as the end of life is a natural time to reflect, reminisce, and reexamine the past (Hilliard, 2005a; Sato, 2011; Wlodarczyk, 2009; Wylie, 1990). Sato (2011) explains that reminiscence, while part of the life review process, refers only to the recalling of memories. Conversely, life review implies an evaluation process that may lead to the resolution of conflicts or the discovery of insights to be passed on to future generations. Sato (2011) proposed a Musical Life Review Model that structures this intervention into four elements: stimuli (e.g., songs, pictures, etc.), theme (e.g., major life events, relationships, hobbies, etc.), response (appreciation, nostalgia, regret, etc.), and evaluation (verbal and musical processing). Musical life review can involve (a) song choice, (b) lyric analysis, (c) song writing paired with storytelling, and (d) both verbal and musical processing (Bailey, 1984; Belgrave et al., 2011; Hilliard, 2001, 2005a; Krout, 2005; Magill, 2009; Nguyen, 2003; Sato, 2011; West, 1994; Wlodarczyk, 2009).

Music therapists often write life review songs, a process that involves interviewing patients and setting their life stories to music, in order to preserve memories and life lessons. Performing these life review songs for the patient and family can provide an opportunity to celebrate the patient's life and strengthen bonds with family members (Nguyen, 2003). These songs can also aid family members in the bereavement process once the patient has died (Magill, 2009; O'Callaghan, 2013; Wlodarczyk, 2009). Due to the short-term nature of music therapy for hospitalized EOL patients, there may not be adequate time for a lengthy life review process. The music therapist is urged to create and perform life review songs quickly in these situations.

Relationship completion. The need for closure is a ubiquitous theme at the end of life. In order for EOL patients to achieve closure, they may need to feel that their lives have had meaning, that they have left a legacy for future generations, and that they have left nothing unsaid to loved ones. We have a human need to develop and maintain significant relationships, which results in emotional turmoil when those relationships are threatened or concluded (Worden, 2009). It follows that the state of these significant relationships would be of high concern to a patient facing the end of life. Clements-Cortes (2011) describes relationship completion as achieving closure with significant relationships at the end of life, including relationships with (a) self, (b) loved ones, or (c) a higher power.

After identifying key relationships in patients' lives, music therapists can provide support for relationship completion though musical (a) life review, (b) lyric analysis, (c) song writing, (d) song dedications, and (e) clinical improvisation (Belgrave et al., 2011; Clements-Cortes, 2011; Hilliard, 2005a; Magill, 2009; Wlodarczyk, 2009). Byock (2004) affirms that relationship completion at the end of life can be facilitated through the following five sentiments shared by patients and family members:

- "Please forgive me."

- "I forgive you."

- "Thank you."

- "I love you."

- "Goodbye."

These sentiments can be communicated through song writing and song dedication (Belgrave et al., 2011; Clements-Cortes, 2011; Wlodarczyk, 2009). Although working toward relationship completion can be difficult for patients and family members, particularly with an unexpected critical illness, the result can lead to a more peaceful death for the patient and better bereavement outcomes for the family (Clements-Cortes, 2011; Magill, 2009; O'Callaghan, 1996a, 1997, 2008, 2013; Wlodarczyk, 2009).

Caregiver bonding. Aside from the more active process of relationship completion, EOL patients also have a basic need to simply spend quality time with loved ones. Music therapy is effective, in part, due to the interpersonal relationship and rapport that is built between therapist and patient. Additionally, music therapists can assist in facilitating bonding between patient and family.

However, meaningful interaction and communication between patient and others is difficult if the patient is drowsy or confused. Thus, music therapists can use the iso-principle to bring patients to the most alert state possible in order to better facilitate these interactions. Interventions to promote caregiver bonding include (a) song choice, (b) music-assisted reminiscence, (c) singing together, or (d) playing instruments together (Belgrave et al., 2011; Magill, 2009).

Instrument play gives the patient's loved ones something active and meaningful to do at a time when they may feel helpless or like they are in the way. The use of tone chimes for instrument play is highly recommended to promote caregiver bonding with patients and family members in EOL care. They are easy to play, have a soothing sound, and allow a large number of loved ones to gather around the patient's hospital bed, making music together under the direction of the music therapist.

Music therapy sessions with patients and their significant others can promote authentic communication and emotional intimacy, which can, in turn, strengthen their ability to support each other during hospitalization (Hinman, 2010). Familiar songs can normalize the environment, increase relaxation, and support the sharing of memories and feelings. Encouragement of expressive touch (e.g., holding hands, arms around each other, etc.) during the music may further enhance the interaction between patients and caregivers (Belgrave, 2009).

Music therapy interventions for spiritual goals. The desire to search for spiritual meaning in life is a universal one. As individuals face the end of life, they may feel spiritual certainty, spiritual confusion, or something in between. EOL patients may question their beliefs, the reason for their illness, or the existence of an afterlife. The need for answers to these questions may result in patients experiencing spiritual distress, which may, in turn, increase anxiety and physical discomfort (Wlodarczyk, 2007). The music therapist is not expected to provide these answers; yet, akin to the life review process, music can provide a forum within which patients can possibly uncover their own answers.

Researchers have examined the effects of music therapy on spirituality in several studies with promising results (Aldridge, 1995; Cook & Silverman, 2013; Foxglove & Tyas, 2000; Hilliard, 2005b; Lipe, 2002; Okamoto, 2004; Ryan, 1996; Salmon, 2001; Wlodarczyk, 2007). Live music making and clinical improvisation can provide opportunities for spiritual exploration, expression, or worship. Additionally, lyric analysis and song writing offer active interventions to address spiritual questions. Finally, prayer or meditation can be enhanced through live music, adding another supportive dimension to the experience. Patient outcomes of music therapy intervention in this goal area include an increased sense of spiritual well-being (Wlodarczyk, 2007), an increased sense of faith and peace, increased feelings of closeness to God, and elevated mood (Cook & Silverman, 2013). Interestingly, in studies by Cook and Silverman (2013) and Wlodarczyk (2007), patients did not exclusively request traditional spiritual or religious music during music therapy sessions, suggesting that patient-preferred secular music may also promote spiritual well-being (Cook & Silverman, 2013). Table 12.3 provides a summary of possible interventions to address physical, psychosocial, and spiritual goals for hospitalized EOL patients.

Table 12. 3. Music Therapy Interventions for Hospitalized EOL Patients		
Physical	**Psychosocial**	**Spiritual**
Iso-principle for symptom management	Music-assisted life review	Music-assisted worship
Music-assisted PMR	Song writing	
Music-assisted terminal extubation	Music-assisted relationship completion	
	Music-assisted caregiver bonding	

A word about self-care. Medical music therapists can play an integral role in meeting the multidimensional needs of EOL patients in the hospital. Yet, working with EOL patients is not easy. Witnessing patients and family members at their most vulnerable moments, while absorbing their intense emotions, can take a toll on the music therapist, making the need for self-care vital to the ability to work long-term in this area. The absence of self-care practices can result in unresolved compound grief, which is a contributing factor to compassion fatigue and burnout (Wlodarczyk, 2013). The music therapist is encouraged to make time for self-care practices such as journaling, meditation, exercise, and making music for pleasure.

Conclusion

This chapter outlined three types of EOL patients that a music therapist will encounter in the hospital: hospice patients, non-hospice palliative care patients, and non-palliative EOL patients. Although reasons for hospitalization will differ, these patients are likely to experience similar acute symptoms at the end of life. Music therapists are encouraged to develop a basic understanding of EOL symptoms, advance directives, and life support options in order to better relate to the patient and the palliative care team. The use of music therapy to mitigate physical, psychosocial, and spiritual symptoms has been well documented in the literature for EOL patients (Belgrave et al., 2011; Bradt & Dileo, 2010; Hilliard, 2005a, 2005b; O'Callaghan, 2009). Music therapists can use the iso-principle and music for distraction to reduce physical symptoms such as (a) pain, (b) discomfort, (c) anxiety, (d) nausea and (e) vomiting (Belgrave et al., 2011; Groen, 2007; Hilliard, 2001, 2005a, 2005b; Horne-Thompson & Grocke, 2008; Krout, 2001; O'Callaghan, 1996b, 2009). Musical life review, lyric analysis, song writing, and song dedications can address psychosocial goals, such as processing anticipatory grief, relationship completion, and enhanced caregiver bonding (Clements-Cortes, 2004, 2011; Hilliard, 2005a; Krout, 2005; Magill, 2009; Nguyen, 2003; O'Callaghan, 1996a, 1997, 2008, 2009; Sato, 2011). Additionally, music therapists can facilitate opportunities for worship, decrease spiritual distress, and increase spiritual well-being for EOL patients (Cook & Silverman, 2013; Foxglove & Tyas, 2000; Hilliard, 2005b; Lipe, 2002; Wlodarczyk, 2007). Finally, music therapists are encouraged to practice diligent self-care to combat burnout and compassion fatigue, ensuring that they can continue this meaningful work for future patients (Wlodarczyk, 2013).

References

Abbott, C. M. (1995). *The effects of music therapy on the perceived quality of life of patients with terminal illness in a hospice setting* (Unpublished master's thesis). Western Michigan University, Kalamazoo.

Aging with Dignity. (2012). *Five Wishes.* Retrieved from http://www.agingwithdignity.org/five-wishes.php

Aldridge, D. (1995). Spirituality, hope and music therapy. *The Arts in Psychotherapy, 22*, 103–109.

American Cancer Society. (2013a). *Advance directives.* Retrieved from http://www.cancer.org/treatment/findingandpayingfortreatment/understandingfinancialandlegalmatters/advancedirectives/index

American Cancer Society. (2013b). *Nearing the end of life.* Retrieved from http://www.cancer.org/treatment/nearingtheendoflife/nearingtheendoflife/nearing- the- end-of-life-death

American Thoracic Society. (2013a). *Mechanical ventilator.* Retrieved from http://www.thoracic.org/clinical/critical-care../patient-information/icu-devices-and-procedures/mechanical-ventilator.php

American Thoracic Society. (2013b). *Withdrawal of life sustaining treatments*. Retrieved from http://www.thoracic.org/clinical/critical-care../patient-information/withdrawal-of-life-sustaining-treatments.php

Anderson, W. G., Kools, S., & Lyndon, A. (2013). Dancing around death: Hospitalist-patient communication about serious illness. *Qualitative Health Research, 23*(1), 3–13.

Bailey, L. M. (1984). The use of songs in music therapy with cancer patients and their families. *Music Therapy, 4,* 5–17.

Bailey, L. M. (1986). Music therapy in pain management. *Journal of Pain and Symptom Management, 1*(1), 25–28.

Beck, S. C. (1991). The therapeutic use of music for cancer-related pain. *Oncology Nursing Forum, 18*(8), 1327–1337.

Belgrave, M. (2009). The effect of expressive and instrumental touch on the behavior states of older adults with late-stage dementia of the Alzheimer's type and on music therapist's perceived rapport. *Journal of Music Therapy, 46*, 132–146.

Belgrave, M., Darrow, A. A., Walworth, D., & Wlodarczyk, N. (2011). *Music therapy and geriatric populations: A handbook for practicing music therapists and healthcare professionals.* Silver Spring, MD: American Music Therapy Association.

Berger, J. S. (2006). *Music of the soul: Composing life out of loss.* New York: Brunner-Routledge.

Bradt, J., & Dileo, C. (2010). Music therapy for end-of-life care. *Cochrane Database of Systematic Reviews, 1,* 1–32. doi:10.1002/14651858.CD007169.pub2

Byock, I. (2004). *The four things that matter most: A book about living.* New York, NY: Simon & Schuster.

Callanan, M., & Kelly, P. (1992). *Final gifts: Understanding the special awareness, needs and communications of the dying.* New York, NY: Simon & Schuster.

Calovini, B. S. (1993). *The effect of participation in one music therapy session on state anxiety in hospice patients* (Unpublished master's thesis). Case Western Reserve University, Cleveland, OH.

Campbell, M. L., Bizek, K. S., & Thill, M. (1999). Patient responses during rapid terminal weaning from mechanical ventilation: A prospective study. *Critical Care Medicine, 27*(1), 73–77.

Centers for Medicare & Medicaid Services. (2013). *Medicare hospice benefits* [Brochure]. Retrieved from http://www.medicare.gov/Pubs/pdf/02154.pdf

Chen, Y. Y., & Youngner, S. J. (2008). "Allow natural death" is not equivalent to "do not resuscitate": A response. *Journal of Medical Ethics, 34*, 887–888.

Chlan, L., Engeland, W., Anthony, A., & Guttormson, J. (2006). Acute effects of music on stress in patients receiving mechanical ventilatory support. *American Journal of Critical Care, 15*(3), 328–328.

Chlan, L., & Heiderscheit, A. (2009). A tool for music preference assessment in critically ill patients receiving mechanical ventilatory support. *Music Therapy Perspectives, 27*, 42–47.

Chlan, L., Tracy, M. F., Nelson, B., & Walker, J. (2001). Feasibility of a music intervention protocol for patients receiving mechanical ventilation support. *Alternative Therapies, 7*(6), 80–83.

Choi, Y. K. (2010). The effect of music and progressive muscle relaxation on anxiety, fatigue, and quality of life in family caregivers of hospice patients. *Journal of Music Therapy, 47*, 53–69.

Clements-Cortes, A. (2004). The use of music in facilitating emotional expression in the terminally ill. *American Journal of Hospice and Palliative Medicine, 21*(4), 255–260.

Clements-Cortes, A. (2011). Portraits of music therapy in facilitating relationship completion at the end of life. *Music and Medicine, 3*, 31–39.

Cook, E. L., & Silverman, M. J. (2013). Effects of music therapy on spirituality with patients on a medical oncology/hematology unit: A mixed-methods approach. *The Arts in Psychotherapy, 40*, 239–244.

Curtis, S. L. (1986). The effect of music on pain relief and relaxation of the terminally ill. *Journal of Music Therapy, 23,* 10–24.

D'Amico, T. A., Krasna, M. J., Krasna, D. M., & Sade, R. M. (2009). No heroic measures: How soon is too soon to stop? *The Annals of Thoracic Surgery, 87*, 11–18.

DiMaio, L. (2010). Music therapy entrainment: A humanistic music therapist's perspective of using music therapy entrainment with hospice clients experiencing pain. *Music Therapy Perspectives, 28*, 106–115.

Foxglove, T., & Tyas, B. (2000). Using music as a spiritual tool in palliative care. *European Journal of Palliative Care, 7*(2), 63–65.

Gerstel, E., Engleberg, R. A., Koepsell, T., & Curtis, J. R. (2008). Duration of withdrawal of life support in the intensive care unit and association with family satisfaction. *American Journal of Respiratory and Critical Care Medicine, 178,* 798–804.

Gfeller, K. (2008). Music therapy, medicine, and well-being. In W. B. Davis, K. E. Gfeller, & M. H. Thaut (Eds.), *An introduction to music therapy theory and practice* (3rd ed.) (pp. 305–342). Silver Spring, MD: American Music Therapy Association.

Groen, K. M. (2007). Pain assessment and management in end of life care: A survey of assessment and treatment practices of hospice music therapy and nursing professionals. *Journal of Music Therapy, 44,* 90–112.

Haskins, J., Reilly, K., & Wlodarczyk, N. (2007, November). *When death is imminent: Hospice music therapy interventions for families.* Paper presented at The American Music Therapy Association National Conference, Louisville, KY.

Hilliard, R. E. (2001). The use of music therapy in meeting the multidimensional needs of hospice patients and families. *Journal of Palliative Care, 17*(3), 161–166.

Hilliard, R. E. (2003). The effects of music therapy on quality of life and length of life of hospice patients diagnosed with terminal cancer. *Journal of Music Therapy, 40*, 113–137.

Hilliard, R.E. (2005a). *Hospice and palliative care music therapy: A guide to program development and clinical care.* Cherry Hill, NJ: Jeffrey Books.

Hilliard, R. E. (2005b). Music therapy in hospice and palliative care: A review of the empirical data. *Evidenced-based Complementary and Alternative Medicine, 2*(2), 173–178.

Hinman, M. L. (2010). Our song: Music therapy with couples when one partner is medically hospitalized. *Music Therapy Perspectives, 28*, 29–36.

Hite, C. A., & Weiss, G. L. (2003). Do not resuscitate. In *Macmillan encyclopedia of death and dying.* (Vol. 1, pp. 240–243). New York, NY: Macmillan Reference USA.

Horne-Thompson, A., & Grocke, D. (2008). The effect of music therapy on anxiety in patients who are terminally ill. *Journal of Palliative Medicine, 11*(4), 582–590.

Hunter, B. C., Oliva, R., Sahler, O. J. Z., Gaisser, D., & Salipante, D. M. (2010). Music therapy as an adjunctive treatment in the management of stress for patients being weaned from mechanical ventilation. *Journal of Music Therapy, 47*, 198–219.

Jacobs, L. M., Burns, K. J., & Jacobs, B. B. (2010). Nurse and physician preferences for end-of- life care for trauma patients. *Journal of Trauma and Acute Care Surgery, 69*, 1567–1573.

Jones, D. A., Bagshaw, S. M., Barrett, J., Bellomo, R., Bhatia, G., Bucknall, T. K., . . . Parr, M. J. (2012). The role of the medical emergency team in end-of-life care: A multicenter, prospective, observational study. *Critical Care Medicine, 40*(1), 98–103.

Kenny, D. T., & Faunce, G. (2004). The impact of group singing on mood, coping, and perceived pain in chronic pain patients attending a multidisciplinary pain clinic. *Journal of Music Therapy, 41*(3), 241–258.

Kim, S. A. (2006). *The effect of music listening on mood state and relaxation of hospice patients and caregivers* (Unpublished master's thesis). Florida State University, Tallahassee.

Korhan, E. A., Khorshid, L., & Uyar, M. (2011). The effect of music therapy on physiological signs of anxiety in patients receiving mechanical ventilatory support. *Journal of Clinical Nursing, 20*, 1026–1034.

Krout, R. E. (2001). The effects of single-session music therapy interventions on the observed and self-reported levels of pain control, physical comfort, and relaxation of hospice patients. *American Journal of Hospice and Palliative Medicine, 18*(6), 383–390.

Krout, R. E. (2003). Music therapy with imminently dying hospice patients and their families: Facilitating release near the time of death. *American Journal of Hospice & Palliative Care, 20*(2), 129–134.

Krout, R. E. (2005). The use of therapist-composed songs in end of life music therapy care. In C. Dileo & J. V. Loewy (Eds.), *Music therapy at the end of life* (pp. 129–140). Cherry Hill, NJ: Jeffrey Books.

Kwekkeboom, K. L. (2003). Music versus distraction for procedural pain and anxiety in patients with cancer. *Oncology Nursing Forum, 30*, 433–440.

Lee, H. J. (2005). *The effect of life music via the iso-principle on pain management in palliative care as measured by self- report using a graphic rating scale (GRS) and pulse rate* (Unpublished master's thesis). Florida State University, Tallahassee.

Lee, O. K. A., Chung, Y. F. L., Chan, M. F., & Chan, W. M. (2005). Music and its effect on the physiological responses and anxiety levels of patients receiving mechanical ventilation: A pilot study. *Journal of Clinical Nursing, 14*, 609–620.

Limehouse, W. E., Feeser, V. R., Bookman, K. J., & Derse, A. (2012). A model for emergency department end-of-life communications after acute devastating events—part I: Decision-making capacity, surrogates, and advance directives. *Academic Emergency Medicine, 19*, 1068–1072.

Lipe, A. W. (2002). Beyond therapy: Music, spirituality, and health in human experience: A review of literature. *Journal of Music Therapy, 39*, 209–240.

Longfield, V. (1995). *The effects of music therapy on pain and mood in hospice patients* (Unpublished master's thesis). Saint Louis University, St. Louis, MO.

Magill, L. (2001). The use of music therapy to address the suffering in advanced cancer pain. *Journal of Palliative Care, 17*(3), 167–172.

Magill, L. (2009). The meaning of the music: The role of music in palliative care music therapy as perceived by bereaved caregivers of advanced cancer patients. *American Journal of Hospice and Palliative Medicine, 26*(1), 33–39.

Magill-Levreault, L. (1993). Music therapy in pain and symptom management. *Journal of Palliative Care, 9*(4), 37–42.

Mandel, S. (1993). The role of the music therapist on the hospice/palliative care team. *Journal of Palliative Care, 9*(4), 37–39.

Mayo Clinic. (2013). *Living wills and advance directives for medical decisions*. Retrieved from http://www.mayoclinic.com/health/living-wills/HA00014

Michel, D. E., & Chesky, K. S. (1995). A survey of music therapists using music for pain relief. *The Arts in Psychotherapy, 22*(1), 49–51.

Mitchell, L. A., & MacDonald, R. A. R. (2006). An experimental investigation of the effects of preferred and relaxing music listening on pain perception. *Journal of Music Therapy, 43*, 295–316.

Mitchell, L. A., MacDonald, R. A. R., Knussen, C., & Serpell, M. G. (2007). A survey investigation of the effects of music listening on chronic pain. *Psychology of Music, 35*(1), 37–57.

Mosenthal, A. C., & Murphy, P. A. (2003). Trauma care and palliative care: Time to integrate the two? *Journal of the American College of Surgeons, 197*, 509–516.

Mosenthal, A. C., Murphy, P. A., Barker, L. K., Lavery, R., Retano, A., & Livingston, D. H. (2008). Changing the culture around end-of-life care in the trauma intensive care unit. *Journal of Trauma and Acute Care Surgery, 64*, 1587–1593.

Munro, S., & Mount, B. M. (1978). Music therapy in palliative care. *Canadian Medical Association Journal, 119*, 1029–1034.

National Cancer Institute. (2013). *Advance directives*. Retrieved from http://www.cancer.gov/cancertopics/factsheet/Support/advance-directives

National Hospice and Palliative Care Organization. (2001). *Hospital-hospice partnerships in palliative care: Creating a continuum of service* [Brochure]. Retrieved from http://www.nhpco.org/sites/default/files/public/NHPCO-CAPCreport.pdf

National Hospice and Palliative Care Organization. (2013a). *Hospice and palliative care.* Retrieved from http://www.nhpco.org/about/hospice-and-palliative-care

National Hospice and Palliative Care Organization. (2013b). *The Medicare Hospice Benefit.* Retrieved from http://www.nhpco.org/sites/default/files/public/communications/Outreach/The_Medicare_Hospice_Benefit.pdf

National Institute of Nursing Research. (2009). *Palliative care: The relief you need when you're experiencing the symptoms of serious illness* [Brochure]. Retrieved from http://cancer.ucsf.edu/_docs/sms/PalliativeCare.pdf

National Institutes of Health. (2008, October). Prolonging the withdrawal of life support in the ICU affects family satisfaction with care. *NIH News.* Retrieved from http://www.nih.gov/news/health/oct2008/ninr-15.htm

Nguyen, J. T. (2003*). The effect of music therapy on end-of-life patients' quality of life, emotional state, and family satisfaction as measured by self-report* (Unpublished master's thesis). Florida State University, Tallahassee.

Nissim, R., Rennie, D., Fleming, S., Hales, S., Gagliese, L., & Rodin, G. (2012). Goals set in the land of the living/dying: A longitudinal study of patients living with advanced cancer. *Death Studies, 36,* 360–390.

O'Callaghan, C. (1996a). Lyrical themes in songs written by palliative care patients. *Journal of Music Therapy, 33,* 74–92.

O'Callaghan, C. (1996b). Pain, music creativity and music therapy in palliative care. *American Journal of Hospice and Palliative Medicine, 13*(2), 43–49.

O'Callaghan, C. (1997). Therapeutic opportunities associated with the music when using song writing in palliative care. *Music Therapy Perspectives, 15,* 32–38.

O'Callaghan, C. (2008). Lullament: Lullaby and lament therapeutic qualities actualized through music therapy. *American Journal of Hospice and Palliative Medicine, 25*(2), 93–99.

O'Callaghan, C. (2009). Objectivist and constructivist music therapy research in oncology and palliative care: An overview and reflection. *Music and Medicine, 1*(1), 41–60.

O'Callaghan, C. (2013). Music therapy preloss care through legacy creation. *Progress in Palliative Care, 21*(2), 78–82.

Okamoto, M. (2004). *The effects of music therapy interventions on grief and spirituality of family members of patients in a hospice setting* (Unpublished master's thesis). Florida State University, Tallahassee.

O'Kelly, J. (2007). Multidisciplinary perspectives of music therapy in adult and palliative care. *Palliative Medicine, 21,* 235–241.

Orellano, S. H. (2009). *The effect of music therapy on the length of life of extubated hospice patients: A post-hoc analysis* (Unpublished master's thesis). Florida State University, Tallahassee.

Quinn, J. R., Schmitt, M., Baggs, J. G., Norton, S. A., Dombeck, M. T., & Sellers, C. R. (2012). Family members' informal roles in end-of-life decision making in adult intensive care units. *American Journal of Critical Care, 21*(1), 43–51.

Reed, J. B. (2009, March 2). 'Do not resuscitate' vs. 'allow natural death.' *USA Today*. Retrieved from http://usatoday30.usatoday.com/news/health/2009-03-02-DNR-natural-death_N.htm

Ryan, K. L. (1996). *Developing an approach to the use of music therapy with hospice patients in the final phase of life: An examination of how hospice patients from three religious traditions use music and respond to music therapy* (Unpublished master's thesis). Case Western Reserve University, Cleveland, OH.

Salmon, D. (2001). Music therapy as psychospiritual process in palliative care. *Journal of Palliative Care, 17*(3), 142–146.

Sato, Y. (2011). Musical life review in hospice. *Music Therapy Perspectives, 29*, 31–38.

Standley, J. (2000). Music research in medical treatment. In *Effectiveness of music therapy procedures: Documentation of research and clinical practice* (3rd ed., pp. 1–64). Silver Spring, MD: American Music Therapy Association.

Temel, J. S., Greer, J. A., Muzikansky, A., Gallagher, E. R., Admane, S., Jackson, V. A., . . . Lynch, T. J. (2010). Early palliative care for patients with metastatic non-small-cell lung cancer. *The New England Journal of Medicine, 363*, 733–742.

Trauger-Querry, B., & Haghighi, K. R. (1999). Balancing the focus: Art and music therapy for pain control and symptom management in hospice care. *The Hospice Journal, 14*(1), 25–38.

Venneman, S. S., Narnor-Harris, P., Perish, M., & Hamilton, M. (2006). "Allow natural death" versus "do not resuscitate": Three words that can change a life. *Journal of Medical Ethics, 34*, 2–6.

Walker, K. A., Nachreiner, D., Patel, J., Mayo, R. L., & Kearney, C. D. (2011). Impact of standardized palliative care order set on end-of-life care in a community teaching hospital. *Journal of Palliative Medicine, 14*(3), 281–286.

Walker, K. A., Peltier, H., Mayo, R. L., & Kearney, C. D. (2010). Impact of writing "comfort measures only" orders in a community teaching hospital. *Journal of Palliative Medicine, 13*(3), 241–245.

Walling, A. M., Asch, S. M., Lorenz, K. A., Roth, C. P., Barry, T., Kahn, K. L., & Wenger, N. S. (2010). The quality of care provided to hospitalized patients at the end of life. *Archives of Internal Medicine, 170*, 1057–1063.

Walworth, D. D. (2005). Procedural-support music therapy in the healthcare setting: A cost-effectiveness analysis. *Journal of Pediatric Nursing, 20*(4), 276–284.

West, T. M. (1994). Psychological issues in hospice music therapy. *Music Therapy Perspectives, 12*, 117–124.

Whitall, J. (1991). Songs in palliative care: A spouse's last gift. In K. Bruscia (Ed.), *Case studies in music therapy* (pp. 603–610). Phoenixville, PA: Barcelona.

Willms, D. C., & Brewer, J. A. (2005). Survey of respiratory therapists' attitudes and concerns regarding terminal extubation. *Respiratory Care, 50*(8), 1046–1049.

Wlodarczyk, N. (2007). The effect of music therapy on the spirituality of persons in an in-patient hospice unit as measured by self-report. *Journal of Music Therapy, 44*, 113–122.

Wlodarczyk, N. (2008, November). *The effect of a live music interaction on the stress levels of hospice staff workers during a hospice interdisciplinary team meeting.* Unpublished paper presented at the American Music Therapy Association National Conference, St. Louis, MO.

Wlodarczyk, N. (2009). The use of music and poetry in life review with hospice patients. *Journal of Poetry Therapy, 22*(3), 133–139.

Wlodarczyk, N. (2011, April). *The use of ritual in group music therapy for grief and loss.* Paper presented at the Midwestern Regional American Music Therapy Association Conference, Overland Park, KS.

Wlodarczyk, N. (2013). The effect of a group music intervention for grief resolution on disenfranchised grief of hospice workers. *Progress in Palliative Care, 21*(2), 97–106.

Wong, E. H. (2004). *Clinical guide to music therapy in adult physical rehabilitation settings.* Silver Spring, MD: American Music Therapy Association.

Worden, J. W. (2009). *Grief counseling and grief therapy: A handbook for the mental health practitioner* (4th ed.). New York, NY: Springer.

Wylie, M. E. (1990). A comparison of the effects of old familiar songs, antique objects, historical summaries, and general questions on the reminiscence of nursing home residents. *Journal of Music Therapy, 27*, 2–12.

Zanartu, C., & Matti-Orozco, B. (2013). Comfort measures only: Agreeing on a common definition through a survey. *American Journal of Hospice & Palliative Medicine, 30*(1), 35–39.

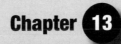

Chapter 13

Music Therapy and the Psychosocial Care of Medical Patients
Lori F. Gooding, PhD, MT-BC

Medical patients face a variety of challenges during all stages of the treatment process, from initial detection and diagnosis, to treatment and rehabilitation, and beyond into continuing care (Livneh & Antonak, 2005; Rainey, Wellisch, Fawzy, Wolcott, & Pasnau, 1983). It is important to recognize that the majority of patients, when given appropriate support, cope fairly well with the challenges of the treatment process. For some patients, however, illness can lead to (a) physical, (b) psychological, (c) social, (d) educational, (e) financial, and (f) vocational obstacles (Livneh & Antonak, 2005). These barriers can negatively impact patients' quality of life and well-being, placing them at increased risk for poor psychosocial health (Rainey et al., 1983).

Psychosocial functioning can be influenced by a number of variables, including (a) personality, (b) coping, (c) social support, and (d) disease-related cognitive appraisals (Janowski, Steuden, & Kurylowicz, 2010). Common psychosocial needs frequently seen in medical patients include:

- lack of information, knowledge, and/or skills to manage illness;

- anxiety, depression, and other emotional distress (anger, guilt, etc.);

- spiritual/existential issues involving personal faith;

- developmental problems;

- impaired work/school roles (e.g., inability to work);

- financial problems (reduced employment, lack of health insurance, etc.);

- lack of logistical and/or social supports (often due to high levels of stress in family members) (Adler & Page, 2008); and

- family conflicts (Zabora, BrintzenhofeSzoc, Curbow, Hooker, & Piantadosi, 2001).

The growing emphasis on patient-centered care as well as the increasing number of individuals with chronic illnesses has led to increased attention on patients' psychosocial needs. However, many providers still fall short in addressing psychosocial needs, either by failing to recognize and treat these needs or by lacking knowledge of appropriate resources (Adler & Page, 2008). According to Adler and Page (2008), effective psychosocial care must promote patient management (i.e., coping) of the psychological, behavioral, and social aspects of illness. Just as importantly, psychosocial care should enable patients' families and health care providers to promote better health, in themselves and their patients.

Psychosocial interventions were developed to help individuals with difficulty adjusting to or coping with illness (de Ridder, Geenen, Kuijer, & van Middendorp, 2008). These strategies have been shown to be effective in improving individuals' psychological and behavioral adjustment (i.e., coping) (Burns, 2001). Music therapy-based psychosocial interventions have been used effectively with children regardless of their level of functioning (Kennelly & Brien-Elliot, 2001). Music therapy has also been shown to ameliorate stress and mood dysfunction associated with specific conditions and has contributed to improvements in patients' affect and decreases in agitated behaviors (Rafieyan & Ries, 2007). Perhaps most importantly, music therapy has the ability to address a variety of needs simultaneously (Robb, 1996). Table 13.1 (children and adolescents) and Table 13.2 (adults) highlight research on the use of music therapy to address psychosocial needs in a variety of settings.

Table 13.1. Music Therapy to Address Psychosocial Needs in Children and Adolescents			
Reason for Referral	**Setting/Diagnosis**	**Outcome**	**Research Study**
Anxiety/Stress	Hematology/Oncology	Significant improvement in children's self-ratings of feelings	Barrera, Rykov & Doyle, 2002
Anxiety/Stress	Hospitalized children	Significant decreases in pain and anxiety	Colwell, Edwards, Hernandez, & Brees, 2013
Anxiety/Stress	NICU infants	Significantly fewer infant stress behaviors	Whipple, 2000
Anxiety/Stress	Preoperative pediatric patients	Significant decreases in anxiety	Chetta, 1981; Robb, Nichols, Rutan, Bishop, & Parker, 1995
Behavioral distress	Hospitalized infants and toddlers	Reduction of stress-related behaviors	Marley, 1984
Behavioral distress	Needle insertion procedures	Significantly less behavioral distress	Malone, 1996; Yinger, 2013
Behavioral distress	Procedural support	Successful completion of procedures without significant behavioral distress responses	Walworth, 2005
Coping	Oncology patients during 1st radiation treatment	0% of MT group used social withdrawal as a coping strategy compared to 67% of the control group	Barry, O'Callaghan, Wheeler, & Grocke, 2010
Coping	Oncology	Higher levels of coping-related behaviors (positive affect, behavioral engagement, initiation)	Robb, 2000; Robb et al., 2008
Enjoyment (increase enjoyment during CPT to increase adherence)	Cystic Fibrosis	Significant increases in child and parent enjoyment with music therapist-composed music	Grasso, Button, Allison, & Sawyer, 2000
Psychosocial care	Epilepsy	835 patients over a 4-year period successfully underwent video electroencephalogram without the use of sedation or medical controls	Mondanaro, 2008
Verbalizations	Pediatrics	More involved verbalizations during MT than medical play therapy (child life approach)	Froehlich, 1984
Well-being (family-centered)	Pediatrics	Provided psychosocial support	Ayson, 2008
Quality of life (family- centered)	Pediatric palliative care	Parents noted improvements in physical and communication scales of the Peds QOL in contrast to diminishing QOL in cognitive/daily activity domains	Lindenfelser, Hense, & McFerran, 2012
Resilience/Quality of life (family-centered)	Adolescent/Young Adult Oncology	Parents were able to articulate helpful/meaningful aspects of music therapy intervention	Docherty et al., 2013

Table 13.2. Music Therapy to Address Psychosocial Needs in Adults			
Reason for Referral	**Setting/Diagnosis**	**Outcome**	**Research Study**
Affective and Quality of Life components	Multiple sclerosis	Significant improvements in MT group for self-esteem, depression, and anxiety	Schmid & Aldridge, 2004
Anxiety	Terminally ill inpatients	Significant reduction in anxiety	Horne-Thompson & Grocke, 2008
Anxiety	Transplant patients	Significant improvements in self-reported levels of anxiety and relaxation	Madson & Silverman, 2010
Anxiety	Procedural support	Improved positive affective states and decrease in negative affect	Ghetti, 2013
Depression/Improved mood	Oncology (stem cell transplantation)	Significant decrease in anxiety, depression, and mood disturbance	Cassileth, Vickers, & Magill, 2003
Emotional distress	Radiation therapy	Lower anxiety and treatment-related distress with higher doses leading to greater decline	Clark et al., 2006
Emotional distress	Parkinson's disease	Improved emotional functioning and quality of life	Pacchetti et al., 2000
Mood state	Oncology (group)	Improved mood state	Waldon, 2001
Mood/Life quality	Oncology	Improved mood and QOL	Burns, 2001
Quality of Life (QOL)	Oncology	Increases in QOL	Hilliard, 2003
Quality of Life	Brain surgery	Improved QOL indicators (anxiety, perception of hospitalization/procedure, relaxation, stress levels)	Walworth, Rumana, Nguyen, & Jarred, 2008
Social functioning	TBI/stroke	Significant improvement in social interactions; increased active involvement and motivation	Nayak et al., 2000
Well-being	Transplant patients	Significant increases in positive affect and significant decreases in negative affect	Ghetti, 2011

Reasons for Referral/Expected Outcomes

According to the 2010 *Complementary and Alternative Medicine Survey of Hospitals* (Samueli Institute, 2011), music therapy is the third most prevalent integrative modality (complementary medicine) offered in inpatient settings. Patients are most often referred to complementary therapies to address psychosocial needs like *anxiety* and *depression*, as well as *pain* (Samueli Institute, 2011). A number of studies from the literature support the use of music therapy to address both anxiety and depression. In addition, patients are also referred to music therapy for other common psychosocial objectives, including (a) fear; (b) stress; (c) grief; (d) poor social engagement; (e) poor relationships with family and/or staff; (f) decreased stimulation, motivation, and self-esteem; (g) poor self-expression and communication; and (h) limited support. Expected outcomes include:

- Reduction of fear, stress, and grief

- Promotion of social objectives like increased interaction/engagement, verbalization, independence, and cooperation

- Enhanced family relationships

- Enhanced relationships with health care personnel

- Increased stimulation (Standley & Hanser, 1995)

- Increased motivation

- Increased self-esteem and self-expression (Kennelly & Brien-Elliot, 2001)

- Increased support for patients who lack support systems

- Increased communication for patients who cannot engage in verbal psychotherapy (Rafieyan & Ries, 2007)

Components of Music Therapy-Based Psychosocial Treatment

While there are a number of important factors to consider during music therapy treatment, two components, in particular, are necessary for effective psychosocial care. Those factors include use of evidence-based practices, and the development of effective therapeutic relationships.

Evidence-Based Music Therapy Practices

In order to promote effective coping and successful patient adjustment, music therapists implement evidence-based music therapy strategies targeting patients' specific needs. A review of the literature indicates a number of commonly used interventions and techniques:

- *Active music engagement:* Colwell, Edwards, Hernandez, and Brees (2013) suggest that there are different ways of being actively engaged in music therapy. Patients can be *cognitively active* via *song writing* and *composition*. Patients can also be *physically active* through *singing, chanting, playing instruments,* or *movement*. A number of studies, including Mondanaro (2008), Robb (2000), Robb et al. (2008), and Schmid and Aldridge (2004) found positive effects when patients were actively engaged in music therapy. It has been suggested that these music therapy experiences function as distracting events, serving to normalize and/or provide opportunities for interaction and self-expression (Colwell et al., 2013).

- *Age appropriate interventions:* Zebrack and Isaacson (2012), in their article on psychosocial care of adolescents and young adult patients, highlight the need for age-appropriate care. Standley and Hanser (1995) also promote age-appropriate activities, stating that music therapy can promote self-expression and self-concept through successful, age-appropriate activities. Examples of effective, age-appropriate interventions found in the literature include (a) *music-based psychoeducation* and *music-based distraction techniques* in young children (Chetta, 1981; Mondanaro, 2008; Yinger, 2013); (b) *song parody, music relaxation/imagery, instrument learning,* and *song writing* in adolescents (Abad, 2003; Robb, 1996); and (c) *improvisation* (Schmid & Aldridge, 2004) and *music-assisted relaxation/distraction* (Clark et al., 2006) in adults.

- *Live, patient-preferred music:* Research strongly supports the use of both live and patient-preferred music to effectively meet patient needs, and the use of live, patient-preferred music to address psychosocial needs is no exception. Cassileth, Vickers, and Magill (2003), Madson and Silverman (2010), Walworth, Rumana, Nguyen, and Jarred (2008), and Ghetti (2013) all used *live, patient-preferred music* to address the psychosocial needs of their patients.

- *Music listening: Passive music listening* has been shown to be effective in decreasing stress. However, more active approaches, often termed *music-assisted relaxation,* pair music listening with other therapeutic elements, such as verbal suggestion, vibrotactile stimulation, and progressive relaxation. These techniques have been shown to have greater effect in reducing anxiety, even more so than Guided Imagery and Music (GIM) or passive listening (Pelletier, 2004).

In addition to the above interventions and techniques, there are a number of therapeutic practices supported in the music therapy literature. A list of common practices can be found in Table 13.3.

Table 13.3. Competent Music Therapy Services	
Practices	**Related Source**
Provide a supportive, therapeutic presence	Kennelly & Brien-Elliot, 2001; Mandel, Davis, & Secic, 2013
Focus on positive patient attributes	Fagen, 1982; Rafieyan & Ries, 2007
Offer the patient opportunities for control and choice	Lindenfelser, Hese, & McFerran, 2012; Rafieyan & Ries, 2007
Use of ongoing assessment to facilitate responsiveness to patient needs	Rafieyan & Ries, 2007
Use of verbal processing (i.e., counseling-based verbal communication) during and in response to music making or listening to increase patient awareness, understanding, and decision making abilities	Nolan, 2005
Flexibility (as related to session frequency, duration, use of patient-directed activities, etc.)	Colwell et al., 2013; Fagen, 1982
Provide a nonthreatening, nonjudgmental, "nonmedical" presence	McDonnell, 1983
Incorporate patient- and family-centered care	Docherty et al., 2013; Gooding & Yinger, 2013; Lindenfelser, et al., 2012; O'Callaghan, Baron, Barry, & Dun, 2011; Stouffer, Shirk, & Polomano, 2007; Yinger, 2013

Development of Effective Therapeutic Relationships

Music plays an important role in the development of the therapeutic relationship. A number of authors, including Clements-Cortes (2004), Magill (2008), and Mondanaro (2008), suggest that music can facilitate therapeutic interactions during psychosocial care. Figure 13.1 highlights ways in which music can be used to facilitate effective therapeutic relationships.

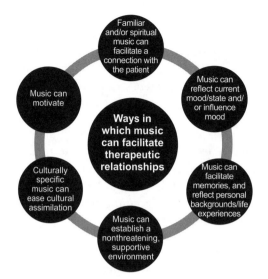

Figure 13.1. Uses of music to facilitate effective therapeutic relationships.

While the music itself is an important part of music therapy's effectiveness, it is also crucial to recognize the role of the therapist. A 2004 study by Kain et al. found significant therapist effects in relation to children's preoperative anxiety; that is, children treated by one therapist were significantly less anxious than those treated by another therapist. This suggests that the therapist's interactions with the patient do, in fact, matter. Magill (2008) points out that the presence of the music therapist is fundamental, and that music therapy is an interactive process between the therapist and participants. More specifically, Robb (2000) suggests that support counseling provided by the music therapist within the context of music therapy interventions like song writing, lyric analysis, and/or video production can be highly effective in addressing psychosocial needs.

In addition to using the contextual support counseling approach, music therapists can foster effective therapeutic relationships by incorporating evidence-based counseling techniques. Microskills, a "set of skills, strategies and concepts of intentional interviewing and counseling" (Ivey & Ivey, 2007, p. 399) have been shown to be effective tools for fostering culturally sensitive, helping relationships. Microskills are tools for effective communication that can be divided into three sets of counseling or helping skills: (a) attending skills (focusing on the patient), (b) responding skills (providing feedback), and (c) influencing skills (promoting change). Skill usage often varies based on the therapist's theoretical orientation and the patient's cultural norms; however, microskills are considered to be "universal to good counseling" (Blonna, Loschiavo, & Watter, 2011, p. 37), regardless of theoretical orientation. The skills are somewhat hierarchical in nature, that is, the "basic" skills in the "Attending" and "Responding" skill sets represent more fundamental counseling interactions. The advanced skills (Influencing) can be more difficult to apply, although training in the use of microskills has been shown to increase effective implementation (Kuntze, van der Molen, & Born, 2010).

Table 13.4 provides an overview of commonly used microskills as identified by Ivey and Ivey (2007) and Blonna, Loschiavo, and Watter (2011). Kuntze, van der Molen, and Born (2010) point out that the use of microskills has been shown to positively impact counselor ratings, patient satisfaction, and patient self-disclosure, and to establish credible relationships. Implementing the skills found in Table 13.4 can help the music therapist facilitate productive therapist–client interactions.

Table 13.4 Microskills			
Skill Area	**Purpose**	**Specific Skills**	**Requirements of the Therapist**
Attending behaviors/skills	Build rapport; Communicate empathy; Focus on the patient	Eye contact	Culturally appropriate
		Vocal qualities	Intentionally varying pitch, volume, and speed of speech
		Verbal tracking (*Active/ Responsive Listening*)	Following patients' stories; staying on-task/ attending to the patient
		Body language/Nonverbal communication	Open, approachable Professional appearance Appropriate use of silence Appropriate use of touch (haptics) Appropriate use of space
Responding Skills	Encourage patient's verbal engagement; Facilitate clarification when needed; Communicate therapist's understanding of patient's stories	Open-ended questions	Asking questions that cannot be answered with a simple yes/no
		Closed-ended questions	Yes/no questions
		Minimal encouragers	Providing minimal verbal (e.g., "Go on"; "Umm") or nonverbal (head nod) feedback to encourage discussion
		Mirroring	Restating patients' words or imitating patients' body posture
		Paraphrasing	Restating an individual idea or specific content using key words from the patient's statements; often followed by a check-out phrase to make sure the paraphrase was accurate
		Summarizing	Synopsis of patients' statements with some interpretation; covers more information than paraphrasing
		Reflection of feeling	Interpreting patients' emotions and paraphrasing them back to the patient ("It sounds like...": "It seems that...")
Influencing skills	Influence the patient to make needed changes	Reframing	Providing an alternate frame of reference from which to view situations/events
		Confrontation/Supportive challenge	Help patients identify/ understand discrepancies in their stories
		Feedback	Providing information to the patient that helps them see how they appear to others

Recommendations for Clinical Practice

Targeted Areas

Patients report the need for both emotional and informational support (Legg, 2011). While pediatric patients receive some support from child life services, adult patients often lack access to the same type of supportive services. Music therapy, with its ability to provide a "unique form of nurture and psychosocial support in a hospital setting" (McDonnell, 1983, p. 29), has been shown to be effective across all ages and settings. As a result, music therapy can be an ideal candidate to fill this supportive role for adults. This is not to say that music therapy cannot and should not be used in pediatric psychosocial care; on the contrary, it can be highly effective. However, addressing psychosocial needs in adults is an area that has been largely untapped and may be an excellent starting place for music therapy-based psychosocial services.

Discussions with administrators and service line personnel can be another possibility when identifying target areas for music therapy-based psychosocial care. For example, discussions with administrators and staff at UK HealthCare, a teaching hospital in Lexington, Kentucky, identified six specific areas of need:

- patients receiving palliative/hospice services;

- patients with chronic and/or long-term illnesses;

- patients with complex needs (i.e., medical and mental health needs);

- patients with mental disorders (especially those first diagnosed in childhood, e.g., autism);

- patients with difficult situations (e.g., limited social support); and

- pediatric patients with anxiety. (Gooding & Rushing, 2013)

As can be seen in this listing, areas of need were included in both specific units (e.g., hospice) and specific patient situations (e.g., patients with complex needs). Discussions with administration and service line staff allowed the music therapists at UK HealthCare to best identify where (and how) they could be most effective for the enterprise and its patient population.

Targeted Objectives

With growing significance placed on (a) patient satisfaction, (b) quality of care, and (c) patient-centered care, objectives that improve the patient experience may be of particular importance to hospital administrators. Psychosocial care, by definition, is geared toward improving an individual's experience throughout the treatment process. As a result, any number of objectives may be appropriate. However, though appropriate, meeting all psychosocial needs may not be feasible with limited staffing and time constraints. Selecting specific objectives may help focus services.

Figure 13.2 identifies objectives targeted within the overall goal of improving psychosocial wellness at UK HealthCare during a 6-month period in 2013. As can be seen in the figure, 254 patients were seen during this period. Of these 254 patients, 227 or 89% were seen for psychosocial care. The largest percentage of patients were referred for mood and/or anxiety (47%), followed by quality of life objectives at 24%. Patients were also often referred for coping (15%). These data can serve as a guide for planning possible music therapy-based psychosocial services.

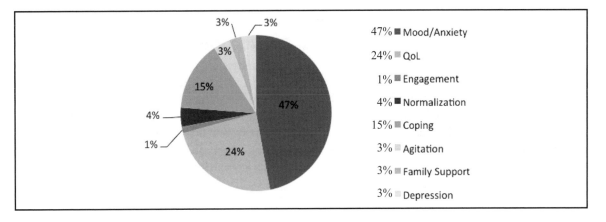

Figure 13.2. Psychosocial Referrals for Music Therapy Services

Improving Patient Satisfaction

Patient satisfaction. Patient satisfaction is often measured using HCAHPS (Hospital Consumer Assessment of Healthcare Providers and Systems) scores (PRWeb, 2013). HCAHPS scores are directly connected to hospital reimbursements through the Affordable Care Act; as a result, many hospitals are actively seeking ways to improve satisfaction scores. Research suggests that patient satisfaction can be enhanced by addressing psychosocial needs (Walker, Ristvedt, & Haughey, 2003). Yinger and Standley (2011) examined patient satisfaction scores in patients who did and did not receive music therapy at a Southeastern hospital. Participants who received music therapy were referred primarily for quality of life and mood improvement, two common psychosocial objectives. Results indicated that patient satisfaction scores were 3.4 points higher for those who received music therapy. It is important to document ways in which music therapy-based psychosocial services can improve patient satisfaction, and music therapists are encouraged to work with service excellence staff to facilitate data collection from standardized formats like the HCAHPS.

Patient feedback. It is also important to present patients and their families with opportunities to provide other types of feedback about music therapy services. A retrospective review of a pilot pediatric pre-surgical music therapy program targeting patient anxiety found that 100% of parent comments ($n = 56$) were positive (Gooding & Yinger, 2013) (see example comments below.) This type of data can also be used to provide support for music therapy services and should be communicated to hospital administration on a regular basis. While these data are often more anecdotal, they can nonetheless be extremely valuable.

Comment 1: *"Great surprise. My wife was very nervous before. Totally relaxed after. She was not the patient, by the way."* *Comment 2:* *"We really enjoyed music therapy as a family. It helped ease my anxiety as well as my son's."*

Conclusion

Psychosocial care should address the quality of life and well-being of patients, their families, and their professional caregivers in order to yield better disease-related management (Jacobsen, Holland, & Steensma, 2012). Psychosocial therapies improve coping, and music therapy with its broad appeal and ability to meet diverse needs simultaneously can be a highly effective psychosocial therapy. Music therapists address a variety of psychosocial needs, including (a) depression, (b) anxiety, (c) quality of life, and (d) behavioral distress. Music therapists use evidence-based interventions like active music engagement and age-appropriate interventions, combined with fundamental counseling skills, to promote adjustment and coping in patients. Data increasingly support the effectiveness of music therapy in psychosocial care.

References

Abad, V. (2003). A time of turmoil: Music therapy interventions for adolescents in a paediatric oncology ward. *Australian Journal of Music Therapy, 14*, 20–37.

Adler, N. E., & Page, A. K. E. (2008). *Cancer care for the whole patient: Meeting psychosocial health needs*. Washington, DC: National Academies Press. Retrieved from http://www.ncbi.nlm.nih.gov/books/NBK4015/pdf/TOC.pdf

Ayson, C. (2008). Child-parent wellbeing in a paediatric ward. *Voices: A World Forum for Music Therapy*, 8. Retrieved from https://voices.no/index.php/voices/article/viewArticle/449/367

Barrera, M. E., Rykov, M. H., & Doyle, S. L. (2002). The effects of interactive music therapy on hospitalized children with cancer: A pilot study. *Psycho-Oncology, 11*, 379–388.

Barry, P., O'Callaghan, C., Wheeler, G., & Grocke, D. (2010). Music therapy CD creation for initial pediatric radiation therapy: A mixed methods analysis. *Journal of Music Therapy, 47*, 233–263.

Blonna, R., Loschiavo, J., & Watter, D. N. (2011). *Health counseling: A microskills approach for counselors, educators, and school nurses* (2nd ed.) Sudbury, MA: Jones & Bartlett Learning.

Burns, D. S. (2001). The effect of the Bonny Method of Guided Imagery and Music on the mood and life quality of cancer patients. *Journal of Music Therapy, 38*, 51–65.

Cassileth, B. R., Vickers, A. J., & Magill, L. A. (2003). Music therapy for mood disturbance during hospitalization for autologous stem cell transplantation. *Cancer, 98*, 2723–2729.

Chetta, H. D. (1981). The effect of music and desensitization on preoperative anxiety in children. *Journal of Music Therapy, 18*, 74–87.

Clark, M., Isaacks-Dowton, G., Wells, N., Redlin-Fraizer, S., Eck, C., Hepworth, J. T., & Chakravarthy, B. (2006). Use of preferred music to reduce emotional distress and symptom activity during radiation therapy. *Journal of Music Therapy, 43*, 247–265.

Clements-Cortes, A. (2004). The use of music in facilitating emotional expression in the terminally ill. *Journal of Hospice & Palliative Medicine, 21*, 255–260.

Colwell, C. M., Edwards, R., Hernandez, E., & Brees, K. (2013). Impact of music therapy interventions (listening, composition, Orff-based) on the physiological and psychosocial behaviors of hospitalized children: A feasibility study. *Journal of Pediatric Nursing, 28*, 249–257.

de Ridder, D., Geenen, R., Kuijer, R., & van Middendorp, H. (2008). Psychosocial adjustment to chronic disease. *The Lancet, 372,* 246–255.

Docherty, S. L., Robb, S. L., Phillips-Salimi, C., Cherven, B., Stegenga, K., Hendricks-Ferguson, V., Roll, L., Stickler, M. D., & Haase, J. (2013). Parental perspectives on a behavioral health music intervention for adolescent/young adult resilience during cancer treatment: Report form the children's oncology group implications and contribution. *Journal of Adolescent Health, 52,* 170–178.

Fagen, T. S. (1982). Music therapy in the treatment of anxiety and fear in terminal pediatric patients. *Music Therapy, 2,* 13–24.

Froehlich, M. A. (1984). A comparison of the effect of music therapy and medical play therapy on the verbalization behavior of pediatric patients. *Journal of Music Therapy, 21,* 2–15.

Ghetti, C. M. (2011). Active music engagement with emotional-approach coping to improve well-being in liver and kidney transplant recipients. *Journal of Music Therapy, 48,* 463– 485.

Ghetti, C. M. (2013). Effect of music therapy with emotional-approach coping on preprocedural anxiety in cardiac catheterization: A randomized controlled trial. *Journal of Music Therapy, 50,* 93–122.

Gooding, L. F., & Rushing, J. L. (2013). *UK HealthCare music therapy statistics.* Unpublished raw data.

Gooding, L. F, & Yinger, O. S. (2013). Pre-operative music therapy for pediatric patients: A retrospective study. Manuscript submitted for publication.

Grasso, M. C., Button, B. M., Allison, D. J., & Sawyer, S. M. (2000). Physiotherapy in infants and toddlers with cystic fibrosis. *Pediatric Pulmonology, 29,* 371–381.

Hilliard, R. E. (2003). The effects of music therapy on the quality and length of life of people diagnosed with terminal cancer. *Journal of Music Therapy, 40,* 113–137.

Horne-Thompson, A., & Grocke, D. (2008). The effect of music therapy on anxiety in patients who are terminally ill. *Journal of Palliative Medicine, 11,* 582–590. doi:10.1089/jpm.2007.0193

Ivey, A. E., & Ivey, M. B. (2007). *Intentional interviewing and counseling: Facilitating client development in a multicultural society* (6th ed.). Pacific Grove, CA: Brooks/Cole.

Jacobsen, P. B., Holland, J. C., & Steensma, D. P. (2012). Caring for the whole patient: The science of psychosocial care. *Journal of Clinical Oncology, 30,* 1–3.

Janowski, K., Steuden, S., & Kurylowicz, J. (2010). Factors accounting for psychosocial functioning in patients with low back pain. *European Spine Journal, 19,* 613–623.

Kain, Z. N., Caldwell, A. A., Krivutza, D. M., Weinberg, M. E., Gaal, D., Wang, S. M., Mayes, L. C. (2004). Interactive music therapy as a treatment for preoperative anxiety in children: A randomized controlled trial. *Anesthesia & Analgesia, 98,* 1260–1266.

Kennelly, J., & Brien-Elliot, K. (2001). The role of music therapy in paediatirc rehabilitation. *Pediatric Rehabilitation, 4,* 137–143.

Kuntze, J., van der Molen, H. T., & Born, M. P. (2010). Increase in counseling communication skills after basic and advanced microskills training. *British Journal of Educational Psychology, 79,* 175–188.

Legg, M. J. (2011). What is psychosocial care and how can nurses better provide it to adult oncology patients. *Australian Journal of Advanced Nursing, 28*(3), 61–67.

Lindenfelser, K. J., Hense, C., & McFerran, K. (2012). Music therapy in pediatric palliative care: Family-centered care to enhance quality of life. *American Journal of Hospice & Palliative Medicine, 29,* 219–226.

Livneh, H., & Antonak, R. F. (2005). Psychological adaptation to chronic illness and disability: A primer for counselors. *Journal of Counseling & Development, 83,* 12–20.

Madson, A. T., & Silverman, M. J. (2010). The effect of music therapy on relaxation, anxiety, pain perception, and nausea in adult solid organ transplant patients. *Journal of Music Therapy, 47,* 220–232.

Magill, L. (2008). The meaning of the music: The role of music in palliative care music therapy as perceived by bereaved caregivers of advanced cancer patients. *American Journal of Hospice & Palliative Medicine, 26,* 33–39.

Malone, A. B. (1996). The effects of live music on the distress of pediatric patients receiving intravenous starts, venipunctures, injections, and heel sticks. *Journal of Music Therapy, 33,* 19–33.

Mandel, S. E., Davis, B. A., & Secic, M. (2013). Effects of music therapy and music-assisted relaxation and imagery on health-related outcomes in diabetes education: A feasibility study. *The Diabetes Educator.* doi:10.1177/0145721713492216

Marley, L. S. (1984). The use of music with hospitalized infants and toddlers: A descriptive study. *Journal of Music Therapy, 21,* 126–132.

McDonnell, L. (1983). Music therapy: Meeting the psychosocial needs of hospitalized children. *Children's Health Care, 12,* 29–33.

Mondanaro, J. F. (2008). Music therapy in the psychosocial care of pediatric patients with epilepsy. *Music Therapy Perspectives, 26,* 102–109.

Nayak, S., Wheeler, B. L., Shiflett, S. C., & Agostinelli, S. (2000). Effect of music therapy on mood and social interaction among individuals with acute traumatic brain injury and stroke. *Rehabilitation Psychology, 45,* 274–283.

Nolan, P. (2005). Verbal processing within the music therapy relationship. *Music Therapy Perspectives, 23,* 18–27.

O'Callaghan, C., Baron, A., Barry, P., & Dun, B. (2011). Music's relevance for pediatric cancer patients: A constructivist and mosaic research approach. *Support Care Cancer, 19,* 779–788.

Pacchetti, C., Mancinin, F., Aglieri, R., Fundaro, C., Martignoni, E., & Nappi, G. (2000). Active music therapy in Parkinson's disease: An integrative method for motor and emotional rehabilitation. *Psychosomatic Medicine, 62,* 386–393.

Pelletier, C. L. (2004). The effect of music on decreasing arousal due to stress: A meta-analysis. *Journal of Music Therapy, 41*, 192–214.

PRWeb. (2013). *PPCAC hospital reimbursements impacted by HCAHPS patient satisfaction: RateHospitals.com empowers patients to define healthcare's future.* Retrieved from http://www.prweb.com/releases/HOSPITAL/HCAHPS/prweb11059500.htm

Rafieyan, R., & Ries, R. (2007). A description of the use of music therapy in consultation-liaison psychiatry. *Psychiatry, 4,* 47–52.

Rainey, L. C., Wellisch, D. K., Fawzy, I. F., Wolcott, D. L., & Pasanu, R. (1983). Training health professionals in psychosocial aspects of cancer. *Journal of Psychosocial Oncology, 1,* 41–60.

Robb, S. (1996). Techniques in song writing: Restoring emotional and physical wellbeing in adolescents who have been traumatically injured. *Music Therapy Perspectives, 14,* 30–37.

Robb, S. L. (2000). The effect of therapeutic music interventions on the behavior of hospitalized children in isolation: Developing a contextual support model of music therapy. *Journal of Music Therapy, 37,* 118–146.

Robb, S. L., Clair, A. A., Watanabe, M., Monohan, P. O., Azzouz, F., Souffer, J. W., . . . Harmon, A. (2008). Non-randomized controlled trial of the active music engagement (AME) intervention on children with cancer. *Psycho-Oncology, 1,* 699–707.

Robb, S. L., Nichols, R. J., Rutan, R., Bishop, B. L., & Parker, J. C. (1995). The effects of music assisted relaxation on preoperative anxiety. *Journal of Music Therapy, 32,* 2–21.

Samueli Institute. (2011). *2010 Complementary and Alternative Medicine Survey of Hospitals: Summary of results.* Retrieved from http://www.samueliinstitute.org/File%20Library/Our%20Research/OHE/CAM_Survey_2 010_oct6.pdf

Schmid, W., & Aldridge, D. (2004). Active music therapy in the treatment of multiple sclerosis patients: A matched control study. *Journal of Music Therapy, 41*, 225–240.

Standley, J. M., & Hanser, S. B. (1995). Music therapy research and applications in pediatric oncology treatment. *Journal of Pediatric Oncology Nursing, 12*, 3–8.

Stouffer, J. W., Shirk, B. J., & Polomano, R. C. (2007). Practice guidelines for music interventions with hospitalized pediatric patients. *Journal of Pediatric Nursing, 22*, 448–456.

Waldon, E. G. (2001). The effects of group music therapy on mood states and cohesiveness in adult oncology patients. *Journal of Music Therapy, 38*, 212–238.

Walker, M. S., Ristvedt, S. L., & Haughey, B. H. (2003). Patient care in multidisciplinary cancer clinics: Does attention to psychosocial needs predict patient satisfaction? *Psycho- Oncology, 12*, 291–300.

Walworth, D., Rumana, C., Nguyen, J., & Jarred, J. (2008). Effects of live music therapy sessions on quality of life indicators, medications administered and hospital length of stay for patients undergoing elective surgical procedures for brain. *Journal of Music Therapy, 45*, 349–359.

Walworth, D. D. (2005). Procedural-support music therapy in the healthcare setting: A cost-effectiveness analysis. *Journal of Pediatric Nursing, 20*, 276–284.

Whipple, J. (2000). The effect of parent training in music and multimodal stimulation on parent-neonate interactions in the neonatal intensive care unit. *Journal of Music Therapy, 37*, 250–268.

Yinger, O. S. (2013). *Music therapy as procedural support for young children undergoing immunizations: A randomized controlled study*. Manuscript submitted for publication.

Yinger, O. S., & Standley, J. M. (2011). The effects of medical music therapy on patient satisfaction: As measured by Press Ganey Inpatient Survey. *Music Therapy Perspectives, 29,* 149–155.

Zabora, J., BrintzenhofeSzoc, K., Curbow, B., Hooker, C., & Piantadosi, S. (2001). The prevalence of psychological distress by cancer site. *Psycho-Oncology, 10*, 19–28.

Zebrack, B., & Isaacson, S., (2012). Psychosocial care of adolescent and young adult patients with cancer and survivors. *Journal of Clinical Oncology, 30*, 1221–1126.

Section 4: Student Training

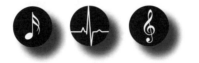

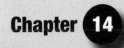

Chapter 14

Pre-Intern Clinical Fieldwork in a Medical Setting
Michelle Pellito, MM, MT-BC

Clinical fieldwork is a journey. It requires the student to learn through experience and involves observation and direct contact with patients outside of the classroom. The music therapy student will gain some of the greatest career lessons during this time, and make leaps and bounds with regard to his or her education. However, the student does not have to travel the journey alone. The music therapy supervisor guides the student along the way, and gives him or her tools necessary to successfully reach the end of training. At times, the student may feel overwhelmed or frustrated by the rush of new information. The student will be entering a period of rapid learning and experience, but should not be overwhelmed or frustrated by lulls along the learning curve. In order to succeed, the student must understand the bigger picture and approach clinical training as though it is a pathway from classroom to career.

This chapter is a general guide to what can be expected during pre-intern clinical fieldwork in a medical setting. It speaks to both the student and the supervisor, as the two roles are connected and both play an integral part in the growth of the music therapy student. It discusses expectations of the student; a general timeline of events; documentation; the process of giving and receiving feedback; relationships with patients, families, and coworkers; and what to do when the original plan is not working. The student should reflect on all the information provided and realize that clinical fieldwork is never the same for every student. There will be challenges and difficulties, but there always exists a way to overcome obstacles. This chapter will provide students with a general idea of what to expect from training, so that they may be better equipped to travel the journey with the supervisor as guide.

Current Practices in Supervision

General Practices
Students and supervisors work closely together during the period in which a student enters clinical fieldwork. The supervisor fills a number of roles, including modeling, facilitating, and evaluating student skills (McClain, 2001). The supervisor provides knowledge of the clinical field and facilitates learning and development for the student. A 2008 article published in the *Journal of Music Therapy* examined the role of the clinical supervisor across registered American Music Therapy Association (AMTA) internship directors throughout the United States. According to survey responses received from the study, supervisors use a rich number of methods to teach and nurture the growth of students during their clinical fieldwork. Those most commonly used by supervisors are (a) co-leading, (b) live observation, and (c) review of assignments and projects. Others may include, but are not limited to, (a) oral instruction, (b) reflection, or (c) practice of musical skills (Tanguay, 2008). The music therapy student and supervisor will use several techniques when it comes to training the student to work effectively within a music therapy setting.

Pre-Internship Practica Expectations

The goal of the both the university and clinical site is to ready students for the professional world and to produce a clinically effective music therapist. An interview of internship directors in one region revealed an expectation that students come into their internship with some degree of mastery in the areas of piano, guitar, and vocal performance, as well as related academic fields. Additionally, students are expected to demonstrate personal qualities of professionalism and independency and to be able to demonstrate the communication skills necessary to work within a team (Brookins, 1984). The development of a music therapist begins long before the student ever enters clinical fieldwork.

Pre-internship clinical fieldwork experiences give students a realistic idea of how a music therapy session functions, and they allow students a chance to explore the role of the music therapist firsthand. Such experiences allow students time to familiarize themselves with all the necessary components required to lead a session, as well as to hone their musical and personal skills to suit client needs. An interesting study conducted by Darrow, Johnson, Ghetti, and Achey (2001) analyzed the effectiveness of practicum students with various amounts of practica experience. Practicum students spent nearly 40% of music therapy sessions providing musical experiences, in which they played an instrument, sang, or facilitated playing or singing by the client. The greater part of the session was spent engaging in verbal behavior. There was no significant difference between practicum students in regard to how their time was used related to their overall clinical effectiveness. It was concluded, however, that the quality of the interactions was very important (Darrow et al., 2001). A student needs to demonstrate good musical skills and rapport-building in order to be an effective clinician.

Specific Techniques Used to Facilitate Student Clinical Training

Supervision includes (a) modeling, (b) observing, (c) shaping, (d) coaching, and (e) evaluating student behaviors (McClain, 2001). A supervisor's primary roles include modeling, facilitating, and evaluating student skills, and methods to accomplish these tasks include (a) observation, (b) feedback, (c) supervision conferences, and (d) written evaluation forms (McClain, 2001). Therefore, being a supervisor often requires a little creativity. The table below outlines some of the creative methods used in clinical fieldwork to facilitate student learning.

Table 14.1. Supervision Strategies		
Strategy	**Purpose**	**Source**
Collaborative peer lyric writing	Develop self-reflection skills	Baker & Krout, 2011
Reflexive journal writing	Generate insight and understanding	Barry & O'Callaghan, 2008
Exploring other musical cultures	Integrate new techniques/musical styles	Shapiro, 2005
Role-playing	Practice interaction with clients	Tanguay, 2008
Audio/videotape review	Self-observe and analyze behavior	Tanguay, 2008
Strengths-based/music centered focus	Provide culturally centered supervision	Swamy, 2011
Use of structured forms and written self-analysis	Improve communication, observation, feedback, and coordination	Farnan, 1996

Student Requirements

By the time most music therapy students reach clinical training, their education has been nurtured through several years of college. They have a good working knowledge of music theory, ear training, performance, and music therapy, and they may have already taken classes in the fields of medicine and psychology. In regard to their personality, these students typically exhibit motivation and drive to attain the status of music therapy professional. More than likely, they love music and people and are interested in merging the two together. All of these combined are necessary tools for the start of a wonderful music therapy career.

Guitar and Vocal Skills

While it takes almost no prior knowledge about a guitar to pick one up and play a single note, it takes a great deal of knowledge to use a guitar effectively in a music therapy intervention. Much of this knowledge is gained long before individuals become music therapy students. Elements like rhythm and pitch are fixed in the mind for years before students start their clinical fieldwork. During the fieldwork experience, there may be times when a supervisor needs to review basic music theory to correct what students have overlooked in learning a song. It may even be necessary for the supervisor to teach certain musical tasks, such as how to restring or tune a guitar, or find music resources. But perhaps the most common issue that a supervisor will have to address is the memorization of chords and lyrics.

Music therapists keep a collection of music that can easily be retrieved from their music books, folders, or electronic device. Typically, therapists will read music directly from the page during an intervention, as long as they can maintain good eye contact and not let the music tool distract from the therapy. However, at times the music therapist needs to abandon the music tool completely and be prepared with a generous inventory of memorized music.

Unexpected events can and will arise during a music therapy work week. Music folders can be lost and electronic devices can be broken. A music therapist may be required to walk with a patient, playing the guitar or continuous music, which does not allow time for page turning. In these instances, music therapists should be able to retrieve a list of songs directly from memory. Students are often required to begin memorizing music when they enter clinical fieldwork.

However big the assignment—whether the task is to learn 1 song or 30, memorizing music can be daunting. If many songs are to be learned across a period of time, the student should distribute the learning evenly from week to week, rather than attempting the overwhelming task of memorizing all the songs at once. Generally, the more complicated the chord progression and the greater the number of chords and lyrics, the harder it will be to memorize. The student and supervisor should strategize to ensure the student is successful. The student may learn one difficult and two easy songs per week, or two difficult songs one week and four easy songs the next week. Everyone approaches music memorization in a different way and must find the way that works best. The supervisor will likely check frequently to see how music memorization is progressing. If the student is repeatedly unsuccessful, a new plan of action should be formed. Once a song is memorized, it should be played often. With more practice, retrieving it from memory will become natural.

Regarding vocal skills, some music therapy students enter clinical fieldwork with only a little voice training. Some may struggle to perform in front of others or to stay on pitch. Again, the supervisor and student need to develop a strategy for tackling these issues. Many times more practice and performance are beneficial, as well as helpful techniques such as (a) plucking the first note, (b) playing a common chord progression from the song as the intro, or (c) humming softly before singing to find the pitch. With patience and dedication to practice, the student can overcome hurdles related to guitar and voice. These basic skills are essential for the music therapist and should be emphasized during clinical fieldwork.

Personality and Interest in the Field

No definitive rules govern what personality traits an individual must have to qualify as a music therapist. In research to identify traits most prevalent among music therapists, results from the Myers Briggs Type Indicator (MBTI), a personality test, showed that music therapists tend to be "warmly enthusiastic, high-spirited, ingenious, [and] imaginative." Also notable among music therapy students is the high rate of volunteerism and service during their high school years (Steele & Young, 2008). Music therapists come from all different backgrounds and display many qualities that make them successful. Other traits that are helpful to the music therapy student and professional include (a) mental stability, (b) good interpersonal skills, and (d) confidence.

Mental stability. Medical music therapists are often faced with difficult situations that are both mentally and emotionally taxing. To be successful in the workplace, the music therapist should have a number of coping mechanisms in place. It is not reasonable for an individual to "switch off" or "bottle" emotions. Instead, the therapist must find an appropriate way to handle emotions before, during, and after an event so as not to interfere with work or personal life. Often, effective coping mechanisms include engaging in a hobby, bettering nutrition and exercise, and maintaining a healthy social life. A survey of music therapists explored career-sustaining behaviors and found the most common ones included (a) maintaining a sense of humor, (b) spending time with a partner or family, (c) maintaining self-awareness, (d) reflecting on positive experiences, and (e) maintaining a professional identity (Swezey, 2013). A combination of these is probably the best coping mechanism of all and can help a music therapist through challenging times or feelings of "burnout." Positivity and problem solving are also helpful traits when dealing with mentally and emotionally challenging situations. Good mental health may at times require the help of professionals. If the stress of work or personal life feels constantly beyond one's control, the music therapy student or professional should not be ashamed to seek a mental health expert for further advice.

Interpersonal skills. Music therapists are typically experts at maintaining good interpersonal skills. An established music therapy program with a full-time program director, part-time music therapist, part-time graduate assistant, and four full-time interns per year have the capacity to visit thousands of patients annually (Standley & Walworth, 2005). Good introductions and first impressions are a necessity. Great interpersonal skills will enable the therapist to build rapport and interact with the patients and their families. Building rapport is critical to the therapeutic relationship, developing respect and trust between the patient and the therapist. Without it, achieving established goals and objectives will be very difficult, if not impossible. Later in the chapter, the practice of building rapport with patients will be discussed in further detail.

Confidence. Confidence does not come easily for everyone, yet it is an important trait possessed by great music therapists. Confidence allows the professional to (a) approach new patients, (b) develop a relationship of trust and respect, and (c) provide a music therapy intervention designed to meet the patient's needs. Even individuals who lack confidence can learn to be confident, or, at the very least, act as if they are. Music therapists who wish to develop more confidence should reflect on the traits that a confident person embodies, think about how that person would act in a professional situation, and then strive to exhibit those qualities. With time and practice, confidence will become more natural. As long as the music therapist remains humble and genuine as well, confidence is a superior quality that will enhance his or her career.

A General Timeline for Student Expectations

The supervisor determines goals for music therapy students to help them develop into music therapy professionals. Often a goal is for the student to independently carry out an effective music therapy intervention, with little to no facilitation from the supervisor. The process to this point is usually gradual, with thoughtful instructions from the supervisor to help the student meet the goal over time. The performance of the student at the end of clinical fieldwork is in part a product of the supervisor's instruction over past weeks or months. The supervisor's role changes as the student's needs change, and it is important to identify clinical, academic, and personal growth throughout the preinternship practice experience (McClain, 2001). Outlined below is a very general but common structure that supervisors may follow to ease the student into the responsibility of independently carrying out a music therapy intervention.

Observation

For the first few sessions, the student may be asked to simply observe a session as a board-certified music therapist facilitates a music therapy intervention. During this time, the student may be asked to practice identifying (a) the patient's needs, (b) appropriate goals and objectives, (c) applicable music interventions, and (d) the patient's responses to an intervention. The student may also begin learning music or the documentation process during this time.

Assistance

Following a period of observation, the student may be asked to provide one or two songs during a music therapy intervention. Assisting the music therapy professional in a small way provides a realistic stepping stone between observations and co-leading, setting the student up for success and building confidence. The supervisor will likely provide feedback regarding guitar and vocal performance, as well as elements of basic interaction with the patient, such as eye contact and proximity.

Co-leading

Eventually the student will be tasked with more responsibilities during the session and will enter a period of co-leading, in which the student and the professional work together to carry out a music therapy intervention. They may take turns during the session, or the supervisor may provide help only if the student struggles. The student will receive feedback in a number of areas and will be expected to more accurately identify goals and interventions appropriate to the patient's needs.

Independence

The end stage of pre-intern clinical fieldwork will require the student to be more independent, carrying out most, if not all, of the music therapy intervention. The supervisor may do little to facilitate during the session but will continue to provide feedback to the student on his or her therapeutic effectiveness. The student will more easily identify patient needs and appropriate interventions without assistance from the supervisor.

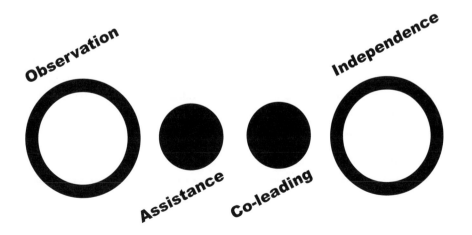

Figure 14.1 Student Training Timeline

Documentation

Data collection or documentation, when implemented systematically, allows students to develop both strong observation and decision-making skills (Hanser, 2001). The music therapy student will learn to recognize patient responses to evidence-based musical interventions and will learn how to share the results with the interdisciplinary team through documentation. In the medical setting, interdisciplinary teams rely on this information to maintain the best care possible for the patient across all disciplines.

The music therapy student should realize that documentation takes many different forms and varies between facilities and populations served. While the student may be familiar with the particular documentation methods of his or her own clinical fieldwork facility, the documentation methods will likely change upon entering a different workplace, even if the content remains the same.

The AMTA Standards of Clinical Practice (2013b) outline the basic elements of documentation for a number of settings, including medical settings. Medical documentation is likely to describe (a) the patient's problem, (b) the decided goal or objective, (c) the applied intervention, and (d) the patient's response to the intervention. Because the medical setting deals with evidence-based practices, the information documented should not be based on speculation, but should be as quantifiable as possible. The student will learn to be very observant of the duration and frequency of a behavior, as both are measurable outcomes that can be useful in documenting changes over time. As the student grows more skilled in documenting the music therapy session, he or she may find that growth also occurs in the areas of identifying patient needs, applying the appropriate intervention, and recognizing patient responses. All of these go hand in hand, and the skill with which they are carried out and documented are good markers of the student's accomplishments over the course of the clinical fieldwork.

Providing Feedback

Feedback is one of the most basic and important aspects of clinical fieldwork. It allows students to recognize their strengths and weaknesses in order to improve as music therapists. Providing feedback is one of the greatest ways to shape a student, so it must be honest, prompt, and constructive. According to McClain (2001), pre-intern students have the right to receive feedback that (a) is regular in nature, (b) is ethical and respectful in nature, (c) clearly defines expectations, and (d) clearly defines problem areas and establishes a clearly defined remediation plan.

Honest feedback is not always easy to give, especially when it involves an uncomfortable subject, such as appropriateness of clothing. The supervisor may find it easy to overlook an area of needed improvement in order to help resolve bigger issues in a student's work. Some supervisors may have difficulty giving honest feedback if students perceive it as an attack on their character. However, the supervisor must move beyond these concerns in order to be a teacher. Unless problems are addressed, students may never fully understand what it takes to be the best music therapist possible. Although difficult, it is more important to constructively critique than to avoid the topic. Thus, the supervisor must be honest when giving feedback to cultivate success in students.

Feedback should also be prompt. Typically, the supervisor gives feedback immediately following a session. Fewer details are missed and the student can better apply the feedback to what just occurred. The student and the supervisor can then create a plan of action for the areas of needed improvement. The supervisor may assign a task to help the student prepare for the following visit. It is best practice for the student to review the feedback after some time has passed, ideally before entering the next session. When the supervisor provides feedback promptly, the student has time to process his or her work and consider techniques to maintain or improve in the next session.

Not only should feedback be honest and prompt, but the best feedback is constructive, delivered with positivity. It is often easy to dwell on areas of needed improvement, especially if quite a few are identified. However, the supervisor should also highlight what students do well in their sessions. In fact, it may be even more important to nurture the positives, as students will remember what went well and strive to repeat those actions in future sessions. Some researchers recommend a 3:1 ratio of positive to negative reinforcement in the classroom; three instances of praise for every one correction is the ideal feedback ratio needed for students to "flourish" (Fredrickson & Losada, 2005). Constructive feedback may also include students identifying their own areas of strength and those needing improvement, which encourages students to think independently and begin a habit of self-critique that will last beyond the clinical fieldwork. In this approach, the supervisor should ensure that students are able to consistently identify positive moments in their practice, as individuals can often be their own worst critic. Positivity in feedback is absolutely essential in motivating students to become music therapy professionals.

When the Plan Is Not Working

Even the best laid plans can go awry. However, there is more than one path to a destination. The supervisor works with students to help them arrive at the end of training, adapting plans as necessary to meet their personal needs. In turn, students must trust the supervisor to guide them to success, working hard to be the best student possible.

The efforts of just one person cannot ensure a successful clinical education. The supervisor and each individual student must come together to determine the best learning methods and how to implement them. Some individuals work best by being thrown into situations and working them out alone. Others need careful and thoughtful guidance throughout training. In a study by Wheeler (2002), practicum students in a university music therapy program voiced their concern that a clinical supervisor needed to be flexible concerning student training. Two students will never be the same, and their individual learning styles may call for new and different approaches.

The following suggestions can guide supervisors when the plan is "not working." Regardless of the avenue chosen, it is important to address issues as soon as possible. The quicker the student is set on the correct path, the more success he or she will achieve by the end of the journey.

When the plan is not working, try a new method of teaching. The supervisor and student should be creative in their approach to accomplishing a difficult task. For example, if students lack confidence when singing, they can practice filling a big room (or a small room like a bathroom) with a booming voice. Using a decibel meter to measure volume, students can practice increasing the volume of their voice until they have to scale it back (it is probably easier to decrease voice volume than increase it). The point is to have more than one technique to address an issue, so that students can find at least one that works. Practicing voice volume through various exercises is an effective way for students to gain more self-awareness.

When the plan is not working, practice more. The supervisor and student may arrange to increase the number of hours spent in the practicum experience. The student may also need to spend more hours practicing at home. Sometimes it may be necessary to put in more time than one's peers in order to achieve the same goal. Although a student may struggle to keep up with other individuals in one area, he or she may excel in another.

When the plan is not working, simplify it. If the student struggles so much in one area that it is impossible to reach the next step of training, the supervisor may need to change the goals, intensely focusing on any deficits until the student is successful. The student may need to work harder or longer to catch up to peers in the future, but it is important to set achievable goals. The supervisor does a disservice to pass the student along without addressing the root of the issue, which may cause the student even bigger problems in the future.

When the plan is not working, turn to available resources. The resources in Table 14.2 provide guidelines for practice and useful tools for clinical supervisors.

Table 14.2. Helpful Resources for Music Therapy Supervision	
Source	**Author**
AMTA National Roster Internship Guidelines	AMTA (2013a)
AMTA Standards of Clinical Practice	AMTA (2013b)
Music Therapy: A Fieldwork Primer	Borczon (2004)
Music Therapy Clinical Training Manual	Boyle & Krout (1988)
Music Therapy Supervision	Forinash (2000)
Music Therapy Education and Training: From Theory to Practice	Goodman (2011)
Clinical Training Guide for the Student Music Therapist	Wheeler, Shultis, & Polen (2005)

Conclusion

The music therapy student does not have to journey alone through clinical fieldwork. In fact, the supervisor is with the student every step of the way, and communication between the two is absolutely essential to the success of the student. The student enters clinical fieldwork with a set of tools gained from years of musical training and education in music therapy and its related fields. Clinical training allows a safe place for the student to put these learned ideas into practice through direct contact and interaction with patients. Usually the student will progress through training by a gradual increase in responsibilities, beginning with observation of the supervisor and ending with the student independently leading the session. The supervisor provides feedback throughout the entire process, allowing the student to recognize his or her own areas of strengths and weaknesses. Just as communication with the supervisor is essential, communication with the interdisciplinary team is equally important, as it allows for the best patient care across all disciplines. Thus, the student will learn skillful documentation of patient problems, goals and objectives, music interventions, and patient responses. As the student and supervisor advance through clinical training, it may be necessary to alter plans according to the student's needs. Communication in this situation is absolutely vital, as the success of the student does not rely solely on the work of the supervisor. Instead, a combination of lessons taught and the student's effort determines the success of the therapist at the end of clinical fieldwork. With the knowledge and expectations gained from reading this chapter, the student is more prepared for the exciting journey from classroom to professional career.

References

American Music Therapy Association. (2013a). *AMTA national roster internship guidelines*. Retrieved from http://www.musictherapy.org/careers/national_roster_internship_guidelines/

American Music Therapy Association. (2013b). *AMTA standards of clinical practice*. Retrieved from http://www.musictherapy.org/about/standards/

Baker, F., & Krout, R. (2011). Collaborative peer lyric writing during music therapy training: A tool for facilitating students' reflections about clinical practicum experiences. *Nordic Journal of Music Therapy, 20,* 62–89.

Barry, P., & O'Callaghan, C. (2008). Reflexive journal writing: A tool for music therapy student clinical practice development. *Nordic Journal of Music Therapy, 17,* 55–66.

Borczon, R. M. (2004). *Music therapy: A fieldwork primer.* Gilsum, NH: Barcelona.

Boyle, M. E., & Krout, R. E. (1988). *Music therapy clinical training manual.* St. Louis, MO: MMB Music.

Brookins, L. M. (1984). The music therapy clinical intern: Performance skills, academic knowledge, personal qualities, and interpersonal skills necessary for a student seeking clinical training. *Journal of Music Therapy, 21,* 193–201.

Darrow, A. A., Johnson, C. M., Ghetti, C. M., & Achey, C. A. (2001). An analysis of music therapy student practicum behaviors and their relationship to clinical effectiveness: An exploratory investigation. *Journal of Music Therapy, 38,* 307–320.

Farnan, L. A. (1996). Issues in clinical training: The mystery of supervision. *Music Therapy Perspectives, 14,* 70–71.

Forinash, M. (2000). *Music therapy supervision.* Gilsum, NH: Barcelona.

Fredrickson, B., & Losada, F. (2005). Positive affect and the complex aspects of human flourishing. *American Psychologist, 60*(7), 678–686.

Goodman, K. D. (2011). *Music therapy education and training: From theory to practice.* Springfield, IL: Charles C. Thomas.

Hanser, S. (2001). A systems analysis approach to music therapy practica. In M. Forinash (Ed.), *Music therapy supervision* (pp. 69–86). Gilsum, NH: Barcelona.

McClain, F. J. (2001). Music therapy supervision: A review of the literature. In M. Forinash (Ed.), *Music therapy supervision* (pp. 9–18). Gilsum, NH: Barcelona.

Shapiro, N. (2005). Sounds in the world: Multicultural. *Music Therapy Perspectives, 23,* 29–35.

Standley, J. M., & Walworth. D. (2005). Cost/Benefit analysis of the total program. In J. M. Standley (Ed.), *Medical music therapy* (pp. 31–40). Silver Spring, MD: American Music Therapy Association.

Steele, A. L., & Young, S. (2008). A descriptive study of Myers-Briggs personality types of professional music educators and music therapists with comparisons to undergraduate majors. *Journal of Music Therapy, 48,* 55–73.

Swamy, S. (2011). "No, she doesn't seem to know anything about cultural differences!" Culturally centered music therapy supervision. *Music Therapy Perspectives, 29,* 133–137.

Swezey, S. (2013). *What keeps us well? Professional quality of life and career sustaining behaviors of music therapy professionals* (Unpublished master's thesis). University of Kentucky, Lexington.

Tanguay, C. L. (2008). Supervising music therapy interns: A survey of AMTA national roster internship directors. *Journal of Music Therapy, 45*, 52–74.

Wheeler, B. L. (2002). Experiences and concerns of students during music therapy practica. *Journal of Music Therapy, 39,* 274–304.

Wheeler, B. L., Shultis, C. L., & Polen, D. W. (2005). *Clinical training guide for the student music therapist.* New Braunfels, TX: Barcelona.

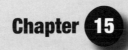

Chapter 15

Medical Music Therapy Internships: Facilitating Effectiveness
Alexandra Fields, MS, MT-BC, and Jessica Rushing, MM, MT-BC

Many music therapists choose to supervise students because they want to bring more diversity into their professional lives. Others may also desire to give back and contribute to the music therapy community and help better the future of our field. Regardless of the reason, choosing to provide clinical supervision to music therapy interns is one of the most important roles we take on as clinicians. By supervising interns, we are stewarding the next generation of music therapy clinicians and impacting the future of our field.

In the field of music therapy, internships differ in terms of structure and setting. Internships can be university-affiliated or approved by the American Music Therapy Association (AMTA). They may be part- or full-time, offered in one or more settings, or last for varying time frames. Students enter internship with an individualized plan and must complete a minimum of 900 hours of internship experiences, which can include (a) observation, (b) assisting, (c) co-leading and leading, and (d) independent work. All internships, regardless of structure, must meet AMTA standards for clinical training and clinical supervision (AMTA, 2014).

Internship supervisors themselves must hold an appropriate credential, have a bachelor's degree or its equivalent in music therapy, and have at least 2 years of full-time experience. Supervisors must have sufficient experience in the internship setting. They must also demonstrate competency and effectiveness as clinicians. Likewise, they must pursue relevant continuing education. In terms of supervision, AMTA requires that all supervisors demonstrate "a general understanding of the supervisory needs of internship students" as well as "established skills in supervision" (AMTA, 2014, 6.2.2). While there are training courses on music therapy supervision available during national and regional conferences and some online courses, training for music therapy supervision, in general, is scarce (Tanguay, 2008). Research is limited, and resources on how to provide effective music therapy supervision are not as readily provided in our field as in others. Music therapy clinical supervisors often must turn to other fields, such as clinical psychology, social work, and psychotherapy, to find resources on how to provide effective supervision. As a result, for many music therapists, learning to provide effective supervision happens on the job (Tanguay, 2008). The purpose of this chapter is to provide guidance on some common issues facing supervisors in the medical setting.

Creating a Positive and Successful Internship Experience

The main task of a supervisor is to model, teach, and evaluate professional-level competencies (McClain, 2001). In order to do these things effectively, supervisors must recognize that a significant transition occurs within music therapy students when they move from practicum student to intern. Knight (2008) stated that "internship is understood as a transition point in one's career because of the new relationship dynamic of Intern/Supervisor" (p. 78). Most interns prefer and function more effectively in a relationship where the dynamic between intern and supervisor is more of a consultant–colleague as opposed to a teacher–student or counselor–client relationship (Knight, 2008).

The most successful and positive internship experiences occur when there is some common ground between the music therapy supervisor and intern. Memory, Unkefer, and Smeltekop (1987) state that supervision should be a "partnership between students and supervisor" (p. 161). Ideally, the intern enters into a collaborative, open, and safe environment where the supervisor is knowledgeable, competent, and insightful, and is also a lifelong learner. This creates a level of comfort between both members of the supervisory relationship, where trust can be built and both members can grow and learn. One way to establish this collaborative, open, and safe environment is to set up clear expectations at the beginning of internship. While fluctuation and daily alternations are inevitable in the medical setting, creating a framework for expectations at the onset can decrease confusion and establish a baseline if issues or concerns arise. Items to discuss, write down, and clearly identify at the beginning of internship include:

- The time the intern should arrive and leave from work;

- Project timelines and due dates;

- Expectation of direct client contact, planning time, and office time;

- Approximate timeline of transition from observing to independent clinical work;

- Tracking system to log internship hours;

- Vacation, sick days, and conference attendance policies;

- Any office cleaning or equipment management systems;

- Infection control policies.

Effective interpersonal relations are also important for intern success (Brookins, 1984). Some basic interpersonal skills identified by the National Research Council (2011) that music therapists use every day in their work include:

- Clear communication;

- Flexibility/adaptability;

- Collaboration;

- Respect for cultural differences;

- Guidance of others toward goals.

These skills readily transfer to the supervisory relationship; in fact, the skills needed to be an effective therapist and those needed to become an effective music therapy intern supervisor are very similar. The relationship created is, in a sense, "once-removed" from the traditional patient–therapist therapeutic relationship; the supervisor nurtures, recognizes, and builds on interns' strengths and skills. One way that supervisors can foster growth is to provide interns with strength-identifying exercises as they begin their journey. Such exercises aid interns in (a) identifying, (b) utilizing, and (c) owning their unique strengths across the internship. Providing this tool at the beginning offers initial insight for the team as a whole, as well as a foundation to foster self-reflection throughout the process. Many resources are available to help interns and team members identify their strengths. *StrengthFinders 2.0* (Rath, 2007) is one option. Another option is the *VIA Survey of Character Strengths* (2014) offered through the Positive Psychology website titled "Authentic Happiness." Similarly, self-awareness activities are helpful when considering how to engage in self-care practices.

The intern learns from the skills, perspective, and knowledge of the supervisor; and the supervisor is involved in a process of refining his/her knowledge and relearning it from new angles.

(Deming, 2005, p. 1)

It is important to constantly evaluate the effectiveness of the supervisory relationship. Examples of effective and ineffective supervision styles and outcomes can be found in Table 15.1.

Table 15.1. Supervision Styles and Outcomes	
Effective/Positive Supervision	**Ineffective/Poor Supervision**
Supervisor provides a warm, safe, inviting environment that fosters a music therapy intern's unique skills, perspective, and growth.	Supervisor creates an unsafe environment where criticism is readily provided with little to no support or respect for music therapy intern's unique skills/perspective.
Results in building competency, support in taking calculated risks, and development of therapists unique clinical voice.	Results in intern feeling uncomfortable in session, overwhelmed by his/her caseload, unprepared for a future as an independent, competent music therapist.

Ideally interns in a medical setting must be able to work independently in a fast-paced, ever-changing environment while collaborating with the treatment team when possible and appropriate. Interns should also be self-directed and comfortable educating medical staff about their important role within the treatment team. It is important to identify these skills, as well as other success-promoting behaviors, prior to internship. Five important areas to consider, with related sample internship interview questions, are provided in Appendix O. Topics include (a) personality, (b) learning style, (c) music therapy knowledge, (d) clinical scenarios, and (e) music skills.

It is important for supervisors to maintain high professional expectations while interns are completing their internship. High expectations are a major factor in a successful music therapy internship experience for both intern and supervisor. Establishing these expectations at the beginning of the internship experience can help prevent problems from arising as the internship progresses. Some of these expectations include:

• Be prompt and punctual at all times.

• Respond to all emails, calls, and pages within 24–48 hours.

• If you do not know the answer or cannot meet an expectation, say so, and delineate a concrete plan for following up as soon as possible.

• Receive constructive criticism and feedback with openness.

• Consult and collaborate with peers and colleagues.

• If conflict arises, communicate it immediately to your internship director/supervisor.

• When approaching your supervisor with a problem, come prepared with at least one potential solution.

- Assume responsibility for completing your own tasks and addressing personal concerns.

- Respect organizational structure and hospital hierarchy.

- Take calculated risks.

Differences in Theoretical Orientation/Approach

The music therapy field is unique in its approach to theoretical orientation. Choi (2008) compares similar helping fields such as psychotherapy, counseling, or clinical psychology to music therapy and finds that the literature does not always distinguish between specific theoretical approaches with clear boundaries. "Many music therapy literatures mix models and approaches because they are not mutually exclusive" (Choi, 2008, p. 95).

Sometimes our theoretical approach combined with our life experiences can make us prone to "blind spots" or areas that the intern or supervisor typically underassess or do not notice. What makes therapists vulnerable to "blind spots" (Deming, 2005, p. 40)? Possibilities include:

- An issue that the clinician has no experience treating.

- An issue that the clinician is not familiar with in his or her own life.

- An issue that, for any reason, causes the clinician to minimize or rationalize as unimportant.

- An issue that the clinician fears will be inappropriate to broach in treatment.

- Culture, personal values, and lifestyle differences.

Regardless of the number of years of experience, all therapists are capable of having blind spots. If supervisors can recognize and manage blind spots, they will be less likely to miss clinically significant information from their interns. In addition, they will be more aware of their surroundings and less likely to miss important events, signs, symptoms, etc., from patients.

It can be a challenge for many music therapy intern supervisors to balance their own theoretical perspective with conflicting or different perspectives of interns. Particularly disabling are issues of transference and countertransference, or strong emotional reactions and/or negative automatic cognitions (Prasko et al., 2010). Supervisors may be unsure how to address these issues within the supervisory relationship. The following questions can help keep the topic client-centered when an intern raises the issue of countertransference or automatic thoughts or feelings:

- When did you notice the countertransference?

- What did you do in the session as a result of noticing these feelings in yourself?

- How did your feelings alter the dynamic of that session?

- What would help you to keep the session client-centered when you notice yourself having that reaction? (Deming, 2005, p. 41).

Generally, regardless of the theoretical orientation/approach, the supervisor's goal is to help interns find creative methods of managing countertransference to reduce its impact on the session (Deming, 2005).

Working Through Challenges in Supervision

One issue that is infrequently discussed is how to deal with interns who are more challenging to supervise. These students may be stubborn, disorganized, or lacking in skills, or they may be experiencing stressors outside the hospital, making it difficult to adequately focus on their training as a music therapy intern. *What should be done in these scenarios?* Internship contracts established by AMTA, university affiliations, and the facilities themselves establish clear guidelines regarding professional behavior and the supervisor's right to terminate the supervisory relationship should inappropriate behavior arise. Not all such behaviors, however, warrant termination. Often, even challenging issues can be resolved, but it is important to first identify the actual problem. Deming (2005) organizes such challenging issues by identifying typical "types" of interns who display problematic behaviors:

- "It Won't Work, Know-It-All" Supervisee

- Defensive Supervisee

- "Bad Client Syndrome" Supervisee

- Clingy Supervisee

- "Yes-man" Supervisee

- "No One Told Me" Supervisee

Supervisors should seek additional support and guidance from administrators or colleagues when faced with challenging interns. Tips on how to work with challenging interns can be found in Table 15.2.

Table 15.2. Strategies for Problematic Supervisees/Interns			
Supervisee Style	**Traits**	**Supervisor Goal**	**Supervisor Strategies**
"It Won't Work, Know-It-All"	Difficulty with authority figures and taking directions. Will give drawbacks to every suggestion. Dwells on drawbacks of ideas/interventions.	Increase openness and flexibility	Role-plays Confront distortions Brainstorming Self-disclosure Direct supervision Tape supervision Prescribing symptom "I-focus"
Defensive	Always has a rationalization for what went wrong in a session, why what he/she did was exactly what the patient needed. Resistant to supervisor's suggestions.	Reduce personalizations Increase flexibility	2:1 feedback Role-plays Self-disclosure Direct supervision Tape supervision Process comments "I- focus on…"
Bad-Patient Syndrome	Takes no responsibility for anything happening in the session – it's the patient's fault. Gives his/her power away to the client.	Increase comfort with presenting new interventions	Role-plays Self-disclosure Direct supervision Prescribing symptom Process comments "I-focus on…"
"No One Told Me"	Helpless Blameless Takes everything very literally. Difficulty coping with change.	Increase confidence Reduce cognitive distortions	Brainstorming Modeling Explore what worked Prescribe dependence Assign reading
Yes-man	Never has any problems, all patients are progressing well. Wants to appear cooperative and successful. Tends to minimize problems of the patient to report success vs. truth.	Create comfort with bringing up issues/challenges from sessions	Brainstorming Self-disclosure 2:1 feedback Process comments
Clingy	Wants constant feedback. Difficulty taking initiative. Executes interventions in non-authentic ways. Always wants to "run something by the supervisor." Relies on styles of other clinicians.	Create/increase confidence and sufficiency	Modeling 2:1 feedback Exploring Assign reading

Adapted from Deming, 2005, pp. 49–55

Music therapy supervisors should communicate to their interns that the goal of supervision is not for the intern to emulate or "copy" the supervisor's exact approach and therapeutic style. Corey (2005) explains that "the therapist's role is to assist clients in making decisions that are congruent with the clients' worldview, not to convince clients to live by the therapist's values" (p. 23); this is likewise true for intern supervisors. Supervisors should support interns in finding their own clinical voice, style, and approach to medical music therapy. Interns need to authentically integrate their life experiences and educational training to find their own unique way to make their mark on patients and the field of music therapy as a whole.

The Internship Process

Internships are often set up along a continuum, with interns moving through observation, assisting, co-leading, leading, and independent work. For many music therapy students, the music therapy internship can be the hardest and yet most rewarding aspect of their educational training. Internship is a time of great growth, learning, and formation, both personally and professionally. Grant and McCarty (1990) followed 59 interns through their 6-month internships, analyzing the professional and personal emotional stages they went through. The authors used Likert-type scales to evaluate feeling states at the beginning of internship, each month within internship, and the conclusion. Ten items were geared toward professional growth and 10 toward personal growth. (See Table 15.3 for more information.)

Table 15.3. Assessment of Feelings During Internship	
Personal	**Professional**
Unhappy – Happy Uncreative – Creative Stagnant – Growing Unaccepted – Accepted Lonesome – Befriended Discontent – Content Bored – Excited Unloved – Loved Misunderstood – Understood Depressed – Elated	Insecure – Confident Incompetent – Competent Incapable – Capable Disorganized – Organized Unaccepted – Accepted Inadequate – Adequate Uncreative – Creative Frustrated – Relaxed Unsure – Sure Unprofessional – Professional

Results suggested that professional growth steadily increased across the internship, with significant growth in months 1 and 2, and then again in months 5 and 6. Personal growth appeared to remain steady through month 3, followed by a slight drop, and then significant increases in months 5 and 6. Whether interns received their first choice of an internship site was the only variable affecting both professional and personal growth, though this appeared to even out by the conclusion of internship. While comments on feelings of growth were present across the internship, other themes arose as well. Feelings such as frustration, inadequacy, self-doubt, or insecurity were reported by 80% of participants at the end of the first month. Comments related to struggle with identity were present following the second month. The fourth month emerged as a particular turning point, with steady increases from then on, and comments related to increased work and responsibilities. The fifth and sixth month comments were almost completely positive. Awareness of interns' professional and emotional growth stages can help supervisors strategically plan the music therapy internship progression, creating a continuum that is structured for student success.

In conjunction with emotional stages, interns appear to move through what some would consider to be overarching transitions. The timing and amount of guidance needed to journey through transitions varies greatly from intern to intern. By recognizing transition periods, the supervisor will be better equipped to provide positive and constructive feedback while facilitating growth along the way. Furthermore, the supervisor who can identify when interns need guidance and can acknowledge their growth will be better equipped to provide individualized feedback based on interns' personal learning styles. Ultimately, these transitions culminate as the intern assumes a new role as a professional music therapist. Consider the following transitions:

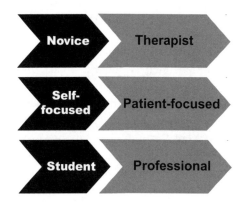

Figure 15.1. Intern transitions.

Often there are cues that indicate an intern's readiness to transition to a new role. Challenges arise when eagerness precedes readiness, thus creating barriers to learning. In this case, interns may push themselves forward before mastering foundational skills, leaving gaps in their skill set and leading to confusion when things do not go as well as anticipated. Another challenge occurs when an intern has moved through most of the internship without showing signs of readiness to transition to these new roles. Internship supervisors walk a fine line, pushing just hard enough to simultaneously prompt success and growth while limiting feelings of frustration. Watching for cues helps the supervisor know when an intern is ready to be pushed or needs more support.

Table 15.4 provides examples of common transition cues interns give. *Guidance Is Needed* cues demonstrate an intern may need additional support or intervention. *Signs of Growth* cues represent an intern's capacity for more complex instruction. To the right of each cue are concrete options for effective supervision. These transitions are not expected to occur in the beginning of internship. As suggested by Grant and McCarty (1990), major shifts are likely in the fifth and possibly sixth months. The supervisor should focus on each intern individually, as his or her growth patterns may differ.

Table 15.4 Common Transition Cues			
Signs that Further Guidance Is Needed	Supervisor Responses	Signs of Growth	Supervisor Responses
Novice → Therapist			
Places excessive weight on mood elevation outcomes when mood is not the primary objective.	Celebrate value of this skill and collaborate in brainstorming what else might be possible when someone is in a good mood. Try taking sessions one specific step further. Follow up.	**Uses mood elevating techniques to prepare patients for more difficult tasks.**	Point out specific things intern did well. Have intern describe how to teach someone how to do what the intern has done.
"This is a problem…I don't know what to do."	Have intern talk through details of problem. Collaborate in brainstorming options. Follow up regularly celebrating independently developed solutions.	**"This is a problem…I have an idea!"**	Support ideas to the fullest extent possible. Create through leading questions and role-play opportunities for the intern to work out ideas. Provide specific expertise at times.
Self-Focused → Patient-Focused			
Daily reports revolve around "I" statements and have an absence of patient focused statements.	Validate shared insights and inquire as to what the patient did, how the patient responded or how the patient may have been affected.	**Reports on the day, excited about patient's personal victories and/ or by brainstorming how to approach challenging patients.**	Provide encouragement as needed. Follow up on challenging patients. Assign intern challenging patients highlighting successes with previous ones.
Intern tends to fall into patterns of clinical comfort zone.	Discuss one specific thing to try over a specific time frame. Follow up across time frame.	**Intern notices patient's good mood is incongruent with patient's verbalizations.**	Collaborate with intern to plan appropriate assessment and interventions.
Student → Professional			
Struggles to identify solutions outside of music therapy resources or is hesitant to ask questions of others.	Model interdisciplinary communications. Collaborate in this way with intern. Have intern take charge independently.	**Solves clinical problems that require consulting with non-music therapy staff independently.**	Set up or have intern set up opportunities to co-treat with other therapies.
Intern takes limited initiative.	Design a project for intern to spearhead requiring expansion of comfort zone while utilizing strengths. Contribute to process as much as is needed for intern to conclude with sense of independent accomplishment.	**Intern develops new ideas and moves forward with them.**	Support ideas from afar. Have intern share details of projects regularly. Address any gaps or potential challenges as needed.

The Light Bulb Moments

Those who have walked with an intern through this process will relate that, for the intern, it suddenly "just clicked." This happens early on for some interns, but for many it may be after the midterm evaluation when they begin to fully take charge of their new roles. Still others will struggle until, finally, around the end of month 5, it just clicks. Supervisors should remain patient, observant, and responsible for their own role in interns' lives, providing consistent guidance and support. Red flags, however, should not go unaddressed. Contacting university directors may necessary at times if issues persist, if competencies are not being met, or if skills are lacking. This is especially true in cases where the intern does not accept or implement feedback.

Tip: When issues arise, consider the use of written contracts with the intern and other involved parties, such as a counselor or university advisor. In the contract, outline specific concerns, what has been done so far, specific steps that are to be taken, who is responsible for those steps, and a specific time frame for expected completion of outlined actions or reevaluation. If necessary, contingencies may include termination or extension of internship.

Feedback

Gigante, Dell, and Sharkey (2011) highlight the separation of feedback from encouragement and evaluation. Feedback is specifically identified as an objective tool to improve clinical skills. The authors recommend that feedback (a) provide reassurance about achieved competency, (b) guide future learning, (c) reinforce positive actions, (d) identify and correct areas for improvement, and (e) promote reflection (p. 205). They identify **STOP** as a tool for giving effective feedback:

Specific – **T**imely – **O**bjective – **P**lan for improvement

If a method such as **STOP** is integrated from the beginning of internship, interns will then have a model to for independently giving themselves feedback. From modeling feedback to daily logistics, many guidelines can be set up from the start of internship. In addition to the **STOP** method, other specific techniques can be used to deliver feedback:

- Observation with feedback

- Meetings, conferences, discussions

- Modeling

- Written or form evaluations (McClain, 2001)

- Self-analysis vs. supervisor analysis

- Immediate or live feedback

- Video tape analysis

Internship supervisors must choose a feedback technique that works best for them and the specific intern. What is unquestionable is that some type of feedback is necessary. According to Feiner (2001), "If interns are not given sufficient information and feedback, if they do not get the opportunity to regularly observe their supervisor's work, they often flounder unproductively. They become extremely anxious and focused on 'doing good' to meet elusive expectations" (p. 102). Marital therapy research suggests that the ideal relationship of positive to negative feedback is 5 to 1 (Gottman, 1999), and studies support this "magic ratio" in work relationships as well (Losada & Heaphy, 2004). The supervisor must keep in mind that *it is just as important to acknowledge progress as it is to acknowledge things that are still to be learned.*

Self-Care

Internship supervisors take on many roles—educator, administrator, and supporter (Feiner, 2001), to name a few. Demands of a supervisory position coincide with the need for self-care. Not only is this important for supervisors to realize, but it should be modeled and taught to interns as well. Richards, Campenni, and Muse-Burke (2010) define self-care as "anything one does to feel good about oneself" (p. 253). They highlight four areas to consider when addressing self-care and well-being: (a) physical; (b) psychological; (c) spiritual; and (d) support, both professional and personal. They found the more one participates in self-care activities and the higher the importance one places on doing so, the greater the benefits to overall well-being.

Eleven to 12% of music therapists are noted to have high levels of burnout (Oppenheim, 1987; Vega, 2010). Swezey (2013) found that music therapists have higher compassion satisfaction than hospice professionals, counselors, and mental health workers. However, their burnout levels were higher than that of counselors, and music therapists' secondary traumatic stress levels were higher than all the other professions listed. In his 2013 survey, Swezey asked music therapists to identify their most used career-sustaining behaviors. Out of a field of 36, the top 5 reported behaviors were

1. Maintain sense of humor;

2. Spend time with partner/family;

3. Maintain self-awareness;

4. Reflect on positive experiences;

5. Maintain professional identity.

Swezey (2013) found a strong positive correlation between reflecting on positive experiences and compassion satisfaction. Appendix P provides a sample weekly internship log, in which the tasks outlined invite interns to reflect and increase awareness of oneself, goals, accomplishments, and challenges. The log also provides space to describe what self-care activities the interns engaged in during the week and what they plan to do the following week. The internship interview is an early indication of an intern's ability to cope with the fast-paced hospital environment. Does the intern already practice self-care strategies? If not, it is important to encourage interns to develop and practice these healthy habits now to prepare for a successful and healthy career in the future.

Conclusion

Supervising music therapy interns is a challenging, rewarding, and vital task. It directly impacts the current and future health of the music therapy profession. Although at times it may seem to be a daunting task, the foundational clinical skills that intern supervisors have can be recognized and used to support a healthy and safe supervisory relationship. This chapter provides supervisors or potential supervisors with tools to create an environment that empowers interns to develop comprehensive and effective approaches to their clinical work and allows them to be nurtured, guided, and challenged. Intern supervisors have the capacity to do more than just assist students in completing their education and passing their board-certification exam. Supervisors can facilitate the development of healthy, life-long habits, which can lead to an effective, successful, and positive career path. Furthermore, the process of supervising interns is a continuous journey that refines the supervisor's own clinical skills and overall effectiveness as a music therapist.

References

American Music Therapy Association (2014). *AMTA standards for education and clinical training.* Retrieved from http://www.musictherapy.org/members/edctstan/

Brookins, L. M. (1984). The music therapy clinical intern: Performance skills, academic knowledge, personal qualities and interpersonal skills necessary for a student seeking clinical training. *Journal of Music Therapy, 21,* 193–201.

Choi, B. (2008). Awareness of music therapy practices and factors influencing specific theoretical approaches. *Journal of Music Therapy, 45,* 93–109.

Corey, G. (2005). *Theory and practice of counseling and psychotherapy* (7th ed.). Pacific Grove, CA: Thomson Learning.

Deming, S. (2005). *Clinical supervision: Legal, ethical, and clinical considerations in the supervisory relationship* [Online course training manual]. Los Angeles, CA: Gerry Grossman Seminars.

Feiner, S. (2001). A journey through internship supervision: Roles, dynamics, and phases of the supervisory relationship. In M. Forinash (Ed.), *Music therapy supervision* (pp. 100–115). Gilsum, NH: Barcelona.

Gigante, J., Dell, M., & Sharkey, A. (2011). Getting beyond "good job": How to give effective feedback. *Pediatrics, 127*(2), 205–207.

Gottman, J. (1999). *The marriage clinic: A scientifically based marital therapy.* New York, NY: W.W. Norton.

Grant, R. E., & McCarty, B. (1990). Emotional stages in the music therapy internship. *Journal of Music Therapy, 27,* 102–118.

Knight, A. J. (2008). Music therapy internship supervisors and preinternship students: A comparative analysis of questionnaires. *Journal of Music Therapy, 45,* 75–92.

Losada, M., & Heaphy, E. (2004). The role of positivity and connectivity in the performance of business teams: A nonlinear dynamics model. *American Behavioral Scientist, 47,* 740–765.

McClain, F. J. (2001). Music therapy supervision: A review of literature. In M. Forinash (Ed.), *Music therapy supervision* (pp. 10–13). Gilsum, NH: Barcelona.

Memory, B. C., Unkefer, R., & Smeltekop, R. (1987). Supervision in music therapy: Theoretical models. In C. D. Maranto & K. E. Bruscia (Eds.), *Perspectives on music therapy education and training* (pp.161–168). Philadelphia, PA: Temple University.

National Research Council (2011). *Assessing 21st century skills: Summary of a workshop.* Washington, DC: The National Academies Press.

Oppenheim, L. (1987). Factors related to occupational stress or burnout among music therapists. *Journal of Music Therapy, 24,* 97–106.

Prasko, J., Divkey, T., Grambal, A., Kamaradova, D., Mozny, P., Sigmundova, Z., Slepecky, M., & Vyskocilova, J. (2010). Transference and countertransference in cognitive behavioral therapy. *Biomedical Papers of the Medical Faculty of the University Palacky, Olomouc Czech Republic, 154,* 189–198.

Rath, T. (2007). *StrengthFinders 2.0.* New York: Gallup Press.

Richards, K. C., Campenni, C. E., & Muse-Burke, J. L. (2010). Self-care and well-being in mental health professionals: The mediating effects of self-awareness and mindfulness. *Journal of Mental Health Counseling, 32*(3), 247–264.

Swezey, S. (2013). *What keeps us well? Professional quality of life and career sustaining behaviors of music therapy professionals* (Unpublished master's thesis). University of Kentucky, Lexington.

Tanguay, C. L. (2008). Supervising music therapy interns: A survey of AMTA national roster internship directors. *Journal of Music Therapy, 45*, 52–74.

Vega, V. P. (2010). Personality, burnout, and longevity among professional music therapists. *Journal of Music Therapy, 47,* 155–179.

VIA Survey of Character Strengths. (2014). Retrieved from http://www.authentichappiness.sas.upenn.edu

Chapter 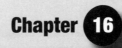 16

Diversity, Culture, and Patient- and Family-Centered Care in the Medical Setting: Implications for Clinicians and Supervisors
Alexandra Fields, MS, MT-BC

Diversity is all around us. It is beautiful and inspiring, yet it can also be one of the most challenging dynamics in our work as music therapists. The unique nature of our role as music therapists is that we can use music to both transcend and break down barriers between multicultural issues, and also amplify the importance of diversity and culture through music. Our interventions can be tailored to work within the patient's and family's culture in unique and creative ways, while maintaining therapeutic boundaries and the therapist's own unique set of beliefs and values. "The way a culture defines and uses music determines whether it is considered relevant to medicine, healing and therapy; and similarly the way a culture views medicine, healing, and therapy determines how relevant music is considered to them" (Bruscia, 1998, pp. 12–13).

The field of medicine and medical music therapy has also diversified tremendously over the past decade, with more and more focus given to employing patient- and family-centered care (Picker Institute, 2013). Along with this focus, there must be a conscious understanding of different cultural backgrounds. The field of medical music therapy has continued to follow suit to align with these changing values and initiatives. These changes affect all clinicians in their individual work and bring a new level of complexity to the supervision of music therapy interns.

Navigating Diversity

What is diversity? It can mean many things within the context of medical music therapy. There is diversity in the different types of medical settings: ambulatory care, outpatient clinics, inpatient rehabilitation, inpatient medical/surgical units, and intensive care units. Diversity also can be seen in the ages of patients served in these settings—infants, toddlers, school-aged children, adolescents, young adults, middle-aged adults, and older adults/geriatric patients. There is diversity in the types of diagnoses, illnesses, injuries, and psychosocial stressors facing patients as well. A great deal of diversity also exists in theoretical approaches, supervision styles, and different musical and clinical strengths.

According to the American Music Therapy Association (2011), diversity is part of the music therapy Standards of Clinical Practice. Music therapists must explore the client's unique diversity and culture during the initial assessment when working in the medical setting. "This can include but is not limited to race, ethnicity, language, religion/spirituality, social class, family experiences, sexual orientation, gender identity, and social organizations" (American Music Therapy Association, 2011).

When supervising music therapy interns in the medical setting, supervisors may encounter difficulties related to diversity. Interns can become understandably overwhelmed with the amount of diversity and change that occurs in medical settings. Music therapy supervisors can also be affected by these factors and can face difficulty in knowing how to manage, guide, and support interns in the most effective way amid so much diversity.

People who wish to understand the place of music in people's lives and its correlates would do well to consider cultural factors. . . . Music not only reflects cultural diversity but also forms an element of intercultural exchange more broadly.

(Werner, Swope, & Heide, 2009, p. 340)

The Development of Personal Identity

A simple way to break down diversity and better understand how to work effectively with culturally diverse patients and families is to look at how personal identity develops in every person. Sue and Sue (2008) discuss the three levels of culture that make up each individual's identity:

- Individual level – "All individuals are, in some respects, like no other individuals."

- Group level – "All individuals are, in some respects, like some other individuals."

- Universal level – "All individuals are, in some respects, like all other individuals." (p. 38)

If music therapists want to effectively help patients and families, no portion of the patient's identity can be discounted. All levels of culture are important and can be significant in successful treatment planning. According to the American Music Therapy Association (2011), part of a music therapist's duty is to explore the patient's culture during the assessment process and throughout the course of music therapy treatment. The Standards of Clinical Practice explain that a patient's culture has no limits to its definition. Culture can include any part of the person's identity or environment that he or she feels is significant. Incorporating the "whole" patient and all aspects of personal identity and culture, as he or she personally defines it, can be a wonderful way to find a point of connection with even the most diverse patients and families.

Cultural Competency

Effective music therapists "understand their own cultural conditioning, the conditioning of their clients, and the sociopolitical system of which they are a part" (Corey, 2005, p. 24). It is also important to understand that culture not only refers to ethnic or racial heritage, but includes gender, religion, age, physical and mental ability, sexual orientation, and socioeconomic status (Corey, 2005).

Some music therapists take the stance that music is universal; therefore, when working with someone from a different cultural background, they may feel it is not important to recognize the cultural difference. While it may be true that music is universal, music therapists are not released from the obligation to recognize the cultural differences in the patients and families they work with. If they choose to ignore patients' cultural differences, they risk missing opportunities to develop more effective treatment strategies. In the medical setting, culture can impact treatment compliance, important decisions about medical care, and the way patients cope with their illness and hospitalization.

Music therapy does not belong to any one culture, race, country, or ethnic tradition; it is global in its conception and manifestation.

(Bruscia, 1998)

Developing Cultural Competency

Music therapists can focus on three goals to actively continue building their cultural competence. "First, a culturally competent helping professional is one who is actively in the process of becoming aware of his or her own assumptions about human behavior, values, biases, preconceived notions, personal limitations, and so forth" (Sue & Sue, 2008, 43–44). Second, the helping professional must actively work to further understand the culturally diverse patient's worldview. Third, the helping professional is actively developing new, creative, relevant, sensitive, and appropriate interventions that meet the unique needs of the culturally diverse patient (Sue & Sue, 2008). Table 16.1 provides general points for consideration when developing cultural competency.

Table 16.1. Cultural Competencies
I. Cultural Competence: Awareness
1. Moved from being culturally unaware to being aware and sensitive to own cultural heritage and to valuing and respecting differences. 2. Aware of own values and biases and of how they may affect diverse clients. 3. Comfortable with differences that exist between themselves and their clients in terms of race, gender, sexual orientation, and other sociodemographic variables. Differences are not seen as deviant. 4. Sensitive to circumstances (personal biases; stage of racial, gender, and sexual orientation identity; sociopolitical influences, etc.) that may dictate referral of clients to members of their own sociodemographic group or to different therapists in general. 5. Aware of their own racist, sexist, heterosexist, or other detrimental attitudes, beliefs, and feelings.
II. Cultural Competence: Knowledge
1. Knowledgeable and informed on a number of culturally diverse groups, especially groups therapists work with. 2. Knowledgeable about the sociopolitical system's operation in the United States with respect to its treatment of marginalized groups in society. 3. Possess specific knowledge and understanding of the generic characteristics of counseling and therapy. 4. Knowledgeable of institutional barriers that prevent some diverse clients from using mental health services.
III. Cultural Competence: Skills
1. Able to generate a wide variety of verbal and nonverbal helping responses. 2. Able to communicate (send and receive both verbal and nonverbal messages) accurately and appropriately. 3. Able to exercise institutional intervention skills on behalf of their client when appropriate. 4. Able to anticipate impact of their helping styles, and limitations they possess on culturally diverse clients. 5. Able to play helping roles characterized by an active systemic focus, which leads to environmental interventions. Not restricted by the conventional counselor/therapist mode of operation.

Adapted from Sue & Sue (2008, p. 47)

Suggestions by music therapists for the development of cultural competency specific to music therapy include developing (a) an awareness of one's own culture of music therapy (Kenny, 2006); (b) an awareness of traditions, rituals, and roles associated with music in various cultures (Brown, 2002; Moreno, 1995); (c) a basic working knowledge of a variety of representative world music genres (Moreno, 1988); and (d) musical flexibility (Chase, 2003).

Individuals who wish to check their cultural competency development, personal awareness, and emotions around cultural issues should consider the following questions:

1. How do I feel working with individuals from different cultural backgrounds?

2. Is it easy or difficult for me to set aside my own biases related to cultural diversity?

3. Do I find myself asking questions and remaining curious about my patient's cultural background, or do I tend to ignore differences?

4. If I am having strong emotional reactions and biases surface in my work, am I reaching out for extra supervision or support from colleagues?

Patient- and Family-Centered Care

Although the values and language around patient- and family-centered care may differ among institutions, patient- and family-centered care consists of the following core concepts:

- *Dignity and Respect* – Patient and family knowledge, values, beliefs, and cultural backgrounds are integrated into delivery of care.

- *Information Sharing* – Practitioners communicate complete and unbiased information to patients and families in useful, affirming ways. Patients and families receive timely, accurate, and complete information to participate in care and decision making.

- *Participation* – Patients and families are encouraged and supported to participate in their care and decision making at the level they choose.

- *Collaboration* – Patients, families, practitioners, and health care leaders are included in all aspects of program development and care. (Adapted from the Institute for Patient- and Family-Centered Care, 2011, p. 4)

According to the Institute for Patient- and Family-Centered Care (2010),

Patient- and family-centered practitioners recognize the vital role that families play in ensuring the health and well-being of infants, children, adolescents, and family members of all ages. They acknowledge that emotional, social, and developmental support are integral components of health care. They promote the health and well-being of individuals and families and restore dignity and control to them . . . [Patient- and family-centered care] leads to better health outcomes and wiser allocation of resources, and greater patient and family satisfaction. (www.ipfcc.org/faq)

Working with Families

Working within the family framework is not always a significant part of music therapy educational or practical training. Therapists are trained to focus more on the patient–therapist relationship as opposed to the family–therapist relationship (McIntyre, 2009). However, with the increased focus on patient- and family-centered care throughout health care institutions, the family must be regarded as a significant part of treatment planning. To further develop their skills, music therapists may challenge themselves to see patients not only as individuals, but also as members of family units. To truly provide patient- and family-centered care, the therapist must understand and acknowledge that when one family member has an injury or illness that results in hospitalization, the entire family unit is affected. Therefore, the family must be included in treatment whenever possible to do what is best for the patient.

Family members are sometimes affected by a hospitalization just as much, if not more so, as the patient. Couples and caregivers of the hospitalized patient often function in crisis mode and are in great need of support that can be provided within the context of a music therapy session (Hinman, 2010). With adult couples, the integrity of the relationship may become stressed and intervention may be necessary to "protect intimate relationships from the negative implications of the hospital experience" (Hinman, 2010, p. 29). Focusing solely on the needs of the hospitalized patient, while pushing aside the needs of other family members, must be resisted. Engaging in this practice does not sufficiently recognize that hospitalization hinders family development. Families can be supported and nurtured through music therapy (Hinman, 2010). While the length of stay for hospitalized couples and families is often unknown, and may be brief, music therapy can quickly enhance positive feelings and connection between family members (Hinman, 2010).

When circumstances allow for only one opportunity to see a patient for music therapy before he or she is discharged, we must look to family involved as a crucial part of treatment planning. If family is present during a session, this opportunity may be used to gain more comprehensive insights into the patient and, potentially, a more effective outcome. Although at times it may appear helpful for a family member to take a "break" from the stress of being at the patient's bedside, this could cause a missed opportunity to involve family in treatment and to introduce applicable, transferable coping strategies that the family can use outside the hospital setting.

Music can serve as a catalyst to bring a family together in a comfortable, familiar way, a way they are all connected—through their unique culture.

(McIntyre, 2009)

Working with Parents

Something that many health care professionals notice when working with children who are hospitalized is that their parents often have difficulty "parenting" the child who is in the hospital. Families are often distressed, anxious, nervous, etc. These emotions can even be heightened due to lack of sleep and physical exhaustion. Empathy for families experiencing this whirlwind of emotions can go a long way, but music therapists must also use their clinical knowledge and judgment to help the family develop healthy skills for maintaining the important structure of the parent–child relationship. Parents do not realize that when this structure is lost, so is the sense of safety and comfort for their children. Many parents may make the excuse that their child is in pain and is having a difficult time, which is why they give in to the child's every demand and the rules of the family no longer apply during hospitalization. This is where the therapist can help by providing psychoeducation about the importance of maintaining structure and parental relationship. Music therapy can be the accessible bridge that connects families back to a healthier state of homeostasis. "When families play music together, a re-establishment of parental roles may occur in a passive yet significant way, one that brings the hierarchy of the family back into order" (McIntyre, 2009, p. 267). When this hierarchy is in place, families are able to support the hospitalized patient and surrounding family members in a more effective way. In turn, patients are more capable of maintaining compliance to various aspects of their treatment.

The issues surrounding some family systems are often complex and, at times, words may fail to express the depth of a family member's emotions. Music—that is, melody, harmony and rhythm—can, however, provide a more immediate route, both to connection and to the processing of these issues.

(McIntyre, 2009, p. 261)

Theoretical Approaches

Many theoretical approaches can incorporate multicultural considerations into practice. However, at times review and integration may be needed. Table 16.2 provides some examples of contributions and limitations of several theoretical approaches related to multicultural practice.

Table 16.2. Theoretical Approaches and Multicultural Music Therapy			
Theoretical Approach	**Techniques/ Interventions**	**Contributions to Multicultural Therapy**	**Limitations in Multicultural Therapy**
Humanistic/Person-Centered Therapy	Work in the "here-and-now" reflection of feelings, and active listening. Does not include diagnostic testing, interpretation, questioning or probing for information.	Focuses on breaking cultural barriers and facilitating open dialogue among culturally diverse populations. Main strengths are respecting patients' values, active listening, welcoming differences, nonjudgmental attitude, understanding, willingness to allow patients to determine what will be explored in sessions and prizing cultural pluralism.	Some of the core values of this approach may not be congruent with the patient's culture. Lack of therapist direction and structure are unacceptable for clients who are seeking help and immediate answer from a knowledgeable professional.
Cognitive-Behavioral Therapy	Uses a variety of cognitive, emotive, and behavioral techniques. Diverse methods to meet individual needs. Active, directive, time-limited, present-centered, structured therapy. Learning new coping skills, debating irrational beliefs, role-playing, homework assignments, etc.	Collaborative approach offers patients opportunities to express their areas of concern. The psychoeducational dimensions are often useful in exploring cultural conflicts and teaching new behavior. The emphasis on thinking (as opposed to expressing feelings) is acceptable to many patients. Patients may value active and directive stance of therapist.	Therapist may attempt to change the beliefs and actions of patients too quickly — it is essential for the therapist to understand and respect the patient's world first. Many patients may have strong reservations about questioning their basic cultural values and beliefs. Clients can become dependent on the therapist for deciding what appropriate ways to solve problems are. There may be a fine line between being directive and promoting dependence.
Behavioral Therapy	Modeling, reinforcement techniques, social skills training. Diagnosis and treatment done first to establish treatment strategies. Asking questions of "what," "how," and "when" (but not "why").	The focus on behavior, instead of feelings, is compatible with many cultures. Strengths include a collaborative relationship, mutually agreed-upon goals, ongoing assessment to measure effectiveness, educational focus, and self-management strategies.	Therapists need to help patients assess the possible consequences of making behavioral changes. Family members may not value patients' newly acquired assertive style, so patients must be taught how to cope with resistance from others.
Family Systems Therapy	Many theoretical approaches can work within this framework (usually cognitive, experiential, and behavioral). Uses genograms, teaching, countertransference, reframing, restructuring, enactments, and setting boundaries.	Many ethnic and cultural groups place value on the role of the extended family. Many family therapies deal with extended family members and support systems. There is a greater chance for individual change if other family members are supportive. Offers ways of working toward health of the family unit and welfare of each member.	Family therapy rests on value assumptions that are not always congruent with the values of patients from some other cultures. Concepts such as individuation, self-actualization, self-determination, and self-expression may be foreign to some patients. In some cultures, admitting problems within the family is shameful. The value of "keeping problems within the family" may make it difficult to explore conflicts openly.

Adapted from Corey (2005, pp. 481–487)

An Integrative/Multimodal Approach

Realizing the different strengths and potential limitations within each theoretical perspective is helpful in making informed clinical decisions within one's own practice and in guiding interns to do the same in their practice. There are ways to cut across domains using more pluralistic approaches to therapy that draw from many theoretical bases and may be more applicable in the unpredictable and fluctuating environment of the medical setting (Okun, 2002). Integrated strategies can be used when the patient's problems or needs do not fall within one domain, but are more complex and "individual, interpersonal and/or related to the person's environment" (Okun, 2002, p. 198). A multimodal approach can use a behavioral strategy for modifying behavior, while also using cognitive restructuring to address negative thinking patterns related to the isolating behavior, while also eliciting the patient's emotion using more affective/humanistic strategies (Okun, 2002). These types of strategies can be used across all cultures, ages, and levels of development (Okun, 2002). These multimodal approaches can combine humanistic/affective, cognitive, and/or behavioral domains creating multimodal, ecological, systems, and multicultural approaches to music therapy (Okun, 2002).

Implications for Clinical Practice

Recognition of Diversity and Culture

We now know that it is important for health care providers to develop knowledge of the diverse health and disease belief systems held by various cultures. We also know that communication plays a significant role in provider–patient interactions and that communication has been linked to patient satisfaction, treatment adherence, and health outcomes (Smedley, Stith, & Nelson, 2003). It is essential that music therapists, like other health care providers, strive to improve cross-cultural communication in order to interact effectively with culturally diverse patients. Berlin and Fowkes (1983) developed a model designed to improve culturally diverse health care by improving cross-cultural communication. This framework, known as the LEARN Model, encourages providers to (a) elicit, (b) discuss, (c) negotiate, and (d) incorporate each patient's cultural, social, and personal information in all health care interactions. Guidelines in this framework are organized around the following mnemonic:

- **L**isten with sympathy and understanding to the patient's perception of the problem.

- **E**xplain your perceptions of the problem.

- **A**cknowledge and discuss differences/similarities.

- **R**ecommend treatment.

- **N**egotiate agreement.

Other models developed to assist health care professionals in providing culturally responsive care include the Explanatory Model (Kleinman, Eisenberg, & Good, 1978), the RESPECT Model (Welch, 1998), and the Four Habits Model of Highly Effective Clinicians (Frankel & Stein, 1999).

Cultural Diversity and Music Therapy

Baker and Grocke (2009) discuss how the following aspects impact the therapeutic relationship when working with culturally diverse groups:

- Language barriers can challenge the development of the therapeutic relationship.

- Cultural empathy is necessary for the development of the relationship.

- People from various cultural groups may feel uncomfortable speaking in English.

- Using culturally appropriate greetings and learning some words in the patient's/family's language can help facilitate rapport building.

- Differences in personal space and boundaries between the therapist and patient can challenge the development of rapport (pp. 47–48).

Baker and Grocke (2009) also discuss how having knowledge of music from a particular culture can be useful; however, this approach can be time-consuming and often a never-ending process. Some of the most effective music therapy techniques that work across several different cultural groups consist of non-language-based and improvisational interventions (Baker & Grocke, 2009). The most successful outcomes occur when the music therapist builds a solid therapeutic relationship with the patient and family. This is commonly done by using the most appropriate repertoire to connect with patients, and, for most patients, this means using songs sung in their native language from their native culture (Baker & Grocke, 2009). In fact, there is an argument that "emphasis be placed on learning repertoire in foreign languages within the music therapy training programs and with more emphasis placed on this as a competency required for AMTA registration" (Baker & Grocke, 2009, p. 49).

Supervision and Diversity, Culture, and Patient- and Family-Centered Care

It is easy to think of multicultural considerations in music therapy practice as secondary—as something that is not as important as other components of clinical work. Therapists may feel that racial, ethnic, or other cultural differences are not important variables that affect patients' lives (Sue & Sue, 2008). However, if they broaden their perspective, they find that culture impacts numerous aspects of medical care, such as patients' methods of coping with their diagnosis, how and when they seek medical care, or even how open patients are to receiving ancillary or adjunctive care such as music therapy. Developing one's own cultural competency as a clinician first is a crucial step to being able to effectively supervise music therapy interns on cultural issues.

When supervising music therapy students, the previously mentioned core concepts of patient- and family-centered care can be interpreted and applied to a healthy relationship between the supervisor and intern. These four principles can be a guide and "check-in" used within supervision to see if both parties are upholding these concepts:

- *Dignity and Respect* – of the supervisor's and intern's unique perspectives, personal experiences, knowledge, values, beliefs, and cultural background, and how these factors inform the intern's experiences and growth.

- *Information Sharing* – the supervisor and intern should openly share information about current patient and family cases, past experiences, personal reflections, struggles, and triumphs in their work.

- *Participation* – the supervisor and intern must reciprocally participate in the supervision process for it to be beneficial and meaningful for either party.

- *Collaboration* – between the supervisor and intern.

Conclusion

Culturally sensitive care ensures dignity and respect. It increases patient, family, and caregiver understanding. It promotes trust, patient satisfaction with provider care, and patient adherence to treatment (Chance, 2014; Tucker et al., 2007). Music therapists, through the unique medium of music, have the opportunity to provide care that is not only culturally sensitive, but also patient- and family-centered. Subsequently, these same principles can be applied to music therapy supervision, ensuring that future music therapists understand the importance of cultural diversity, cultural sensitivity, and patient- and family-centered care.

References

American Music Therapy Association. (2011, November 19). *AMTA standards of clinical practice: Medical settings.* Silver Spring, MD: Author. Retrieved from http://www.musictherapy.org/about/standards/#MEDICAL_SETTINGS

Baker, F., & Grocke, D. (2009). Challenges of working with people aged 60–75 years from culturally and linguistically diverse groups: Repertoire and music therapy approaches employed by Australian music therapists. *Australian Journal of Music Therapy, 20,* 30–55.

Berlin, E., & Fowkes, W. A. (1983). A teaching framework for cross-cultural health care. *Western Journal of Medicine, 139,* 934–938.

Brown, J. M. (2002). Towards a culturally centered music therapy practice. *Voices: A World Forum for Music Therapy, 2.* Retrieved from https://normt.uib.no/index.php/voices/article/viewArticle/72/62

Bruscia, K. E. (1998). *Defining music therapy* (2nd ed.). Gilsum, NH: Barcelona.

Chance, K. G. (2014). *2014 cultural sensitivity and awareness training.* UK HealthCare Enterprise Learning, University of Kentucky, Lexington, KY.

Chase, K. M. (2003). Multicultural music therapy! A review of literature. *Music Therapy Perspectives, 21,* 84–88.

Corey, G. (2005). *Theory and practice of counseling and psychotherapy* (7th ed.). Pacific Grove, CA: Thomson Learning.

Frankel, R. M., & Stein, T. (1999). Getting the most out of the clinical encounter: The Four Habits model. *The Permanente Journal, 3*(3), 79–88.

Hinman, M. L. (2010). Our song: Music therapy with couples when one partner is medically hospitalized. *Music Therapy Perspectives, 28,* 29–36.

Institute for Patient- and Family-Centered Care. (2010, December 29). *Frequently asked questions.* Retrieved from http://www.ipfcc.org/faq.html

Institute for Patient- and Family-Centered Care. (2011). *Advancing the practice of patient- and family-centered care in primary care in hospitals: How to get started.* Bethesda, MD: Author. Retrieved from http://ipfcc.org/tools/downloads.html

Kenny, C. (2006). *Music and life in the field of play: An anthology.* Gilsum, NH: Barcelona.

Kleinman, A., Eisenberg, L. & Good, B. (1978). Clinical lessons from anthropologic and cross-cultural research. *Annals of Internal Medicine, 88,* 251–288.

McIntyre, J. (2009). Interactive family music therapy: Untangling the system. *Australian & New Zealand Journal of Family Therapy, 30*(4), 260–268.

Moreno, J. (1988). Multicultural music therapy: The world music connection. *Journal of Music Therapy, 25,* 17–27.

Moreno, J. (1995). Ethnomusictherapy: An interdisciplinary approach to music and healing. *The Arts in Psychotherapy, 26*(2), 3–14.

Okun, B. F. (2002). *Effective helping, interviewing and counseling techniques* (6th ed.). Pacific Grove, CA: Brooks/Cole.

Picker Institute. (2013). *Patient-centered care: The road ahead.* Retrieved from http://www.ipfcc.org/pdf/Patient-Centered%20Care%20The%20Road%20Ahead.pdf

Smedley, B. D., Stith, A. Y., & Nelson, A. R. (Eds). (2003). *Unequal treatment: Confronting racial and ethnic disparities in healthcare.* Institute of Medicine Committee on Understanding and Eliminating Racial and Ethnic Disparities in Health Care. Washington, DC: National Academies Press.

Sue, D. W., & Sue, D. (2008). *Counseling the culturally diverse: Theory and practice* (5th ed.). New York: John Wiley & Sons.

Tucker, C. M., Herman, K. C., Ferdinand, L. A., Beato, C., Adams, D., & Cooper, L. (2007). Providing culturally sensitive healthcare: A formative model. *The Counseling Psychologist, 35,* 679–705. doi:10.1177/0011000007301689

Welch, M. (1998). *Enhancing awareness and improving cultural competence in health care. A partnership guide for teaching diversity and cross-cultural concepts in heath professional training.* San Francisco, CA: University of California at San Francisco.

Werner, P. D., Swope, A. J., & Heide, F. J. (2009). Ethnicity, music experience, and depression. *Journal of Music Therapy, 46,* 339–358.

Section 5: Appendices

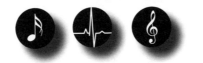

Appendix A Program Development Checklist	
Initial Program and Proposal Planning	
☐ Market research	Local, national, music therapy literature, adjunctive therapies, etc.
☐ Identify Strategic Initiatives	Review hospital's and self-initiatives.
☐ Medical Terminology	Familiarize yourself with buzz words (see Glossary), current issues in healthcare, hospital grades (outcome measurements).
☐ Specific Research	Be as specific as possible. Put it in an easy-to-read-and-disseminate format. Have a copy of 1 to 2 key full-length articles. Study it, know it and anticipate questions.
☐ Prepare Proposal	Bring everything, give them what they need based on your conversation.
☐ Budget	Itemize factors contributing to the cost of music therapy. Include: -Salary -Benefits (percentage of salary varies from 0-37% based on employer) -Equipment (instruments) -Annual fees, certifications -Continuing education -Conferences -Leave time for above 2012 AMTA Workforce Analysis largest response revealed a purchasing budget of $1-$1000
☐ Additional Needs	Up front set the program up for success. Lay out everything an MT program would need, then work with administration to develop an implication plan.
During Initial Service Implication (approximately 6 months)	
☐ Documentation system	Have examples but work within the already established system used.
☐ Referral System	Determine based on unit needs and current flow of communication.
☐ Data Collection System	Census and/or other measurable outcomes used to generate program reports and effectiveness of your program.
☐ Identify Key Contacts	Administration, service line administrators, program managers, nurse managers, charge nurses, lead therapists
Ongoing Tasks and Items to Develop	
Keep updated key research available	
Regular program/story updates to administration	
Policies and procedures -Infection control -Music therapy competencies -Referral guidelines/algorithms -Assessments	
Program evaluation measures	
Staff -Education/Presentations/Support	
Keep a running list of talking points for administrative meetings	
Plan–Do–Check–Act	

Appendix B
Glossary of Common Healthcare Terminology

Ambulatory Care – generally refers to an outpatient care setting that delivers treatment or intervention using advanced medical technology or procedures.

C-Suite Executives – also known as executive team or "corporate"; this is an informal term referring to the senior executives of the hospital.

Census – a term that refers to the count of patients at the setting in question; depending on the setting, it could refer to inpatients actually admitted to inpatient status or an adjusted number accounting for a combination of inpatients and outpatients; it may also refer to a service or unit specific case load.

Center for Medicare and Medicaid Services (CMS) – the United States federal agency that administers Medicare, Medicaid, and the State Children's Health Insurance Program.

Chief positions: CEO, CIO, CAO – the senior executive positions of the hospital or ambulatory setting.

> Examples:
> CEO – Chief Executive Officer
> CAO – Chief Administrative Officer
> CIO – Chief Information Officer

Competencies – the measurable or observable knowledge, skills, abilities, and behaviors critical to successful job performance. These are usually assessed on hire and then annually as they are considered key to judging a person's ability to do a job successfully and safely.

Continuum of Care – an integrated system of health care that serves a patient from inpatient to outpatient to home settings.

Fiscal Intermediary (FI) – a private insurance company that serves as the federal government's agents in the administration of the Medicare.

Fiscal Year (FY) – the financial or budget period used to calculate annual statements for business purposes.

Full Time Equivalent (FTE) – a unit that indicates the workload of an employed person (or student) in a way that makes workloads comparable across settings. An FTE can be made up of more than one worker.

Functional Independence Measure (FIM) – the functional assessment measure used primarily in rehabilitation to objectively grade a patient's abilities, using an 18-item ordinal scale.

HCAHPS – Hospital Consumer Assessment of Healthcare Providers and Systems – provides a standardized survey instrument and data collection methodology for measuring patients' perspectives on hospital care.

Hospital Grades – various systems or websites that provide comparative data for hospitals.

The Joint Commission (TJC) – an independent, not-for-profit organization that accredits and certifies health care organizations and programs in the United States. Joint Commission accreditation and certification is recognized nationwide as a symbol of quality that reflects an organization's commitment to meeting certain performance standards.

Length of Stay (LOS) – a measurement of the time a patient stays in a particular setting. This usually equates to the time period from admission to discharge.

Patient- and Family-Centered Care – active involvement of patients and their families in decision making about individual options for treatment that accounts for the patients' individual and cultural preferences.

Performance Improvement – projects that are focused on improving processes in health care, which, as a result, improve quality of care.

Plan–Do–Check–Act (PDCA) – a four-step cycle for carrying out change and continuous improvement used in both business and health care.

Policy and Procedures (P&P) – a set of policies and guidelines that direct business and health care decisions and action; they are usually available in a book or by computer so that they are easily accessible.

Primary Care – health care that is focused on health promotion and disease prevention. An example may be a class on how to correctly install a child seat restraint system in a car.

Return on Investment (ROI) – a performance measure used to evaluate the efficiency of an investment.

Secondary Care – an intermediate level of health care focused on diagnosis and treatment. This can occur in an outpatient setting or a hospital. An example may be a mammogram.

Service Line Administrator – the job title of a management job that generally includes all services across a similar diagnosis. An example is Orthopedic Service Line Administrator.

Tertiary Care – specialized, highly technical level of health care that includes diagnosis and treatment of disease and disability. This occurs in an inpatient or post-acute setting after a diagnosis such as a stroke

Value Added Service – a non-core or augmentative service.

Value Based Purchasing – a program designed to promote better clinical outcomes for hospital patients, as well as improve their experience of care during hospital stays, by using mandatory hospital reported data.

Appendix C Reimbursement and Budgeting Resources		
Resource	**Details**	**Type of Resource**
CPT Coding Manual	CPT 2014 Professional Edition; American Medical Association. ISBN#: 978-1-60359-844-6	Book
Music Therapy Reimbursement: Best Practices and Procedures	Simpson, J & Burns, D. (2004). Silver Spring, MD: American Music Therapy Association	Book
Reimbursement for Evidence-Based NICU-MT	Standley, J.M. & Walworth, D. (2010). *Music Therapy with Premature Infants: Research and developmental interventions* (2nd ed.)	Book Chapter
Reimbursement	Robertson, A. (2009). *Music, medicine & miracles: How to provide medical music therapy for pediatric patients and get paid for it.* Orlando, FL: Florida Hospital.	Book Chapter
CMTE: Reimbursement Revolution	Jamie George, MM, MT-BC Available at www.musictherapyed.com	Online CMTE course
Music Therapy Reimbursement: Sources and Steps to Success	AMTA Available at www.musictherapy.org	E-course
AMTA Member Survey & Work Force Analysis*	www.musictherapy.org Available at: Member Resources > Job Center > Resources and Links	Membership Statistical Report
Cost Effectiveness of Music Therapy in Research*	www.musictherapy.org Available at: Member Resources > Member Toolkit > under AMTA and CBMT Advocacy Toolkit	
AMTA CPT Code Fact Sheet*	www.musictherapy.org Available at: Member Resources > Job Center > Reimbursement – scroll to the bottom of the page.	Fact Sheet
State Task Forces/Committees	http://www.musictherapy.org/members/ official/com_reimburseme/ Consult the American Music Therapy Association Reimbursement Committee to identify your regional representative	Committee

*Available to current AMTA members.

Appendix D
Arts in Medicine URLs

http://www.nea.gov/news/news03/aihexamples.html.

http://nccam.nih.gov/health/whatiscam

http://www.thesah.org/template/index.cfm

http://cyber.law.harvard.edu/sites/cyber.law.harvard.edu/files/KBWPositiveDevelopmentandSocial-ChangeThroughtheArts2012.pdf

(http://www.thecreativecenter.org/tcc/publications__dvds/online_publications/Colloquium_White_Paper:en-us.pdf

http://www.nea.gov/news/news03/nea_sahconceptpaper.pdf

http://www1074.ssldomain.com/thesah/members/affiliate_list.cfm

http://www.beadsofcourage.org/pages/hospitals.htm

http://www.artmedinsight.org/programs.html

http://www.artsandhealinginitiative.org/

Appendix E
List of Forms Used

The following forms and items are used in the AIMS course:

1. An inventory completed in the on-campus orientation session

2. A hospital experience inventory completed in the on-campus orientation session

3. The Master Schedule completed as students submit schedule requests at the beginning of the semester

4. A weekly Performance documentation form submitted after each performance

5. A weekly Unit Contact documentation form submitted after each unit visit

6. An example of a Weekly Assignment posted on the website submitted each week

7. The Cumulative Log students maintain each week and submit at the end of the semester

8. Questions and directions for writing the Final Essay

9. Brief TMH unit staff survey

Appendix F
Arts in Medicine Student Inventory

Date_____   Semester (Check one): Fall ___ Spring___ Sum ___

1. Name _____

2. Major _____

3. Year in School _____

4. Phone Number (emergency contact, only) _____

5. Number of semesters of previous AIMS course enrollment ____
   Which semesters? _____

6. Number of credits to be earned for AIMS this semester (1, 2, or 3) _____
   Total number of contracted contact hours (Multiply number of credits x 2 x 12 weeks) _____

7. FSU email address _____
   (All AIMS communications will go to your FSU EMAIL ADDRESS)

8. Other email addresses: _____

9. How did you learn about the AIMS course?

10. Why are you taking the AIMS course; i.e., what are your personal objectives?

11. *The ARTS IN MEDICINE program at TMH provides opportunities to interact with people in arts activities without having a specific purpose or goal other than to involve the person in a positive, pleasant, and often entertaining interaction. These opportunities rely on several social skills that you use daily in many other types of settings.* **Please describe on the back of this sheet** *recent experiences related to AIMS, such as other community service volunteering, being in a hospital setting, working with other people in job situations, interacting with new people on a one-to-one basis, babysitting, entertaining people, sharing talents with other people in a casual setting, etc.*

12. Briefly describe your skills, talents, and interests in any of the following: music, drama, visual arts, and computers. (Use back of this sheet.)

13. Do you have access to a computer that can access Blackboard at home? ____

14. Do you use the campus computers in the FSU libraries and centers? _____

15. How often do you use a computer for email? _____

16. How often do you use a computer to access websites on the Internet? _____

17. Approximately how many web-based or web-assisted courses have you taken at FSU? _____
    Did you use the computer on a daily basis in some of the courses? _____

Appendix G
Hospital Experiences as a Patient

1. What is your general attitude about hospital environments? Determine which of the words is more descriptive of your attitude and write an X in a blank somewhere between the two words.

    Negative ____   ____   ____   ____   ____   ____   ____ Positive

2. Approximately how many experiences have you had as an overnight hospital patient?
    Number of experiences: ____

3. Please provide the following information about your most recent overnight hospital experience as a patient, if applicable.

    How old were you? ____ How long did you stay in the hospital? _____

    Please rate your recollection of the experience by determining which of the words is more descriptive of the experience and write an X in a blank somewhere between the two words.

    Peaceful ____   ____   ____   ____   ____   ____   ____ Traumatic

Comments:

Appendix H
MASTER SCHEDULE

Appendix H
MASTER SCHEDULE
ADULT UNITS: Select one hour per unit--one volunteer per hour, 2 volunteers on unit per day

CARDIOLOGY	Monday	Tuesday	Wednesday	Thursday	Friday
3-4					
4-5					
5-6					
ORTHO	Monday	Tuesday	Wednesday	Thursday	Friday
3-4					
4-5					
6-7					
NEURO	Monday	Tuesday	Wednesday	Thursday	Friday
3-4					
4-5					
6-7					
INTERNAL MED	Monday	Tuesday	Wednesday	Thursday	Friday
3-4					
4-5					
6-7					
DIABETES	Monday	Tuesday	Wednesday	Thursday	Friday
3-4					
4-5					
6-7					
ONCOLOGY	Monday	Tuesday	Wednesday	Thursday	Friday
3-4					
4-5					
6-7					

PEDIATRIC UNIT: Attend Pediatric Orientation Session with the Child Life Specialist before your first contact

TWO HOUR MINIMUM	Monday	Tuesday	Wednesday	Thursday	Friday
9am - 12pm (must start at 9am)	max of 2	max of 2	not available	not available	max of 2
12 - 3pm	not available	1 position available	1 position available	not available	1 position available
3 - 6pm	not available	max of 2	max of 2	not available	max of 2

PERFORMANCES: Times will be added as requests are submitted. Specify your preferred time on your schedule request. Music majors: Please schedule a minimum of a weekly 30 minute performance. Select Magnolia if you want to play the piano.

	Monday	Tuesday	Wednesday	Thursday	Friday
MAGNOLIA LOBBY					
ATRIUM					

Appendix I
Weekly Performance Documentation

PERFORMANCES

Arts in Medicine Service – Tallahassee Memorial HealthCare

Week 4   6/3–9

Directions: Complete the form immediately after you perform. Sign the form. Get a staff member to sign the form. Put the completed form in the AIMS Documentation Notebook at the Atrium Desk BEFORE leaving the hospital.

Day of Contact (Circle *one*): *Mon   Tues   Wed   Thurs   Fri   Sat   Sun   Date: ___/___/___*

Unit (Circle *one*):   ATRIUM | MAGNOLIA LOBBY | CAFETERIA | CANCER CENTER |
        Other (specify) _____

Time: What time did you start performing?   *Time In ____: ____ am or pm* (circle one)

    What time did you stop performing?   *Time out ____: _____ am or pm* (circle one)

    What was the total amount of time performing?   *Total Time ____ hours ____ minutes*

Describe Performance (circle): Solo or Group | Music   Dance   Drama   Art

    If the group included people not currently enrolled in AIMS, how many people? _____

    If the group included currently enrolled AIMS students, please write their names:

    _____

Content of Performance: List selections or describe activity (Use back if necessary)

Observations: Estimate the number (#) of people in the blank provided.

Sat near the performance area but engaged in reading, talking with others # _____

Came close to the performance area and listened # ____

Verbally spoke favorably about the performance # _____

Engaged you in conversation # _____

Stopped to listen briefly (maybe smiled, thumbs up) then left the performance area   #___

Other: (specify) _____ #___

Additional Information Relevant to AIM Program

AIMS Volunteer Signature _____ Print Last Name _____

Get signature from a **TMH Staff person**:
TMH Staff Member Signature _____

Appendix J
Weekly Contact Documentation Form

MAIN HOSPITAL UNIT

Arts in Medicine Service – Tallahassee Memorial HealthCare

Week 4   6/3–9

Directions: Complete the form immediately after volunteering in a TMH unit. Sign the form. Get a staff member in the unit to sign the form. ***Complete a different form for each unit***. Put all completed forms in the AIMS Documentation Notebook at the Atrium Desk BEFORE leaving TMH.

Day of Contact (Circle *one*): *Mon   Tues   Wed   Thurs   Fri   Sat   Sun   Date: ___/___/13*

Unit (Circle *one*):   *Peds | Cardio | Oncology | Ortho-Neuron | Pulmonary-Med | Diabetes*
        Other (specify) _____

Time: What time did you start in the unit? *Time in ____:_____ am or pm* (circle one)

    What time did you leave the unit? *Time out ____:_____ am or pm* (circle one)

    What was the total amount of time on the unit? *Total Time _____ hours _____ minutes*

Contacts: How many people in the hospital unit did you contact? _____

    How many of the contacts in this unit did you spend AIMS time with? _____

Rooms Visited: Write the room #. Circle it if AIMS contact was made

Time Spent: How did you spend time in the unit?   (Circle all listed below that apply):

Card Games	Cleaning Play Room	Coloring, Drawing	Computer Games	Conversation
Crafts	Crossword Puzzles	Feeding	Imaginary Play	Jigsaw Puzzles
Making Greeting Cards	Organizing supplies	Origami	Painting	Playing with toys
Playing Board Games, Dominoes	Performing Music	Performing Dance	Performing Skit/ Play	Puppet Play
Reading books, magazines	Rocking, holding infant	Sewing, knitting	Transporting	Tea Cart
Writing letters	Writing poetry	Watching video	Making Scrapbook	Balloon Animals

Other Activity (specify) _____

Who did you interact with while on the unit: (Circle all that apply)

Patients | Parents | Siblings | Other family members | Nurse | Doctor | Therapist | Tech staff

Were you working with another AIMS volunteer during these interactions? *Yes or No*

If Yes, *who?* _____

Brief Description, Observation, Reaction:

AIMS Volunteer Signature _____ Print Last Name _____

Get signature from a **TMH Staff person on the Unit**:
TMH Staff Member Signature _____

Please circle answers: Volunteer (1) followed dress code? YES   NO
(2) Followed hospital protocol? YES   NO

Appendix K
Weekly Assignment

If you did not complete contacts this week, please read the information at the bottom and submit a "no contact" report with the cumulative hours from last week. If you completed contacts this week, as soon as possible after you've completed your contacts at the hospital this week, send one email message with a Week 8 heading containing the following information for each unit (and performance, if applicable):

(1) Unit

(2) Day of Week and Time begin and end

(3) #of hours this week and total cumulative hours including this week

(4) What you did during the time (activities, observations of patients and their reactions, etc.). Write details describing your observations about the people, staff, and patients you interact with during the hours on the unit.

(5) Reflection about what you learned (about yourself, about patients, about connections with other courses and experiences, philosophical questions, etc.).

(6) Did you meet your goal for the week? What did you learn?

(7) Personal goal for next week-something small you can and will change about yourself or your experience that can be reached in a week or during your next visit (short-term, obtainable).

If you were not able to complete contact hours at TMH this week, send a Week 8 report saying "no contact" and include the cumulative number of hours to date. Then record this information on cumulative log and grade points sheet. (You get points for submitting a "no contact" report.) Also answer the "question of the week" if one is asked.

Question of the Week: Please find the "Excerpts from Week 7 reports" item in the Course Library and follow the directions. Add your answers to the questions in your Week 8 report.

Reminders: (1) Keep a copy of your report in your email folders in the event you are asked to resend the original email. (2) Record the information requested on your Cumulative Log. (3) Update the weekly points on your Grade Evaluation Sheet for your personal files. (4) Criteria for total points available for the Weekly Reports are the inclusion of all 7 items in the paragraph above. (Long answers to #4 and thoughtful answers to #5 are evaluated as full credit.) Reports are academic assignments.

Appendix L
MUE4092/5096: ARTS IN MEDICINE SERVICE Cumulative Log

Accountability Log of Volunteer Activity

Maintain this log weekly throughout the semester and turn in the original form with your final essay.

Name _____ AIMS Contract (#of Hours) _____

Week of Course	Date	Unit/Area	Activity	Time begin	Time end	Total # of Hours Completed	Cumulative Number of Hours Completed	Date Weekly Report was Submitted (due Sun., midnight)

Appendix M
FINAL ESSAY DIRECTIONS

The questions below are provided as a structure for reflecting about your AIMS experience this semester. Think about the variety of experiences you have encountered. Read your weekly reports to find trends and learning moments. Think about your personal progress through the semester. Then complete the following directions.

First read all of the questions. Make shorthand notes of how you will you answer each one of them. Then collect and organize your thoughts and answer each of the questions as completely as possible. Details and examples are expected. "More is better" when it comes to responding. You may complete the questions in an essay form or as single numbered items.

For questions 1-9: These questions are personal. Please provide specific examples of situations or reactions to explain your answer. Question 10-15: These questions provide very important and helpful information.

1) What was the most enjoyable part of your experience at the hospital?

2) What was the most challenging part of your experience?

3) What was the most valuable part of your experience?

4) What did you learn about yourself personally?

5) What did you learn about setting goals, meeting goals, structuring your success?

6) What, if any, impact did your experience have on your future plans?

7) What did you learn about the group of patients with whom you worked?

8) What did you learn about the use of the arts in a medical setting?

9) What did you learn about community service for college students?

10) Do you have ideas for implementation of any new arts programs at the hospital?

11) What supplies would be beneficial additions for the programs?

12) What suggestions can you offer for improving the course?

13) Would you recommend this course to other students in your subject area? Why or why not?

14) How often did you access the course web site?

15) Do you have any suggestions for the course website content?

Appendix N
Arts in Medicine Service

Florida State University
TMH Staff Survey

Date _____

How long have you had contacts with Arts in Medicine Service student volunteers? (Check one)

__within the last 36 months

__within the last 24 months

__within the last 12 months

__within the last 6 months

__within the last 3 months

__within the last month

Did you see the student(s) on a weekly basis? Yes   No

Did the student(s) follow the hospital protocol? Yes   No

Please rate your level of support for the Arts in Medicine program. (Circle a number)

Low   Neutral   High

0   1   2   3   4   5   6

Please use this space for additional comments and suggestions.

_____ _____

Position   Unit

Name (optional) _____

Appendix O
Sample Internship Interview Questions

Personality

- What drew you to this internship?

- What do you hope to get out of an internship?

- What strengths would you bring to an internship?

- What sets you apart from other internship candidates?

- What was something that was challenging for you? How did you overcome this challenge?

- What are some areas of growth that you would like to focus on during your internship?

- When working on projects do you prefer to work alone or with a group?

- How have you collaborated with others on group projects/ventures? Can you give an example?

Exploring Learning Style

- Can you please describe a situation in which you had to quickly adapt, music therapy or otherwise.

- Of the practicums listed on your resume what aspects of each did you like? Is there anything you would change/improve upon in any of them?

- What are you looking for in a supervisor?

- What type of feedback/communication styles do you benefit most from?

- How do you handle stress?

- What are your favorite self-care strategies?

Understanding of Music Therapy

- When was the moment that you realized you wanted to be a music therapist?

- What is music as therapy? What is music in therapy?

- What is *your* definition/philosophy of music therapy? What theoretical orientation(s)/approaches do you gravitate toward?

- What is the iso-principle?

- What are two music therapy techniques and a situation in which you might use them?

Clinical Scenarios/Vignettes

- If you were walking into a hospice room and a family member greets you with, "Oh, he is not dying, we don't need any of that," how would you respond?

- In the middle of your session with an agitated patient who has now calmed down and listening with closed eyes, a staff member comes through the door. What would you do?

- A young child presents distressed and withdrawn prior to a procedure. The child is seen looking toward parents when new things happen in the room but turns away when staff talks to the child. What are some strategies to attempt to engage the child with music?

Music Skills

- Play and sing 2–3 songs of varying styles and genres.

- Provide intern with a song recording and 15 minutes to work out playing and singing the song. Option: repeating a 4-chord pop song.

Appendix P
Weekly Log

Name _____ **Week** _____ **Hrs this week** _____ **Total** _____

Goals (Set at the beginning of the week):

Personal:

Clinical:

Day	Monday	Tuesday	Wednesday	Thursday	Friday
I felt accomplished today when...					
How did I celebrate and reflect on this accomplishment?					
I was challenged today when...					
How did I approach the challenge?					
Hours					

This week for self care I...

Next week for self-care I will...